Inflammation in the Pathogenesis of Chronic Diseases

Subcellular Biochemistry
Volume 42

SUBCELLULAR BIOCHEMISTRY

SERIES EDITOR

J.ROBIN HARRIS, University of Mainz, Mainz, Germany

ASSISTANT EDITORS

B.B. BISWAS, University of Calcutta, Calcutta, India

P.QUINN, King's College London, London, U.K

Recent Volumes in this Series

Inflammation in the Pathogenesis of Chronic Diseases

The COX-2 Controversy

Subcellular Biochemistry
Volume 42

Edited by

Randall E. Harris

Director, Center of Molecular Epidemiology and Environmental Health,
College of Medicine and School of Public Health,
The Ohio State University Medical Center,
Columbus, Ohio, USA

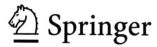 Springer

This series is a continuation of the journal Sub-Cellular Biochemistry. Volume 1 to 4 of which were published quarterly from 1972 to 1975

ISBN 978-1-4020-5687-1 (HB)
ISBN 978-1-4020-5688-8 (e-book)

(BS/DH)

9 8 7 6 5 4 3 2 1

springer.com

CONTENTS

PREFACE

In *"Inflammation in the Pathogenesis of Chronic Diseases: The COX-2 Controversy"*, a panel of leading experts chronicles the evidence supporting the role of inflammation in the pathogenesis of major chronic diseases and discusses the current controversy regarding beneficial versus adverse effects of selective cyclooxygenase-2 (COX-2) inhibitors. Experts in multiple disciplines of medical research provide exciting and enlightening perspectives on COX-2 and related molecular targets in the future of medicine. The book is broadly divided into five sections. We begin with historical perspectives on the discovery and development of aspirin, ibuprofen, and compounds that selectively inhibit COX-2, including discussion of risk versus benefit and the potential for development of new compounds with better efficacy and safety in the 21st century. This is followed by a section illuminating the role of inflammatory mechanisms in the pathogenesis of arthritis, cardiovascular disease, cancer, neurodegenerative disease, diabetes mellitus, obesity, and other life-threatening and debilitating conditions. Specific chapters then explore the "COX-2 controversy" regarding the potential for positive versus negative impact of selective COX-2 inhibitors on the cardiovasculature. Recent findings suggest that cardiovascular risk associated with some COX-2 inhibitors may not be due to a class effect involving COX-2 inhibition, but rather depends upon the molecular structure of specific compounds that have independent effects unrelated to COX-2 and prostaglandin biosynthesis. Important findings are documented in cancer research showing that selective COX-2 inhibitors have powerful antineoplastic effects against major forms of cancer. A special section explores the current evidence supporting the role of COX-2 and inflammation in the development of Alzheimer's disease and other neurodegenerative conditions and the potential benefit of compounds that modulate COX-2 and other inflammatory cytokines. The final section addresses nutritional modulation of inflammation in the pathogenesis of chronic disease and the chemopreventive value of anti-inflammatory nutraceutical agents.

CONTRIBUTORS

Galal A. Alshafie, MD, PhD
College of Medicine and College of Pharmacy, The Ohio State University Medical Center, Columbus, Ohio

Paolo Calabro', MD
Division of Cardiology, Department of Cardiothoracic Sciences, Second University of Naples, Italy, The Brown Foundation Institute of Molecular Medicine for the Prevention of Human Diseases, The University of Texas-Houston Health Science Center, The University of Texas-M.D. Anderson Cancer Center, Houston, Texas

Charles A. Day
Elucida Research LLC, Beverly, MA

Michel de Lorgeril, MD
Laboratoire Nutrition, Vieillissement et Maladies Cardiovasculaires (NVMCV), Faculté de Médecine, Université Joseph Fourier, Grenoble, France

Joanne Beebe-Donk
College of Medicine and School of Public Health, The Ohio State University Medical Center, Columbus, Ohio

Beverley Fermor, PhD
Department of Surgery, Division of Orthopedics, Duke University Medical Center, Durham, North Carolina

Farshid Guilak, PhD
Department of Surgery, Division of Orthopedics, Duke University Medical Center, Durham, North Carolina

Andreas Hald, PhD
Department of Pharmacology and Pharmacotherapeutics, The Danish University of Pharmaceutical Sciences, Universitetsparken, Copenhagen, Denmark

Barbara Shukitt-Hale, PhD
Human Nutrition Research Center on Aging at Tufts University, Boston, MA

Randall E. Harris, MD, PhD
College of Medicine and School of Public Health, The Ohio State University
Medical Center, Columbus, Ohio

Robert F. Jacob, PhD
Elucida Research LLC, Beverly, MA

James Joseph, PhD
Human Nutrition Research Center on Aging at Tufts University, Boston, MA

Frances C. Lau, PhD
Human Nutrition Research Center on Aging at Tufts University, Boston, MA

Julie Lotharius, PhD
Department of Pharmacology and Pharmacotherapeutics, The Danish University of
Pharmaceutical Sciences, Universitetsparken, Copenhagen, Denmark

R. Preston Mason, PhD
Cardiovascular Division, Brigham and Women's Hospital, Harvard Medical
School, Boston, MA; Elucida Research LLC, Beverly, MA

Luisa Minghetti, PhD
Department of Cell Biology and Neurosciences, Istituto Superiore di Sanità, Rome,
Italy

K. D. Rainsford, PhD
Biomedical Research Centre, Sheffield Hallam University, Howard Street Sheffield,
SI 1WB, UK

Bandaru S. Reddy, DVM, PhD
Susan Lehman Cullman Laboratory for Cancer Research, Department of Chemical
Biology, Rutgers, The State University of New Jersey, Piscataway, New Jersey

Christine A. Szekely, PhD
Department of Mental Health, Johns Hopkins Bloomberg School of Public Health,
Baltimore, MD

Terrence Town, PhD
Section of Immunobiology, Yale University School of Medicine, New Haven, CT

Johan van Beek, PhD
Department of Disease Biology, H. Lundbeck A/S, Ottiliavej 9, 2500 Valby, Denmark

Mary F. Walter, PhD
Elucida Research LLC, Beverly, MA; Atlanta VA Medical Center, Atlanta, GA

J. Brice Weinberg, MD
Department of Medicine, Division of Hematology-Oncology, VA and Duke University Medical Centers, Durham, North Carolina

William B. White, MD
Professor of Medicine and Chief, Division of Hypertension and Clinical Pharmacology, Pat and Jim Calhoun Cardiology Center, University of Connecticut School of Medicine, 263 Farmington Avenue, Farmington, Connecticut

Edward T. H. Yeh, MD
The Brown Foundation Institute of Molecular Medicine for the Prevention of Human Diseases, The University of Texas-Houston Health Science Center, and The Department of Cardiology, The University of Texas-M.D. Anderson Cancer Center, Houston, Texas

Peter P. Zandi, PhD
Department of Mental Health, Johns Hopkins Bloomberg School of Public Health, Baltimore, MD

SECTION I

HISTORICAL PERSPECTIVES

CHAPTER 1

ANTI-INFLAMMATORY DRUGS IN THE 21ST CENTURY

K.D. RAINSFORD*

Biomedical Research Centre, Sheffield Hallam University, Howard Street, Sheffield, SI 1WB, UK

Abstract: Historically, anti-inflammatory drugs had their origins in the serendipitous discovery of certain plants and their extracts being applied for the relief of pain, fever and inflammation. When salicylates were discovered in the mid-19th century to be the active components of *Willow* Spp., this enabled these compounds to be synthesized and from this, acetyl-salicylic acid or Aspirin™ was developed. Likewise, the chemical advances of the 19th–20th centuries lead to development of the non-steroidal anti-inflammatory drugs (NSAIDs), most of which were initially organic acids, but later non-acidic

* Biomedical Research Centre, (Faculty of Health & Wellbeing), Sheffield Hallam University, Howard Street, Sheffield SI 1WB, UK.
E-mail: k.d.Rainsford@shu.ac.uk

R. E. Harris (ed.), Inflammation in the Pathogenesis of Chronic Diseases, 3–27.
© 2007 *Springer.*

compounds were discovered. There were two periods of NSAID drug discovery post-World War 2, the period up to the 1970's which was the pre-prostaglandin period and thereafter up to the latter part of the last century in which their effects on prostaglandin production formed part of the screening in the drug-discovery process. Those drugs developed up to the 1980-late 90's were largely discovered empirically following screening for anti-inflammatory, analgesic and antipyretic activities in laboratory animal models. Some were successfully developed that showed low incidence of gastro-intestinal (GI) side effects (the principal adverse reaction seen with NSAIDs) than seen with their predecessors (e.g. aspirin, indomethacin, phenylbutazone); the GI reactions being detected and screened out in animal assays. In the 1990's an important discovery was made from elegant molecular and cellular biological studies that there are two cyclo-oxygenase (COX) enzyme systems controlling the production of prostanoids [prostaglandins (PGs) and thromboxane (TxA_2)]; COX-1 that produces PGs and TxA_2 that regulate gastrointestinal, renal, vascular and other physiological functions, and COX-2 that regulates production of PGs involved in inflammation, pain and fever. The stage was set in the 1990's for the discovery and development of drugs to selectively control COX-2 and spare the COX-1 that is central to physiological processes whose inhibition was considered a major factor in development of adverse reactions, including those in the GI tract. At the turn of this century, there was enormous commercial development following the introduction of two new highly selective COX-2 inhibitors, known as coxibs (celecoxib and rofecoxib) which were claimed to have low GI side effects. While found to have fulfilled these aims in part, an alarming turn of events took place in the late 2004 period when rofecoxib was withdrawn worldwide because of serious cardiovascular events and other coxibs were subsequently suspected to have this adverse reaction, although to a varying degree. Major efforts are currently underway to discover why cardiovascular reactions took place with coxibs, identify safer coxibs, as well as elucidate the roles of COX-2 and COX-1 in cardiovascular diseases and stroke in the hope that there may be some basis for developing newer agents (e.g. nitric oxide-donating NSAIDs) to control these conditions.

The discovery of the COX isoforms led to establishing their importance in many non-arthritic or non-pain states where there is an inflammatory component to pathogenesis, including cancer, Alzheimer's and other neurodegenerative diseases. The applications of NSAIDs and the coxibs in the prevention and treatment of these conditions as well as aspirin and other analogues in the prevention of thrombo-embolic diseases now constitute one of the major therapeutic developments of the this century. Moreover, new anti-inflammatory drugs are being discovered and developed based on their effects on signal transduction and as anti-cytokine agents and these drugs are now being heralded as the new therapies to control those diseases where cytokines and other non-prostaglandin components of chronic inflammatory and neurodegenerative diseases are manifest. To a lesser extent safer application of corticosteroids and the applications of novel drug delivery systems for use with these drugs as well as with NSAIDs also represent newer technological developments of the 21st century. What started out as drugs to control inflammation, pain and fever in the last two centuries now has exploded to reveal an enormous range and type of anti-inflammatory agents and discovery of new therapeutic targets to treat a whole range of conditions that were never hitherto envisaged

1.   HISTORICAL DEVELOPMENTS

The anti-inflammatory analgesic drugs have their origins in the use of extracts of salicylate-containing plants, especially the bark of the willow tree (*Salix alba* and other members of the *Salix* species), in the treatment of fever, pain and inflammatory conditions (Rainsford, 2004a). These treatments date from early Chinese, Indian, African and American eras and were initially described in some detail by Roman and Greek medical authorities. During the 17th–19th centuries, the popularity of these plant extracts became evident following the publication by the Reverend Edward Stone in the 17th century of probably what were the first clinical trials of willow bark extract for the treatment of agues or fever. Isolation of the principally-active salicylate components followed in the early 19th century and with advances in chemistry in Europe and developments in the German chemical industry in the mid-late 19th century, there followed the synthesis or salicylic and acetylsalicylic acids, the latter being highly successfully commercialised by Bayer AG as Aspirin™ over 100 years ago. The historical aspects of the origins and development of aspirin and other salicylates are told in detail elsewhere (Rainsford, 2004a). During the period of the exploitation of the by-products of the coal tar industry in Germany in the 19th century came also the development of antipyretic/analgesic agents, antipyrine, aminopyrine, phenacetin and later following recognition of paracetamol (acetaminophen) as the active metabolite of phenacetin, this was eventually commercially developed for use as an analgesic/antipyretic agent in the 1950's (Prescott, 2001).

1.1. Discovery of NSAIDs

The development of the first of the category of what are now known as the non-steroidal anti-inflammatory drugs (NSAIDs) of which aspirin has now become recognised as the progenitor, was phenylbutazone in 1946 (by JR Geigy, Basel, Switzerland) and later indomethacin in the 1960's (by Merck & Co, Rahway, NJ, USA) (Otterness, 1995). Phenylbutazone was initially employed as a combination with antipyrine in the belief it would enhance the actions of the latter. However, it emerged to have greater anti-inflammatory/analgesic activity than antipyrine and was for the best part of 30 years successfully used for the treatment of arthritic and other painful inflammatory conditions until its popularity progressively waned after associations with life-threatening agranulocytosis and bone marrow suppression (still essentially not conclusively proven today), upper gastrointestinal ulcers and bleeding and subsequent popularity of more advanced NSAIDs.

Ibuprofen was developed by Boots (UK) in the 1950–1960's and after establishing its favourable safety profile at dose ranges for analgesic and anti-pyretic efficacy (up to 1200mg daily) it was the first NSAID (other than aspirin) to be approved for non-prescription (over-the-counter or OTC sale) use in the UK (in 1963), then the USA (in1964) and later in many other countries worldwide (Rainsford, 1999). Just after ibuprofen was developed, a large number of pharmaceutical companies undertook the discovery and development of NSAIDs with a range of chemical and biological properties (Evans & Williamson, 1987; Otterness, 1995; Rainsford, 1999, 2004a; 2005a). The general chemical categorization of these drug classes are shown in Figure 1. Most of these drugs developed in the 1960's were discovered in the pre-prostaglandin era (i.e. before Vane and his

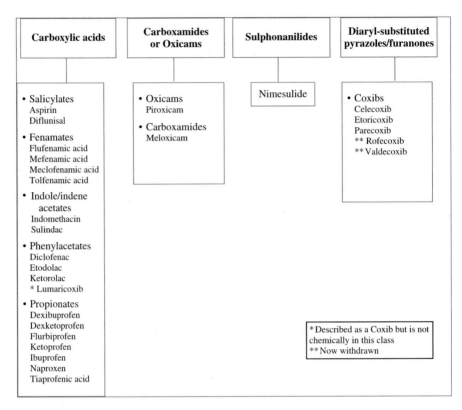

Figure 1. Chemical Classification of the NSAIDs

colleagues had discovered the inhibitory actions of aspirin and related drugs on the production of prostaglandins). Their anti-inflammatory, analgesic and anti-pyretic properties were discovered using animal models with some supportive properties being established in some biochemical systems which were known also to be important in inflammation (e.g. mitochondrial oxidative, intermediary and connective tissue collagen and proteoglycan metabolism; stability of albumin; and later oxyradicals).

2.   COX-2 SELECTIVE AGENTS AND THE COXIBS

Coxibs belong to a class of nonsteroidal anti-inflammatory drugs (NSAIDs) that are used to treat pain and inflammation in a variety of acute and chronic conditions. They have been principally employed for treating rheumatoid and osteo-arthritis, and other arthritic diseases, dental and surgical pain in post-operative settings, dysmenorrhoea, and acute injuries (Kean & Buchanan, 2005). The coxibs have also been explored for the prevention of colorectal and some other cancers (Harris, 2002a; see later section) as well as Alzheimer's disease (Firuzo & Practico, 2006), although the outcomes of these studies have not been particularly favourable largely through lack of efficacy and/or cardiovascular complications. Indeed, the apparent high risk of myocardial infarctions and the exacerbation of symptoms of hypertension and elevation of blood pressure led to the worldwide dramatic withdrawal of one of the leading members of the coxib class, rofecoxib, by the Merck Company on September 29, 2004 (Rainsford, 2005b). This has been followed by the recommendation of the US Food and Drug Administration in April 2005 that Pfizer Inc, the company manufacturing other leading coxibs (celecoxib and valdecoxib) also withdraw valdecoxib from the US market because of the same adverse events. Questions have now been posed whether a cardio-renal syndrome is associated with the entire class of coxibs – a class effect – that may account for the mortality or non-fatal myocardial infarctions and elevation of blood pressure associated with these drugs, possibly in at risk subjects (as yet undetermined). The US FDA has subsequently specified a black box warning on the use of celecoxib and all other coxibs (that remain on the market or in clinical trial) and also a general warning of cardiovascular risk with all other NSAIDs. The European Medicines Evaluation Agency (EMEA), now the European Medicines Agency (EMA) has also re-evaluated the cardiovascular risk with the coxibs and has recommended only restricted use of these drugs. Thus, in somewhat over half a decade since their much-heralded introduction as being safer to the gastrointestinal tract and kidneys than traditional NSAIDs and with rofecoxib and celecoxib having achieved worldwide market domination, they have now plummeted from sales to almost obscurity in the therapeutic armamentarium. There are indications, however, that celecoxib may find its way back onto the world markets but the future of rofecoxib is less certain and maybe it will find applications (e.g. in juvenile rheumatoid arthritis in which it was especially effective) but under very strictly restricted conditions. Another Merck drug, etoricoxib, might not be associated with an excess risk of cardio-renal effects and associated myocardial infarction and exacerbation of hypertension. Likewise, although less adequate data are available with lumiracoxib, there are suggestions this drug may not have the same risks as seen with rofecoxib or other coxibs.

A key factor that has emerged from the analysis of reasons why rofecoxib, valdecoxib, and celecoxib may have led to development of the cardio-renal syndrome thought to underlie myocardial infarction and hypertension appears to have been that these effects were apparent with high dose levels of these drugs. It is possible that in some of the conditions where they were being used (e.g. a colorectal preventative trials of rofecoxib and celecoxib and post-operative coronary bypass in the case of valdecoxib) may have been conditions where there were appreciable manifestations of disease stress that led to pre-disposition to the development of cardio-renal syndromes and myocardial infarction. A major factor was dosage and the data indicates that the cardio-renal syndrome and cardiovascular risks were only evident with high doses of these drugs. Another factor which has emerged is that the principal mode of action of these drugs, to specifically inhibit the enzyme, cyclooxygenase-2 (COX-2) may have been a major factor causing the development of these site effects – this being an example of what is known as "mechanism-based" toxicology.

Coxibs are strictly classed as *functional analogues* since aside from the general chemical features in common with members of this class there are few common specific chemical features that uniformly describe their properties. There are, of course, some features of the biochemical interactions of these with the enzyme, COX-2, which mediates their main pharmacological actions. With the possibly unique exception of lumiracoxib, the other coxibs are tricyclic compounds with high pKa values (pKa 8–9). These contrast with the conventional NSAIDs that are weakly acidic compounds with pKa values of about 3–5, derived from either aryl-carboxylic acids or keto-enolic compounds. The coxibs are diaryl-heterocycles that have a *cis*-stilbene moiety substituted in one of the pendant phenyl rings with a 4-methylsulphone (e.g. rofecoxib) or sulfonamide (e.g. celecoxib) substituent (Figure 2). These moieties are critical together with the diaryl heterocyclic structure in determining their actions as highly specific COX-2 inhibitors.

The odd drug apparent in these chemical associations within the coxibs is lumiracoxib. This drug is an analogue of the traditional acid NSAID, diclofenac, and does not have the tricyclic character of the other coxibs but is an anilino-phenylacetic acid. The 2,6-dichloro-substituents of diclofenac are replaced by 2-chloro, 6-fluoro-moieties in lumiracoxib. There are indications that the COX-2 specificity of lumiracoxib. Perhaps this drug should not be classed as a coxib in view of the lack of associations both chemically and possibly pharmacologically with the other coxibs.

The term coxib derives logically from *cox*-inh**ib**it(or) and appears to have been a marketing ploy by the two major companies that developed these drugs to discriminate them from other NSAIDs. Whether such a pharmacological description is

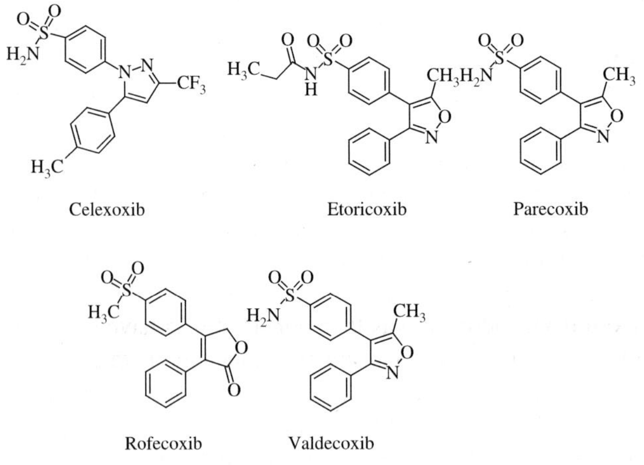

Celexoxib   Etoricoxib   Parecoxib

Rofecoxib   Valdecoxib

Figure 2. The Coxibs

justifiable is debatable especially since the claims for markedly improved GI safety with the coxibs are now being increasingly challenged in relation to at least the risk of serious GI adverse reactions observed with low-risk NSAIDs such as diclofenac or ibuprofen.

2.1. Rationale for the Discovery of Coxibs

The discovery in 1991 of two COX enzymes that are responsible for the synthesis of inflammatory prostaglandins gave a new basis for understanding how these molecules regulate and mediate inflammatory reactions, pain and fever, as well as a number of diverse physiological reactions such as blood flow, thrombosis, and gastrointestinal, renal and reproductive functions (Rainsford, 2004e). About two years previously, a unique COX enzyme was discovered that was produced in response to inflammatory stimuli. In a short while, the genes coding for two separate enzyme proteins were isolated and cloned. By convention the enzyme that is responsible for the production of physiologically important prostaglandins and thromboxane A_2 is termed COX-1. The other enzyme, which is responsible for prostaglandins involved in inflammation and pain and is induced upon stimulation with various inflammatory stimuli (lipopolysaccharide, growth factors etc.), is known as COX-2. Actually the term COX refers to the cyclooxygenase enzyme activity and since peroxidase activity is also present, both enzymatic properties exist in one protein which is termed prostaglandin G/H endoperoxide synthase or PGHS. COX-1 is present in PGHS-1 and COX-2 in PGHS-2. Because the enzymatic activity is the functional response to the gene-regulated and expressed production of prostanoids (prostaglandins and thromboxane A_2) it is usual to term the two isoforms COX-1 and COX-2 for short.

2.1.1. *Prototypes of the coxibs*

Two classes of COX-2 selective inhibitors have, in retrospect, emerged as the prototypes for the development of the coxibs. These are (a) a group of aryl sulfonanilides typified by NS298, nimesulide (R-805), flosulide (CGP28238), diflumidone (R-807), T-614, L-745,337 and FR115068, and (b) the 1,2-diarylheterocyles, DuP697 and SC58125 (De Leval et al., 2000; Rainsford, 2004e). Thus, many COX-2 selective agents have been discovered by taking the sulfonanilide moiety and superimposing this on various diaryl heterocyles. The sulfonanilide could be a 4-methylsulfonyl- or sulphonamide in one of the pendant phenyl rings; the former being attached to a *cis*-stilbene moiety. It has been suggested that the origins of the diaryl-substituted heterocycles are from phenylbutazone, which led to the development of indoxole and oxaprozin. Indoxole was then considered to have been the precursor of DuP697 and SC58125. Some have claimed that indomethacin may have served as a basis for development of diaryl heterocycles with the acetic acid moiety being modified to be replaced by a sulfonanilide.

Probably the first sulfonanilide to be developed which has emerged as a clinically successful COX-2 selective drug was nimesulide. This drug was initially discovered (coded R-805) by Riker in the 1960's as part of a programme to identify anti-inflammatory analgesic drugs based on sulphonamides (Rainsford, 2005a). Clearly, these studies took place and this drug developed as a clinically effective drug some three decades before the COX-isoforms were discovered. Screening for relative COX-1/COX-2 activities of established NSAIDS was initially undertaken by a number of academic groups as well as in the pharma industry after the COX-isoforms were discovered in the early 1990's. Thus, nimesulide emerged from these studies and as well, meloxicam, a derivative of piroxicam was also found to have COX-2 selectivity (Trummlitz & van Ryn, 2002). Meloxicam is different from other COX-2 selective drugs in being an enolcarboxamide although structural studies with COX-isoforms investigated by molecular modelling has confirmed its fit with the active site of COX-2 (Trummlitz & van Ryn, 2002).

The development of nimesulide was predicated on the search for anti-oxidant compounds. The carboxyl group of NSAIDs (then regarded as a prerequisite for anti-inflammatory activity of aromatic drugs, the NSAIDs) was replaced by nitro- and sulphonamides to give putative anti-oxidant compounds with higher pKa values (6.5–7.0) than conventional carboxylates (pKa 2.5–4.0) or keto-enolates (e.g. phenylbutazone) (pKa 4.5–5.5).

In summary, the identification of nimesulide and meloxicam, along with etodolac and oxaprozin as agents having COX-2 selectivity, has emerged long after these drugs were introduced clinically. The search for highly selective COX-2 inhibitors proceeded on the basis that more potent and selective inhibitors of COX-2 would be more effective in controlling pain, inflammation and fever, and with fewer side effects in the gastrointestinal tract and possibly the kidneys than the above mentioned established COX-2 selective NSAIDs as well as others of this class of drugs.

2.1.2.   Development of the coxibs

The chemical development of the coxibs has been comprehensively reviewed by a number of authors, to whom the reader is referred for more detailed information (Dannhardt & Laufer, 2000; De Leval et al., 2000). Here, some of the salient features of the development of the coxibs are outlined (Rainsford, 2004e). The basis for the identification of COX-2 selectively has been the development of *in vitro* assays. These have comprised (a) isolated recombinant enzymes, (b) cell lines with COX-2 and COX-1 activity, (c) primary cells e.g. platelets or platelet rich plasma as a source of COX-1 and stimulated macrophages for COX-2 activities respectively, (d) cell lines (e.g. chinese hamster ovary, (CHO) cells transfected with either human recombinant COX-2 or COX-1 genes, and (e) variants of whole blood assays in which COX-1 activity is determined after 1 hr by measuring thromboxane production, and COX-2 after incubation with lipopolysaccharide (endotoxin of *Escherichia coli*) or interleukin-1 for 24 hr and measuring prostaglandin E_2 production. Each of these assays has its merits and applications. Mostly, assays (a) and (d) were employed in the discovery of relative COX-2/COX-1 activity. The whole blood assay has been regarded as more appropriate for determining the clinically relevant COX-2 selectivity especially in relation to the plasma pharmacokinetics of the drugs.

In determining the structural requirements for COX-2 selectivity, drug modelling of interaction with the COX-isoenzymes has been made possible because of the availability of crystal structures of the ovine COX-1, murine COX-2 and human COX-2, which have been solved to 3 to 3.5 Å resolution (Trummlitz & van Ryn, 2002).

3.   NOVEL NSAIDs AND DERIVATIVES

Over the century or more since the discovery of drugs used to treat inflammation, pain and fever there have been an immense number and variety of chemical analogues and derivatives that have been developed some of which have found successful application in treating inflammatory diseases and some have passed out of favour or use for one reason or another (Adams & Cobb, 1967; Otterness, 1995; Rainsford, 1999a; 1999b; 2004a; 2004e; 2004f; 2005a). Many of the older agents could usefully be employed given understanding that they may have unique modes of action in controlling different pathways or cellular reactions in inflammatory diseases. Their potential for exploitation is phenomenal!

3.1.   Nitric Oxide – Donating NSAIDs

The development of nitric oxide (NO) – donating NSAIDs had its origin in the recognition that nitric oxide has an important role in regulating blood flow and vascular functions and that NO donors could protect the gastro-intestinal (GI) mucosa against injury by NSAIDs and various necrotizing agents (Whittle, 2003). The idea of chemically coupling an NO-donor to an NSAID in the form of an acidic ester, such that upon absorption by the gastric mucosa NO would be released to produce local vasodilatatory effects and protection of the mucosa from injury from the NSAID seemed an elegant means of developing NSAID derivatives that would be notably safer to the GI tract than the parent NSAID. It has been known for over 40 years that simple alkyl or phenyl esters of NSAIDs have less gastro-irritancy than their parent acids (Rainsford, 2004b; 2004f) so that esterification with NO-donating groups would also be expected to confer protection against the injurious effects of the acidic moieties of NSAIDs. To what extent the addition of an NO-donor to the alkyl or other ester adds to the protective effects has not been determined. While much work has been done to establish the actions of different NO-NSAIDs (Keeble & Moore, 2002; Whittle, 2003; Zacharowski et al., 2004; Corazzi et al., 2003, 2005; Dhawan et al., 2005) and many derivatives have been developed (Chiroli et al., 2003; Whittle, 2003; Gao et al., 2005) to date this has not yet clearly translated into clinically useful drugs although many hold promise. The development of nitro-aspirin for prevention of cardiovascular disease (Whittle, 2003; Abrosini et al., 2005) must hold the greatest promise as present. There are, however, exciting prospects for exploiting the pro-apoptotic effects of NO-NSAIDs (Huguenin et al., 2004a, 2004b; Royle et al., 2004; Fabbri et al., 2005; Bolla & Zoli,

2006; Rosetti et al., 2006), pro-oxidant effects (Gao et al., 2005) and inhibition of MAP kinase pathways (Hundley & Rigas, 2006) in the prevention and treatment of a variety of different cancers.

3.2.   Resolvins or Epilipoxins

These products of lipoxygenase (LOX) activities, among them the aspirin-triggered lipoxin (Rainsford, 2004c; Serhan 2005) and the products of omega-3 fatty acid metabolism through the LOX pathways, and stable analogues thereof that have been found to have anti-inflammatory activity now attract much interest as potential therapies not only for treating inflammatory diseases but also the inflammatory components of cancers and many other chronic diseases (Serhan et al., 2004; Petasis et al., 2005; Serhan, 2005; Parkinson, 2006). These fatty acid derivatives hold particular promise because of their structural novelty and unique lipoxin receptor targets.

3.3.   COX-3 as a Therapeutic Target?

There has been much speculation and interest in the possibility that there may be another cyclooxygenase in addition to COX-1 or COX-2 which could be a target for actions of analgesics e.g. paracetamol (acetaminophen) (Berenbaum, 2004; Lucas et al., 2005). Despite earlier discovery of a variant of COX-1 in some regions of the brain and suggestions that paracetamol may act selectively on this variant, it is now clear from recent experimental studies and evaluation of the earlier evidence that COX-3 is actually a splice variant of COX-1 (Figure 3) and that acetaminophen

**COMPARISON OF THE STRUCTURE
OF COX-1 WITH COX-3**

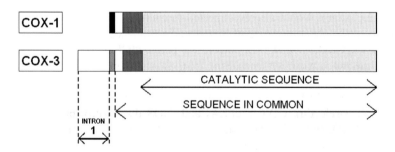

Figure 3. Structure of the genome for cyclooxygenase-3 contrasted with that of COX-1, showing the splice variant nature of COX-3 and its derivation by inclusion on intron-1. Based on information in Berenbaum (2004)

while inhibiting cyclooxygenase activity in intact cells (but not in broken cell preparations) does so by interfering with the oxidant status of cells (Lucas et al., 2005) in a manner that resembles the anti-oxidant actions of phenolic compounds. Thus the search for analgesics that might act on the suggested COX-3 enzyme would appear to be an exercise in futility.

4.   DISEASE-MODIFYING AGENTS & CORTICOSTEROIDS

The term "disease-modifying" agent (involving use of disease-modifying anti-rheumatic drugs, DMARDs) has had particular vogue in the therapy of rheumatic diseases where attempts to achieve control or at best reversal of the chronic inflammatory disease have involved a variety of approaches (Paulus, 1995; Abadie et al., 2004; Simon, 2004). For treatment of rheumatoid arthritis, a whole range of drugs have been employed over the years. Among these are the parenteral and oral gold salts (whose use has been given the term "crysotherapy") and D-penicillamine, whose uses were discovered serendipitously as well as chloroquine or hydroxy-chloroquine, sulphasalazine, cyclosporine A, levamisole, azathioprine, cyclophosphamide, chlorambucil and methotrexate (Brooks et al., 1985; Simon, 2004) as well as combinations of some of these drugs in therapy resembling the approaches employed in cancer therapy (Paulus, 1995). Of these agents, probably methotrexate has now assumed greatest use as a first line therapy having relatively fewer severe adverse reactions, some of which are manageable, compared with many other DMARDs. Likewise, corticosteroids have had considerable popularity since the discovery by Hench at the Mayo Clinic in 1949 that cortisone had a dramatic effect in bed-ridden patients suffering with severe rheumatoid arthritis (Evans & Williamson, 1987; Hirschmann, 1992). Indeed the synthetic developments and large commercial efforts put into the discovery of corticosteroids (or glucocortocoids) made in the 1950s–1980's) (Evans & Williamson, 1987; Hischmann, 1992; Berstein, 1992) only to yield the relatively few drugs used today is a striking reflection of the complex nature of this class of compounds. Indeed, it was originally considered that corticosteroids acted by immunosuppressive activity, an idea arising due to the effects that occurred at the high doses that were given in former times (Brooks et al., 1985). Long after their discovery, advances in the molecular biology of inflammatory mediator production have shown that these drugs act principally through their binding to the specific glucocorticoid receptor (GR*) and consequent inhibition of cellular signalling pathways (especially AP-1 and NFκB) that regulate the production of inflammatory cytokines and chemokines (IL-1, TNF-α, IL-2, IL-5, IFN-γ, GM-CSF, MIP-1, MCP-1, Eotaxin, RANTES), cell adhesion molecules (I-CAM, V-CAM, E-selectin), COX-2, cPLA$_2$ and iNOS that control production of eicosanoids and NO, and the production of joint-destructive metalloproteinases (Vayssiere et al., 1997; Russo-Marie, 2004). The inhibitory effects of corticosteroids on production of acute phase proteins and erythrocyte sedimentation rate (ESR) are indicators of the effectiveness of these drugs on pathognomic biomarkers of chronic disease (Russo-Marie, 2004). In some respects the corticosteroids are ideal anti-inflammatory drugs for use in chronic disease but their side-effects are proven formidable and often severe or irreversible (e.g. bone damage, immunosuppression and propensity to infection, gastrointestinal ulcers and bleeding, skin thinning) and in part their undoing. While low-dose corticosteroids are now used commonly in rheumatoid arthritis, concerns about their long-term use are still a matter of major concern.

In the past two decades, significant advances have been made in the molecular biology of the cells and mediators of chronic inflammatory disease and the biotechnological processes involved in the production of peptides, anti-bodies (including "humanized" monoclonal anti-bodies, or hMAbs, from mouse precursors) and the isolation and cloning of genes regulating the production of endogenous inhibitors or soluble receptors that interact with pro-inflammatory cytokines as well as the production of anti-inflammatory cytokines. These developments have led to a revolution in the therapy of not only rheumatoid arthritis, but also chronic inflammatory diseases affecting a large number of organ systems (e.g. ulcerative colitis, Crohn's disease, psoriasis) (Katz, 2005). Of the principal anti-cytokine biological therapies that have been developed and are now given parenterally in treating rheumatoid arthritis in select patients, the following drugs have specific targets, namely:

1. *Target: TNFα*

Etanercept – Recombinant TNF-R Fc fusion protein.

Infliximab [Remicade™] – Chimeric human-murine anti-TNFα monoclonal antibody. Adalimumab – fully human anti-TNF monoclonal antibody.

2. *Target: IL-1*

Anakinra – recombinant human IL-1Ra protein.

In rheumatoid arthritis, all except infliximab are used as monotherapies; otherwise, drugs are usually given with methotrexate. The outcomes from therapy with these agents can be summarized as follows (see Weaver, 2004; Crum et al., 2005).

(1) Anakinra used alone or with methotrexate reduces clinical signs and symptoms of RA.

(2) TNF inhibitors show similar efficacy and have higher response rates for clinical and radiological parameters than with anakinra.

(3) There is a question of whether long-term therapy produces radiological evidence of reduced joint disease.

(4) There are major issues about infections due to immunosuppression.

The applications of these biological therapies have been considered with much caution following the initial concerns about immunosuppression and consequent predisposition to conditions such as latent tuberculosis. In many countries there are now patient registries for rheumatic patients receiving these biological therapies and this reflects the need for careful therapy and monitoring. What has been learnt from their application is, however, that the respective pro-inflammatory cytokine targets have valid "proof of concept" for their importance in treating rheumatoid arthritis, and where these therapies have also been found effective in other conditions there is also support for the central concept of controlling pro-inflammatory cytokines in these chronic inflammatory diseases.

5. ANTI-CYTOKINE AGENTS AND SIGNAL TRANSDUCTION INHIBITORS

In the light of the above conclusions about the importance of pro-inflammatory cytokines in chronic disease, it is not surprising that the emphasis in recent years has been to develop small molecules to target the processes governing the control of their actions. Several NSAIDs affect the production or actions of cytokines and this property has been considered to be a component of their actions, positive or negative. Thus, indomethacin and some other NSAIDs may increase production of interleukin-1 (IL-1 or tumour necrosis factor-α (TNF-α) and these effects have been considered important in the development of GI ulcers and asthma attributed to these drugs. However, some other NSAIDS such as nimesulide inhibit IL-6 and TNF-α (Rainsford et al., 2005) while ibuprofen inhibits TNF-α (Jiang et al., 1998). TNF-α induction of the NFκB/IκB signalling pathway is inhibited by salicylate at the level of the activity of IKKinase and cAMP-response element binding protein (CREB) (Rainsford 2004b). These effects are considered among the anti-inflammatory effects of these drugs. The inhibitory effects on signalling pathways, especially those involving NFκB/IκB and MAP kinases, may have particular significance in subsequent inhibition of the expression of mRNAs and the proteins of COX-2, iNOS and PLA$_2$ (Rainsford, 2004; Rainsford et al., 2005b). With nimesulide there is also an interesting additional property that this drug activates glucocorticoid receptors leading to down-regulation of a number of cytokines, metalloproteinase enzymes, COX-2, iNOS and PLA$_2$ (Rainsford et al., 2005b). Some NSAIDs also affect the response of T-cells to IL-2 (Hall et al., 1997) and this together with reduction in the effects of PGE$_2$, due to blockade of the production of this prostanoid by NSAIDs, may form a component of their immuno-regulatory effects (Smith et al., 1971; Goodwin et al., 1977, 1978).

The original observations of the inhibitory effects on NFκB activation by high concentrations of salicylates (Koop and Ghosh, 1994) followed by reports of effects on this and other intracellular signalling pathways and subsequent actions in controlling production of COX-2, iNOS etc with other NSAIDs (Paik et al., 2000; Allgayer, 2003; Bryant et al., 2003; Yoon et al., 2003; Rainsford, 2004) and naturally occurring anti-inflammatory agents (e.g. curcumins, ginger, resveratrol, various plant polyphenols) (Pellegatta et al., 2003; Grzanna et al., 2005; Yeh et al., 2005; Yoon & Baek, 2005; Bengmark, 2006) together with other studies on the cellular mechanisms of inflammation (Lo et al., 1998) have provided insight into the potential effects of regulating intracellular signalling as a means of controlling cytokines, COX-2, PLA$_2$, iNOS and metalloproteinases and the actions of reactive oxygen species (ROS; oxyradicals) that are central to the inflammatory processes (Celec, 2004; Saklatvala, 2004; Jimi & Ghosh, 2005; Wu, 2005; Papa et al., 2006; see Figure 4). Thus, much effort has been devoted in recent years to discover and develop specific inhibitors of the various signalling pathways involved in inflammation (Saklatvala, 2004; Miwatashi et al., 2005; Bolos, 2005; Diller et al., 2005; Hynes and Leftheri, 2005; Goldstein and Gabriel, 2005; Kaminska, 2005; Peifer et al., 2006; Goldstein et al., 2006; Lin et al., 2006; Sabat

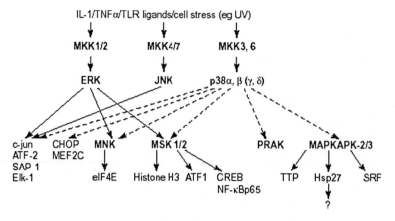

Figure 4. Intracellular Signaling in Inflammation
Source: From Saklatvala (2004)

et al., 2006; Metzger et al., 2006; Kulkarni et al., 2006; Friedmann et al., 2006) many of which have strikingly different chemical structures (e.g. see Figure 5). While many of these agents are in early stages of development there are indications that some (e.g. see Saklatvala, 2004; Miwatashi et al., 2005) are orally active and effective in rheumatoid arthritis and some other chronic inflammatory diseases.

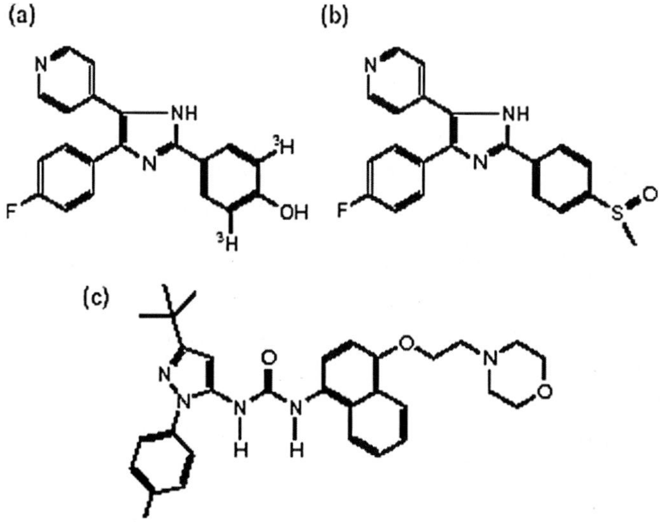

(a)   (b)

(c)

Figure 5. (*Continued*)
Source: (*a*) From Saklatvala (2004)

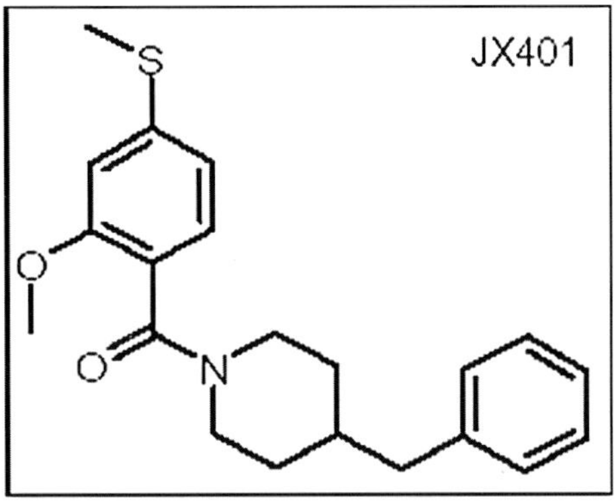

JX401

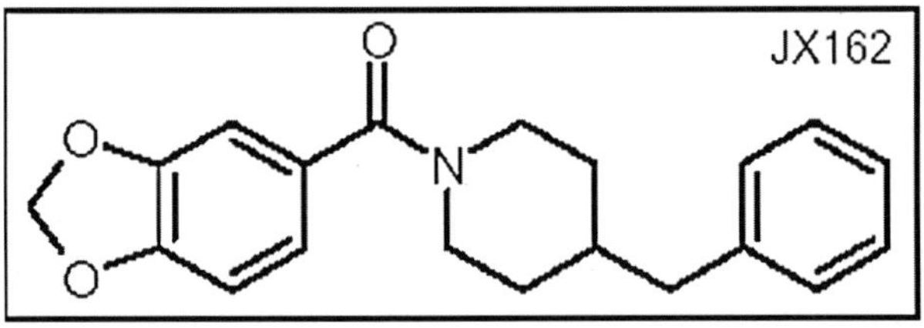

JX162

Source: (b) From Friedman et al., 2006

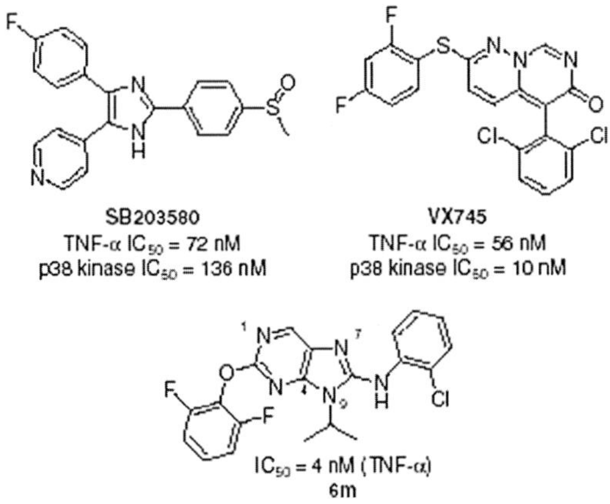

SB203580
TNF-α IC$_{50}$ = 72 nM
p38 kinase IC$_{50}$ = 136 nM

VX745
TNF-α IC$_{50}$ = 56 nM
p38 kinase IC$_{50}$ = 10 nM

IC$_{50}$ = 4 nM (TNF-α)
6m

Figure 5. (Continued)
Source: (c) From Sabat et al. (2006)

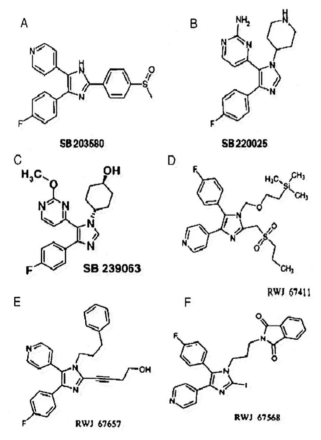

Source: (d) R-130823; from Lin et al. (2006)

Figure 5. Inhibitors of p38
Source: (e) From Kaminska (2005)

Other cell signalling systems that are thought to have potential as targets include the family of nuclear proteins known as **S**ignal **T**ransducers and **A**ctivators of **T**ranscription (STAT), of which STAT1, which controls production of IFN-γ and growth hormone are of particular interest (de Prati et al., 2005). As with all signalling pathways which areso ubiquitous in cells, the specificity of attack by drugs on the components of these pathways will be a determinant of their utility. Any generalised inhibition of signalling pathways may have generic effects, some of which may be undesirable. Already, certain p38 MAP kinase inhibitors have been found to have broad actions that limit their safety in some cases and there has, as a consequence, been a move to develop drugs with inhibitory effects down-stream of post receptor pathways (Saklatvala, 2004).

6. NOVEL NON-ARTHRITIC USES OF NSAIDs

Over the past 3–4 decades, there have been a considerable number of developments involving the use of NSAIDs in conditions other than the treatment of arthritic disease and other painful states. These developments have mostly arisen from investigations of the pharmacological actions of these drugs or from chance pharmaco-epidemiological observations, not necessarily directly related to investigating the associations with NSAIDs. The first of these observations was by O'Brien (1968) who found that aspirin, but not salicylate, caused inhibition of the aggregation of platelets which was initially thought to be, and later confirmed as a factor in promoting bleeding from the gastroduodenal region (Rainsford, 2004b). It was not long before the "antiplatelet" effect of aspirin was exploited not only for its potential anti-inflammatory effects (Rainsford, 2004c) but also for prevention of thromboembolic- and coronary-vascular diseases, which is now legend (Webert & Kelton, 2004).

The initial observations that have lead to aspirin and other NSAIDs being recognized for their tumour-inhibiting and anti-metastatic properties have been somewhat less clear. It was known in the 1970's that aspirin and some other NSAIDs could inhibit the growth and metastasis of tumour cells (Gasic et al., 1972; Wood & Hilgard, 1972; Powles et al., 1973) 1974; LiVolsi, 1973). There were also suggestions that oxyphenbutazone (Tanderil®) could have benefit in radiation treatment of otorhino-laryngeal tumours (JForl, 1976) by ameliorating inflammatory effects of radiation (Dargent, 1969; Klein et al., 1972; Muller-Fassbender et al., 1973). Multiple observations that there were marked increases in the concentrations of prostaglandins in tumours (Sandler et al., 1968; Bennett, 1971, 1976; Bennett & Del Tacca, 1975) as well as in cancer cell cultures (Jaffe et al., 1971; Levine et al., 1972) combined with prostaglandin effects on cell metabolism and proliferation (Makman, 1971; Van Wijk et al., 1972) and bone resorption and metastasis (Harris et al., 1973; Bennett et al., 1975, 1976) gave rise to the recognition that increased prostaglandin production was a major factor in the growth and proliferation of cancer. The recognition at about the same period (early 1970's) that prostaglandin production could be inhibited by aspirin and other NSAIDs (Vane, 1971; Ferriera et al., 1971; Flower, 1974) and reduce the growth of tumours (see above) gave rise to the suggestion that aspirin and other NSAIDs could inhibit growth and proliferation of malignant tumours (Harris, 2003; Rainsford, 2004d; Rigas & Kashfi, 2005; Deans & Wigmore, 2005; Wang & Dubois, 2006).

Extensive investigations have now shown that NSAIDs have protective effects against colorectal cancer (Hull et. Al., 2003; Thun & Henley, 2003; Damjanovic et al., 2004, Sanborn & Blanke, 2005; Abir et al., 2005). NSAIDs have also been found to reduce the incidence of gastric tumours (Dai & Wang, 2006), two common brain tumours (i.e. gliomas and meningiomas) (Nathoo et al., 2004), breast cancer (Saji et al., 2004; Harris, 2004), cholangiocarcinoma of the biliary tract (Wu, 2005) and possibly adenocarcinomas and squamous cell carcinomas of the oesophagus or gastro-oesophageal junction (Tew et al., 2005). A whole range of other cancers are being considered for potential therapy with NSAIDs (Riedl et al., 2004; Claria & Romano, 2005; Kashfi & Rigas, 2005). Indeed the application of the NSAIDs, including those which have novel modes of action (e.g. inhibition of 5-lipoxygenase, production of nitric oxide from NO-NSAIDs) and what are regarded as non-COX-2 models of action are now broadening the focus of therapeutic attack in prevention and possibly even treatment of many pathological types of cancers (Rigas et al., 2003; Claria & Romano, 2005; Kashfi & Rigas, 2005).

NSAIDs have found particular application in the prevention of Alzheimer's disease and other neurodegenerative conditions (Rogers, 2004; Piruzi and Practico, 2006). Their application arose from clinico-epidemiological observations of reduction in the risk of onset and development of Alzheimer's patients taking NSAIDs (Rainsford, 1999b; 2004g; 2005a). Later investigations have found variable effects of different NSAIDs, but with some limited significant benefit from the coxibs or COX-2 selective agents (Rainsford, 2005a; Piruzi & Practio, 20–06) suggesting that there may be non-COX mechanisms important in the putative neuroprotection in this syndrome involving the actions of pro-inflammatory cytokines, oxyradicals and leucocyte activation (Rainsford, 2004g; 2005a).

Aspirin, ibuprofen and some other NSAIDs have been found to have benefit in preventing cataract, especially that attributed to diabetes mellitus, as well as in control of this and other perturbed metabolic states (Rainsford, 2004g).

7.   FUTURE SCOPE

There is now enormous scope for the application of new and established anti-inflammatory agents with various receptors and targets for their actions as well as the development of novel anti-inflammatory drugs in the future. An immense array and variety of inflammatory reactions are now known to underlie serious chronic diseases and conditions which urgently require new therapeutic approaches centering on control of chronic inflammation. These include cardiovascular disease (Elhajj et al., 2004), transplantation reactions (Rocha et al., 2003), skin diseases including difficult conditions such as psoriasis (Lee et al., 2003; Skinner, 2004; Nash & Clegg, 2005), and actinic keratosis (Jorizzo, 2004), neurodegenerative diseases including Alzheimer's disease (Rogers and Lahiri, 2004), sepsis (Rice & Bernard, 2005), ageing [here aspirin has given encouraging results] (Phillips & Leeuwenburgh, 2004), and ophthalmic diseases (O'Brien, 2005). Each of these has a differing spectrum of inflammatory reactions and varying involvement of inflammatory mediators as well as cells of the immune system that regulate the inflammation. NSAIDs, each with differing mechanisms of action on inflammation, will continue to be exploited for therapy of these and other conditions and the design of drug delivery systems may help considerably where there is need to get focussed delivery of the drug at specific body sites e.g. skin, (Skinner, 2004) bone marrow etc. There are a large number of older NSAIDs and derivatives (e.g. see Rainsford, 1999; 2004f) some of which have passed out of fashion, but these may have utility in some conditions where their mechanism of action suits the particular application. There are also the new signal transduction inhibitors that may have specific utility in a wide variety of inflammatory conditions by virtue of their mechanism of action. Anti-cytokine agents may eventually prove to be useful for chronic diseases not only by way of therapeutic benefits and targets for their actions, but also by way of showing "proof of principle" which can serve to encourage development of small molecules to control the action of target cytokines either at the level of cytokine receptors or post-receptor signalling events. Likewise, the successful application of nutraceuticals, a large number of which have been found effective in controlling inflammation (Shay and Banz, 2005), may ultimately lead to isolation of their active components (as shown with the grape component, resveratrol; Pellegatta et al., 2003) and the development of potent derivatives.

8. CONCLUSIONS

Many of the newer anti-inflammatory agents that have been developed since the turn of this century were discovered following the investigations of the mechanisms underlying the control of inflammatory conditions over the past 2–3 decades. We are now beginning to see an immense array of potential for these new drugs as well as the long-established drugs (NSAIDs, corticosteroids, DMARDs) and natural products (nutraceuticals). As better understanding of the mechanisms underlying chronic diseases progresses, so the applications of individual anti-inflammatory agents will be investigated and conditions for their optimal use and delivery established. There is a whole world of new opportunities awaiting the use of anti-inflammatory agents, both established and novel, in the future.

REFERENCES

Abadie E, Ethgen D, Avouac B, Bouvenot G, Branco J, Bruyere O, Calvo G, Devogelaer JP, Dreiser RL, Herrero-Beaumont G, Kahan A, Kreutz G, Laslop A, Lemmel EM, Nuki G, Van De Putte L, Vanhaelst L, Reginster JY; Group for the Respect of Excellence and Ethics in Science. Recommendations for the use of new methods to assess the efficacy of disease-modifying drugs in the treatment of osteoarthritis. Osteoarthritis Cartilage. 2004;12:263–268.

Adams SS, Cobb R. Non-steroidal anti-inflammatory drugs. In: *Progress in Medicinal Chemistry*, 5, GP Ellis, GB West, eds. London: Butterworth, 1967, 59–133.

Allgayer H. Review article: mechanisms of action of mesalazine in preventing colorectal carcinoma in inflammatory bowel disease. Aliment Pharmacol Ther. 2003;18 Suppl 2:10–14.

Ambrosini MV, Mariucci G, Rambotti MG, Tantucci M, Covarelli C, De Angelis L, Del Soldato P. Ultrastructural investigations on protective effects of NCX 4016 (nitroaspirin) on macrovascular endothelium in diabetic Wistar rats. J Submicrosc Cytol Pathol. 2005;37:205–213.

Bengmark S. Curcumin, an atoxic antioxidant and natural NFkappaB, cyclooxygenase-2, lipooxygenase, and inducible nitric oxide synthase inhibitor: a shield against acute and chronic diseases. JPEN J Parenter Enteral Nutr. 2006;30:45–51.

Bennett A, Charlier EM, McDonald AM, Simpson JS, Stamford IF. Bone destruction by breast tumours. Prostaglandins. 1976;11:461–463.

Bennett A. Prostaglandins as factors in diseases of the alimentary tract. Adv Prostaglandin Thromboxane Res. 1976;2:547–555.

Bennett A, McDonals AM, Simpson JS, Stamford IF. Breast cancer, prostaglandins, and bone metastases. Lancet. 1975;31:1218–1220.

Bennett A, Del Tacca M. Proceedings: Prostaglandins in human colonic carcinoma. Gut. 1975;16:409.

Bennett A, Effects of kinins and prostaglandins on the gut. Proc R Soc Med. 1971;64:12–13.

Bernstein S. Historic reflection on steroids: Lederle and personal aspects. Steroids. 1992;57:392–402.

Bolos J. Structure-activity relationships of p38 mitogen-activated protein kinase inhibitors. Mini Rev Med Chem. 2005;5:857–868.

Bolla M, Zoli W. Molecular characterization of cytotoxic and resistance mechanisms induced by NCX 4040, a novel NO-NSAID, in pancreatic cancer cell lines Apoptosis. 2006;11:1321–30.

Brooks PM, Buchanan WW, Rosenbloom D, Bellamy N. Clinical efficacy and responses in therapy with anti-inflammatory and anti-rheumatic drugs. In: *Anti-Inflammatory and Anti-Rheumatic Drugs*, Vol III: Anti-Rheumatic Drugs, Experimental Agents, and Clinical Aspects of Drug Use, K D Rainsford, ed. Boca Raton (Fl): CRC Press, 1985, 167–203.

Bryant CE, Farnfield BA, Janicke HJ. Evaluation of the ability of carprofen and flunixin meglumine to inhibit activation of nuclear factor kappa B. Am J Vet Res. 2003;64:211–215.

Celec P. Nuclear factor kappa B–molecular biomedicine: the next generation. Biomed Pharmacother. 2004;58:365–371.

Chiroli V, Benedini F, Ongini E, Del Soldato P. Nitric oxide-donating non-steroidal anti-inflammatory drugs: the case of nitroderivatives of aspirin. Eur J Med Chem. 2003;38:441–446.

Claria J, Romano M. Pharmacological intervention of cyclooxygenase-2 and 5-lipoxygenase pathways. Impact on inflammation and cancer. Curr Pharm Des. 2005;11:3431–3447.

Corazzi T, Leone M, Roberti R, Del Soldato P, Gresele P. Effect of nitric oxide-donating agents on human monocyte cyclooxygenase-2. Biochem Biophys Res Commun. 2003;311:897–903.

Corazzi T, Leone M, Maucci R, Corazzi L, Gresele P. Direct and irreversible inhibition of cyclooxygenase-1 by nitroaspirin (NCX 4016). J Pharmacol Exp Ther. 2005;315:1331–1337.

Crum NF, Lederman ER, Wallace MR. Infections associated with tumor necrosis factor-alpha antagonists. Medicine (Baltimore). 2005;84:291–302.

Dai Y, Wang WH. Non-steroidal anti-inflammatory drugs in prevention of gastric cancer. World J Gastroenterol. 2006;12:2884–2889.

Damjanovic D, Thompson P, Findlay MP. Evidence-based update of chemotherapy options for metastatic colorectal cancer. ANZ J Surg. 2004;74:781–787.

Dannhardt G, Laufer S. Structural approaches to explain the selectivity of COX-2 inhibitors: is there a common pharmacophore? Curr Med Chem, 2000;7:11-1-1112.

Dargent D. Utilization of tanderil during radium therapy of cancer of the female genital apparatus. Lyon Med. 1969;221:1261–1262.

De Leval X, Delarge J, Somers F, de Tullio P, Henrotin Y, Pirotte B, Dogné J-M. Recent advances in inducible cyclooxygenase (COX-2) inhibition. Curr Med Chem. 2000;7:1041–1062.

de Prati AC, Ciampa AR, Cavalieri E, Zaffini R, Darra E, Menegazzi M, Suzuki H, Mariotto S. STAT1 as a new molecular target of anti-inflammatory treatment. Curr Med Chem. 2005;12:1819–1828.

Dhawan V, Schwalb DJ, Shumway MJ, Warren MC, Wexler RS, Zemtseva IS, Zifcak BM, Janero DR. Selective nitros(yl)ation induced in vivo by a nitric oxide-donating cyclooxygenase-2 inhibitor: a NObonomic analysis. Free Radic Biol Med. 2005;39:1191–1207.

Diller DJ, Lin TH, Metzger A. The discovery of novel chemotypes of p38 kinase inhibitors. Curr Top Med Chem. 2005;5:953–965.

Elhajj II, Haydar AA, Hujairi NM, Goldsmith DJ. The role of inflammation in acute coronary syndromes: review of the literature. J Med Liban. 2004;52:96–102.

Evans D, Williamson WRN. Chemistry of clinically active anti-inflammatory compounds. In: *Anti-Inflammatory Compounds*. New York & Basel: Marcel Dekker, 1987, 193–302.

Fabbri F, Brigliadori G, Ulivi P, Tesei A, Vannini I, Rosetti M, Bravaccini S, Amadori D, Bolla M, Zoli W. Pro-apoptotic effect of a nitric oxide-donating NSAID, NCX 4040, on bladder carcinoma cells. Apoptosis. 2005;10:1095–1103.

Ferriera SH, Moncado S, Vane JR. Indomethacin and aspirin abolish prostaglandin release from spleen. Nature New Biology. 1971;231:237–239.

Firuzi O, Pratico D. Coxibs and Alzheimer's disease: should they stay or should they go? Ann Neurol. 2006;59:219–228.

Flower RJ. Drugs which inhibit prostaglandin synthesis. Pharmacol Rev. 1974;26:33–67.

Franzoso G. The NF-kappaB-mediated control of the JNK cascade in the antagonism of programmed cell death in health and disease. Cell Death Differ. 2006;13:712–729

Friedmann Y, Shriki A, Bennett ER, Golos S, Diskin R, Marbach I, Bengal E, Engelberg D. JX401, a p38{alpha} inhibitor, containing a 4-benzylpiperidine motif, identified via a novel screening system in yeast. Mol Pharmacol. 2006 Jul 17; [Epub ahead of print]

Gao J, Kashfi K, Rigas B. In vitro metabolism of nitric oxide-donating aspirin: the effect of positional isomerism. J Pharmacol Exp Ther. 2005;312:989–997.

Gao J, Liu X, Rigas B. Nitric oxide-donating aspirin induces apoptosis in human colon cancer cells through induction of oxidative stress. Proc Natl Acad Sci U S A. 2005;102:17207–17212.

Gasic GJ, Gasic TB, Murphy S. Anti-metastatic effect of aspirin. Lancet 1972;2:932–933.

Goodwin JS, Bankhurst AD, Messner RP. Suppression of T-cell mitogenesis by prostaglandin. Existence of a prostaglandin producing suppressor cell. J Exp. Med. 1977;146:1719–1734.

Goodwin JS, BankhurstAD, Murphy SA, Selinger DS, Messner RP, Williams RC Jr. Partial reversal of the cellular immune defect in common variable immunodeficiency with indomethacin. J. CLin. Lab. Immunol. 1978;1:197–199.

Goldstein DM, Alfredson T, Bertrand J, Browner MF, Clifford K, Dalrymple SA, Dunn J, Freire-Moar J, Harris S, Labadie SS, La Fargue J, Lapierre JM, Larrabee S, Li F, Papp E, McWeeney D, Ramesha C, Roberts R, Rotstein D, San Pablo B, Sjogren EB, So OY, Talamas FX, Tao W, Trejo A, Villasenor A, Welch M, Welch T, Weller P, Whiteley PE, Young K, Zipfel S. Discovery of S-[5-amino-1-(4-fluorophenyl)-1H-pyrazol-4-yl]-[3-(2,3-dihydroxypropoxy)-phenyl]methanone (RO3201195), an orally bioavailable and highly selective inhibitor of p38 MAP kinase. J Med Chem. 2006;49: 1562–1575.

Goldstein DM, Gabriel T. Pathway to the clinic: inhibition of P38 MAP kinase. A review of ten chemotypes selected for development. Curr Top Med Chem. 2005;5:1017–1029.

Grzanna R, Lindmark L, Frondoza CG. Ginger–an herbal medicinal product with broad anti-inflammatory actions. J Med Food. 2005;8:125–32.

Hall VC, Wolf RE. Effects of tenidap and non-steroidal anti-inflammatory drugs on the response of cultured human T cells to interleukin 2 in rheumatoid arthritis. J. Rheumatol. 1997;24:1467–1470.

Harris M, Jenkins MV, Bennett A, Wills MR. Prostaglandin production and bone resorption by dental cysts. Nature. 1973;245: 213–215.

Harris RE (ed.). COX-2 Blockade in Cancer Prevention and Therapy. Totawa, NJ: Humana Press, 2002a

Harris RE. Epidemiology of breast cancer and nonsteroidal anti-inflammatory drugs. In: *COX-2 Blockade in Cancer Prevention and Therapy*. R.E. Harris, ed. Totawa, NJ: Humana Press, 2002b, 57–68.

Hirschmann R. The cortisone era: aspects of its impact. Some contributions of the Merck Laboratories. Steroids. 1992;57:579–592.

Huguenin S, Fleury-Feith J, Kheuang L, Jaurand MC, Bolla M, Riffaud JP, Chopin DK, Vacherot F. Nitrosulindac (NCX 1102): a new nitric oxide-donating non-steroidal anti-inflammatory drug (NO-NSAID), inhibits proliferation and induces apoptosis in human prostatic epithelial cell lines. Prostate. 2004a;61:132–141.

Huguenin S, Vacherot F, Kheuang L, Fleury-Feith J, Jaurand MC, Bolla M, Riffaud JP, Chopin DK. Antiproliferative effect of nitrosulindac (NCX 1102), a new nitric oxide-donating non-steroidal anti-inflammatory drug, on human bladder carcinoma cell lines. Mol Cancer Ther. 2004b;3:291–298.

Hundley TR, Rigas B. Nitric oxide-donating aspirin inhibits colon cancer cell growth via mitogen-activated protein kinase activation. J Pharmacol Exp Ther. 2006;316:25–34.

Hynes J Jr, Leftheri K. Small molecule p38 inhibitors: novel structural features and advances from 2002–2005. Curr Top Med Chem. 2005;5:967–985

Kashfi K, Rigas B. Non-COX-2 targets and cancer: expanding the molecular target repertoire of chemoprevention. Biochem Pharmacol. 2005;70:969–986.

Jaffe BM, Parker CW, Philpott GW. Immunochemical measurement of prostaglandin or prostaglandin-like activity from normal and neoplastic cultures tissue. Surg Forum. 1971;22:90–92.

JForl J. Trial of Tandearil in prevention of cutaneous and mucosal complications in patients with otoshinolaryngeal neoplasms treated by irradiation. Otorhinolaryngeal Audiophonol Chir Maxillofac. 1976;25:175–178.

Jiang C, Ting AT, Seed B. PPAR-γ agonists inhibit production of monokine inflammatory cytokines. Nature. 1998;391:82–86.

Jimi E, Ghosh S. Role of nuclear factor-kappaB in the immune system and bone. Immunol Rev. 2005;208:80–87.

Jorizzo JL. Current and novel treatment options for actinic keratosis. J Cutan Med Surg. 2004;8 Suppl 3:13–21.

Kaplan EL, Peskin GW. Physiologic implications of medullary carcinoma of the thyroid gland. Surg Clin North Am. 1971;51:125–137.

Kaminska B. MAPK signalling pathways as molecular targets for anti-inflammatory therapy–from molecular mechanisms to therapeutic benefits. Biochim Biophys Acta. 2005;1754:253–262.

Katz S. Update in medical therapy of ulcerative colitis: newer concepts and therapies. J Clin Gastroenterol. 2005;39:557–569.

Kean WF, Buchanan WW. The use of NSAIDs in rheumatic disorders 2005: a global perspective. Inflammopharmacology. 2005;13:343–370.

Keeble JE, Moore PK. Pharmacology and potential therapeutic applications of nitric oxide-releasing non-steroidal anti-inflammatory and related nitric oxide-donating drugs. Br J Pharmacol. 2002;137:295–310.

Klein U, Muller-Fassbender H, Bublath H, Heinze HG. Effects of oxyphenbutazone on radiation fibrosis following irradiation for breast carcinoma. Strahlentherapie. 1972;144:421–429.

Kopp E, Ghosh S. Inhibition of NFkappaB by sodium salicylate and aspirin. Science. 1994;265:956–959.

Kulkarni RG, Achaiah G, Sastry GN. Novel targets for antiinflammatory and antiarthritic agents. Curr Pharm Des. 2006;12:2437–2454.

Lee JL, Mukhtar H, Bickers DR, Kopelovich L, Athar M. Cyclooxygenases in the skin: pharmacological and toxicological implications. Toxicol Appl Pharmacol. 2003;192:294–306.

Levine L, Hinkle PM, Voelkel EF, Tashjian AH Jr. Prostaglandin production by moouse fibrosarcoma cells in culture: inhibition by indomethacin and aspirin. Biochem Biophys Res Commun. 1972;47:888–896.

Lin TH, Metzger A, Diller DJ, Desai M, Henderson I, Ahmed G, Kimble EF, Quadros E, Webb ML. Discovery and characterization of triaminotriazine aniline amides as highly selective p38 kinase inhibitors. J Pharmacol Exp Ther. 2006;318:495–502.

Lindahl F. Intestinal injuries following irradiation for carcinoma of the uterine cervix and vesical carcinoma. Acta Chir Scand. 1970;136:725–730.

LiVolsi VA. Anti-metastatic effect of aspirin. Lancet. 1973;2:263.

Lo CJ, Cryer HG, Fu M, Lo FR. Regulation of macrophage eicosanoid generation is dependent on nuclear factor kappaB. J Trauma. 1998;45:19–23

Makman MH. Conditions leading to enhanced response to glucagons, epinephrine, or prostaglandins by adenylate cyclase of normal and malignant cultured cells. Proc Natl Acad Sci USA. 1971;68: 2127–2130.

Maulik N, Sato M, Price BD, Das DK. An essential role of NFkappaB in tyrosine kinase signaling of p38 MAP kinase regulation of myocardial adaptation to ischemia. FEBS Lett. 1998;429:365–369.

Metzger A, Diller DJ, Lin TH, Henderson I, Webb ML. Successful screening of large encoded combinatorial libraries leading to the discovery of novel p38 MAP kinase inhibitors. Comb Chem High Throughput Screen. 2006;9:351–358.

Miwatashi S, Arikawa Y, Kotani E, Miyamoto M, Naruo K, Kimura H, Tanaka T, Asahi S, Ohkawa S. Novel inhibitor of p38 MAP kinase as an anti-TNF-alpha drug: discovery of N-[4-[2-ethyl-4-(3-methylphenyl)-1,3-thiazol-5-yl]-2-pyridyl]-benzamide (TAK-715) as a potent and orally active anti-rheumatoid arthritis agent. J Med Chem. 2005;48:5966–5979.

Muller-Fassbender H, Klein U, Bablath H, Heinze HG. Effect of oxyphenbutazone on radiation-induced lung diseases. Med Klin. 1973; 68:478–483.

Nash P, Clegg DO. Psoriatic arthritis therapy: NSAIDs and traditional DMARDs. Ann Rheum Dis. 2005 Mar;64 Suppl 2:ii74–7.

Nathoo N, Barnett GH, Golubic M. The eicosanoid cascade: possible role in gliomas and meningiomas. J Clin Pathol. 2004;57:6–13.

O'Brien JR. Effects of salicylates on human platelets. Lancet. 1968; 1(4546), 779–783.

Otterness IG. The discovery of drugs to treat arthritis. A historical view. In: *The Search for Anti-inflammatory Drugs*. VJ Merluzzi, J. Adams, eds. Boston: Birkhäuser, 1995, 1–26.

Paik JH, Ju JH, Lee JY, Boudreau MD, Hwang DH. Two opposing effects of non-steroidal anti-inflammatory drugs on the expression of the inducible cyclooxygenase. Mediation through different signaling pathways. J Biol Chem. 2000;275:28173–28179.

Papa S, Bubici C, Zazzeroni F, Pham CG, Kuntzen C, Knabb JR, Dean K, Peifer C, Wagner G, Laufer S. New approaches to the treatment of inflammatory disorders small molecule inhibitors of p38 MAP kinase. Curr Top Med Chem. 2006;6:113–149.

Parkinson JF. Lipoxin and synthetic lipoxin analogs: an overview of anti-inflammatory functions and new concepts in immunomodulation. Inflamm Allergy Drug Targets. 2006;5:91–106.

Paulus HE. Clinical trial design for evaluating combination therapies. Br J Rheumatol. 1995;34 Suppl 2:92–95

Pellegatta F, Bertelli AA, Staels B, Duhem C, Fulgenzi A, Ferrero ME. Different short- and long-term effects of resveratrol on nuclear factor-kappaB phosphorylation and nuclear appearance in human endothelial cells. Am J Clin Nutr. 2003;77:1220–1228.

Petasis NA, Akritopoulou-Zanze I, Fokin VV, Bernasconi G, Keledjian R, Yang R, Uddin J, Nagulapalli KC, Serhan CN. Design, synthesis and bioactions of novel stable mimetics of lipoxins and aspirin-triggered lipoxins. Prostaglandins Leukot Essent Fatty Acids. 2005;73:301–321.

Phillips T, Leeuwenburgh C. Lifelong aspirin supplementation as a means to extending life span. Rejuvenation Res. 2004 Winter;7(4):243–51.

Powles TJ, Easty DM, Easty GC, Neville AM. Tumor-induced osteolysis. N Engl J Med. 1974;291:105.

Powles TJ, Clark SA, Easty DM, Easty GC, Neville AM. The inhibition by aspirin and indomethacin of osteolytic tumor deposits and hypercalcaemia in rats with Walker tumour, and its possible application to human breast cancer. Br J Cancer. 1973;28:316–321.

Powles TJ, Easty GC, Easty DM, Neville AM. Anti-metastatic effect of aspirin. Lancet. 1973;2:100.

Prescott LF. Paracetamol (Acetaminiphen). A Critical Bibliographic Review. Revised 2nd Edn. London: Taylor & Francis, 2001.

Rainsford KD. History and development of ibuprofen. In: *Ibuprofen. A Critical Bibliographic Review*, K.D. Rainsford, ed. London: Taylor & Francis, 1999a, 1–24.

Rainsford KD. Pharmacology and toxicology of ibuprofen. In: *Ibuprofen. A Critical Bibliographic Review*, K.D. Rainsford, ed. London: Taylor & Francis, 1999b, 145–275.

Rainsford KD. History and development of the salicylates. In: *Aspirin and Related Drugs*, K.D. Rainsford, ed. London & New York: Taylor & Francis, 2004a, 1–23.

Rainsford KD. Side effects and toxicology of the salicylates. In: *Aspirin and Related Drugs*, K.D. Rainsford, ed. London & New York: Taylor and Francis, 2004b, 367–554.

Rainsford KD. Pharmacology and Biochemistry of salicylates and related drugs. In: *Aspirin and Related Drugs*, K.D. Rainsford, ed. London and New York: Taylor & Francis, 2004c, 215–366.

Rainsford KD. Aspirin and NSAIDs in the prevention of cancer, Alzheimer's disease and othe novel therapeutic actions. In: *Aspirin and Related Drugs*, K.D. Rainsford, ed. London and New York: Taylor & Francis, 2004d, 707–756.

Rainsford KD. Inhibitors of eicosanoids. In: *The Eicosanoids*, P Curtis-Prior, ed. Chichester: John Wiley & Sons, 2004e, 189–210.

Rainsford KD. Occurrence, properties and synthetic developments of the salicylates. In: *Aspirin and Related Drugs*, K.D. Rainsford, ed. London & New York: Taylor & Francis, 2004f, 45–95.

Rainsford KD. Aspirin and NSAIDs in the prevention of cancer, Alzheimer's disease and other novel therapeutic actions. In: *Aspirin and Related Drugs*, K.D. Rainsford, ed. London & New York: Taylor & Francis, 2004g, 707–756.

Rainsford KD. The discovery, development and novel actions of nimesulide. In: *Nimesulide – Actions and Uses*, K.D. Rainsford, ed. Basel: Birkhäuser Verlag, 2005a, 1–61.

Rainsford KD. The coxib controversies. Inflammopharmacology. 2005b;13:331–341.

Riedl K, Krysan K, Pold M, Dalwadi H, Heuze-Vourc'h N, Dohadwala M, Liu M, Cui X, Figlin R, Mao JT, Strieter R, Sharma S, Dubinett SM. Multifaceted roles of cyclooxygenase-2 in lung cancer. Drug Resist Updat. 2004;7:169–184.

Rice TW, Bernard GR. Therapeutic intervention and targets for sepsis. Annu Rev Med. 2005;56:225–248.

Rigas B, Kalofonos H, Lebovics E, Vagenakis AG. NO-NSAIDs and cancer: promising novel agents. Dig Liver Dis. 2003;35 Suppl 2:S27–34.

Rocha PN, Plumb TJ, Coffman TM. Eicosanoids: lipid mediators of inflammation in transplantation. Springer Semin Immunopathol. 2003;25:215–227.

Rogers JT, Lahiri DK. Metal and inflammatory targets for Alzheimer's disease. Curr Drug Targets. 2004;5:535–551.

Rosetti M, Tesei A, Ulivi P, Fabbri F, Vannini I, Brigliadori G, Amadori D, Ouyang N, Williams JL, Tsioulias GJ, Gao J, Iatropoulos MJ, Kopelovich L, Kashfi K, Rigas B. Nitric oxide-donating aspirin prevents pancreatic cancer in a hamster tumor model. Cancer Res. 2006;66:4503–4511.

Royle JS, Ross JA, Ansell I, Bollina P, Tulloch DN, Habib FK. Nitric oxide donating nonsteroidal anti-inflammatory drugs induce apoptosis in human prostate cancer cell systems and human prostatic stroma via caspase-3. J Urol. 2004;172:338–344.

Russo-Marie F. Antiinflammatory steroids. In: *The Eicosanoids*. P. Curtis-Prior, ed. Chichester: John Wiley & Sons, 2004, 327–332.

Sabat M, Vanrens JC, Clark MP, Brugel TA, Maier J, Bookland RG, Laufersweiler MJ, Laughlin SK, Golebiowski A, De B, Hsieh LC, Walter RL, Mekel MJ, Janusz MJ. The development of novel C-2, C-8, and N-9 trisubstituted purines as inhibitors of TNF-alpha production. Bioorg Med Chem Lett. 2006;16:4360–4365.

Saji S, Hirose M, Toi M. Novel sensitizing agents: potential contribution of COX-2 inhibitor for endocrine therapy of breast cancer. Breast Cancer. 2004;11(2):129–133.

Saklatvala J. The p38 MAP kinase pathway as a therapeutic target in inflammatory disease. Curr Opin Pharmacol. 2004;4:372–377.

Sanborn R, Blanke CD. Cyclooxygenase-2 inhibition in colorectal cancer: boom or bust? Semin Oncol. 2005;32:69–75.

Sandler M, Karim SM, Williams ED. Prostaglandins in amine-peptide-secreting tumours. Lancet. 1968;2:1053–1054.

Serhan CN. Novel eicosanoid and docosanoid mediators: resolvins, docosatrienes, and neuroprotectins. Curr Opin Clin Nutr Metab Care. 2005;8:115–121.

Serhan CN, Arita M, Hong S, Gotlinger K. Resolvins, docosatrienes, and neuroprotectins, novel omega-3-derived mediators,and their endogenous aspirin-triggered epimers. Lipids. 2004;39:1125–1132.

Shay NF, Banz WJ. Regulation of gene transcription by botanicals: novel regulatory mechanisms. Annu Rev Nutr. 2005;25:297–315.

Simon LS. The treatment of rheumatoid arthritis. Best Pract Res Clin Rheumatol. 2004;18:507–538.

Skinner R. Role of topical therapies in the management of cutaneous disease. J Cutan Med Surg. 2004;8 Suppl 3:22–31.

Smith JW, Steiner AL, Parker CW. Human lymphocyte metabolism. Effects of cyclic and non-cyclic nucleotides, on stimulation by phytohaemagglutinin. J.Clin. Invest. 1971;50:442–448.

Tew WP, Kelsen DP, Ilson DH. Targeted therapies for esophageal cancer. Oncologist. 2005;10:590–601.

Trummlitz G, van Ryn J. Designing selective COX-2 inhibitors: molecular modeling approaches. Curr Opin Drug Discov Devel. 2002;5:550–561.

Thun MJ, Henley SJ. Epidemiology of nonsteroidal anti-inflammatory drugs and colorectal cancer. In: *COX-2 Blockade in Cancer Prevention and Therapy*. R.E. Harris, ed. Totawa, NJ: Humana Press, 2002; 35–55.

Vane JR. Inhibition of prostaglandin synthesis as a mechanism of action of aspirin-like drugs. Nature New Biology. 1971;231:232–235.

Van Wijk R, Wicks WD, Clay, K. Effects of derivatives of cyclic 3′, 5′-adenosine monophosphate on the growth, morphology, and gene expression of hepatoma cells in culture. Cancer Res. 1972;32: 1905–1911.

Vayssiere BM, Dupont S, Choquart A, Petit F, Garcia T, Marchandeau C, Gronemeyer H, Resche-Rigon M. Synthetic glucocorticoids that dissociate transactivation and AP-1 transrepression exhibit antiinflammatory activity in vivo. Mol Endocrinol. 1997;11:1245–1255.

Wang D, Dubois RN. Prostaglandins and cancer. Gut. 2006;55:115–122.

Weaver AL. The impact of new biologicals in the treatment of rheumatoid arthritis. Rheumatology. 2004;43 (Suppl 3): iii17-iii23.

Webert KE, Kelton JG. Acetylsalicylic acid for prevention and treatment of thromboembolic diseases. In: *Aspirin and Related Drugs*, K.D. Rainsford, ed. London & New York: Taylor & Francis, 619–633.

Whittle BJ. Nitric oxide and the gut injury induced by non-steroidal anti-inflammatory drugs. Inflammopharmacology. 2003;11:415–422.

Wood S Jr, Hilgard P. Aspirin and tumour metastasis. Lancet. 1972;2:1416–1417.

Wu KK. Control of cyclooxygenase-2 transcriptional activation by pro-inflammatory mediators. Prostaglandins Leukot Essent Fatty Acids. 2005;72:89–93.

Wu T. Cyclooxygenase-2 and prostaglandin signaling in cholangiocarcinoma. Biochim Biophys Acta. 2005 Jul 25;1755(2):135–150.

Yeh CH, Chen TP, Wu YC, Lin YM, Jing Lin P. Inhibition of NFkappaB activation with curcumin attenuates plasma inflammatory cytokines surge and cardiomyocytic apoptosis following cardiac ischemia/reperfusion. J Surg Res. 2005;125:109–116.

Yoon JH, Baek SJ. Molecular targets of dietary polyphenols with anti-inflammatory properties. Yonsei Med J. 2005;46:585–596.

Yoon JB, Kim SJ, Hwang SG, Chang S, Kang SS, Chun JS. Non-steroidal anti-inflammatory drugs inhibit nitric oxide-induced apoptosis and dedifferentiation of articular chondrocytes independent of cyclooxygenase activity. J Biol Chem. 2003;278:15319–15325.

Zacharowski P, Zacharowski K, Donnellan C, Johnston A, Vojnovic I, Forte P, Del Soldato P, Benjamin N, O'Byrne S. The effects and metabolic fate of nitroflurbiprofen in healthy volunteers. Clin Pharmacol Ther. 2004;76:350–358.

Zheng Z, Yenari MA. Post-ischemic inflammation: molecular mechanisms and therapeutic implications. Neurol Res. 2004;26:884–892.

SECTION II

INFLAMMATORY MECHANISMS OF PATHOGENESIS

CHAPTER 2

NITRIC OXIDE SYNTHASE AND CYCLOOXYGENASE INTERACTIONS IN CARTILAGE AND MENISCUS

Relationships to joint physiology, arthritis, and tissue repair

J. BRICE WEINBERG[1,*], BEVERLEY FERMOR[2]
AND FARSHID GUILAK[2]

Department of Medicine, Division of Hematology-Oncology, VA and Duke University Medical Centers[1]
Department of Surgery, Division of Orthopedics, Duke University Medical Center[2]
Durham, North Carolina

Abstract: Rheumatoid arthritis and osteoarthritis are painful and debilitating diseases with complex pathophysiology. There is growing evidence that pro-inflammatory cytokines (e.g., interleukin-1 and tumor necrosis factor alpha) and mediators (e.g., prostaglandins, leukotrienes, and nitric oxide) play critical roles in the development and perpetuation of tissue inflammation and damage in joint tissues such as articular cartilage and meniscus. While earlier studies have generally focused on cells of the synovium (especially macrophages), there is increasing evidence that chondrocytes and meniscal cells actively

---

* J. Brice Weinberg, MD, VA & Duke University Medical Centers, 508 Fulton Street, Durham, NC 27705.
E-mail: brice@duke.edu

R. E. Harris (ed.), Inflammation in the Pathogenesis of Chronic Diseases, 31–62.
© *2007 Springer.*

contribute to inflammatory processes. In particular, it is now apparent that mechanical forces engendered by joint loading are transduced to biological signals at the cellular level and that these signals modulate gene expression and biochemical processes. Here we give an overview of the interplay of cytokines and mechanical stress in the production of cyclooxygenases and prostaglandins; lipoxygenases and leukotrienes; and nitric oxide synthases and nitric oxide in arthritis, with particular focus on the interactions of these pathways in articular cartilage and meniscus

1.   INTRODUCTION

Rheumatoid arthritis (RA) and osteoarthritis (OA) are frequent and important diseases with complex pathophysiology. There is convincing evidence that cytokines (e.g., IL-1 and TNF), prostaglandins (PG), and nitric oxide (NO) play critical roles in the development and perpetuation of inflammation and cartilage and meniscus damage in RA and OA. While earlier studies have generally focused on cells of the synovium (especially macrophages), there is increasing evidence that cells in cartilage (chondrocytes) and meniscus (fibrochondrocytes) contribute to these processes. We now realize that mechanical force affecting cells is transduced to biological signals that modulate gene expression and biochemical processes. Here we give an overview of the interplay of mechanical stress, cyclooxygenases (COX) and PG, nitric oxide synthases (NOS) and NO, and cytokines in arthritis. We focus on cartilage and meniscus studies. We also refer the reader to some other recent pertinent reviews [1–5].

2.   NO AND NO SYNTHASES

The simple gas NO has many important physiologic and pathologic functions [6]. These include roles in host resistance to tumors and microbes, regulation of blood pressure and vascular tone, neurotransmission, learning, and neurotoxicity, carcinogenesis, and control of cellular growth and differentiation [6, 7]. In the presence of oxygen, NO rapidly (seconds) is converted to nitrite and nitrate, substances which are generally not bioactive (8 for review). NO binds with high affinity to iron in heme groups of proteins such as hemoglobin (Hb) and guanylyl cyclase; Hb is a very effective quencher of NO action. NO also reacts with O_2^-, and SOD prolongs NO life by eliminating O_2^-. On reacting with O_2^-, NO may form peroxynitrite ($OONO^-$), a very reactive molecule. In addition to these NO-related species, S-nitrosothiols (formed by coupling of NO to a reactive cysteine thiol) are very important regulators of physiology and pathology, playing roles in signaling and modulating of cellular and enzyme function [9].

NOS converts L-arginine to L-citrulline and NO (Figure 1). Three forms of the enzyme nitric oxide synthase are encoded by three different genes. Neural NOS (nNOS or NOS1) and endothelial cell NOS (eNOS or NOS3) are constitutive enzymes, demonstrating low level, constant transcription of mRNA. The enzymatic actions of NOS1 and NOS3 are modulated by regulation of cytoplasmic calcium levels, with agents inducing increases in calcium, with subsequent binding

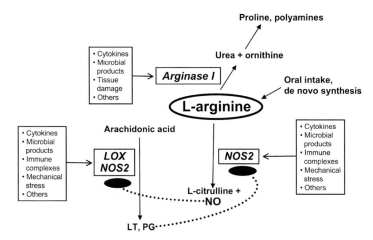

Figure 1. Nitric oxide synthase, cyclooxygenase, arginine, and arginase pathways and interactions. Plasma arginine levels are held relatively constant at approximately 100 to 120 uM by endogenous synthesis by the intestine and kidney, and through absorption of ingested arginine. A variety of factors and signals can activate certain cells (e.g., mononuclear phagocytes, chondrocytes, and meniscal fibro-chondrocytes) for COX2, NOS2, and arginase I (inducible arginase) expression and arginine, PG, and NO production and metabolism. NO may either increase or decrease COX2 activity and PG production, but we have found the effects to be generally inhibitory in macrophages, cartilage, and meniscus. Likewise, PG may either increase NOS expression/NO production. NOS2 can bind and nitrosylate COX2 and consequently enhance its enzymatic activity. PG and NO contribute to the cellular homeostasis and to inflammatory processes. Arginase can deplete arginine and thus limit NO production. Arginase products (proline and polyamines) may influence cell proliferation and collagen formation. The dotted lines with black ovals indicate that NO may modulate (increase or decrease) COX2 and that PG may modulate NOS2 expression and NO production

to calmodulin and activation of the enzyme. Although inducible NOS (NOS2) was described initially in mononuclear phagocytes, it also is found in numerous other cells including synoviocytes, chondrocytes, meniscal cells, smooth muscle cells, hepatocytes, B lymphocytes and others [6, 10].

Regulation of NOS2 mRNA can occur at multiple steps including mRNA transcription, mRNA stability, and mRNA translation, but transcription is the major step of regulation. The promoter region upstream of the 5′ region of the NOS2 gene contains numerous consensus sequences for known DNA-binding proteins [12–15]. These include 2 activating protein 1 (AP-1), 2 NF-κB, 2 TNF-response element (TNFRE), 2 IFN-α stimulatable RE (ISRE), 1 X-box, 3 gamma activated sites (GAS), 1 PU.1/IFN-γ element, NF-IL-6, and 10 IFN-γ RE (γ-IRE). AP-1 (*c-fos/c-jun*) appears to inhibit transcription [16]. Interferon regulatory factor 1 (IRF-1), a protein factor that binds to γ-IRE DNA and initiates gene transcription, is critical for the production of NOS2 transcription and NO production in transgenic mice experiments [17]. STAT factors also are important in the activation of NOS2 gene expression [16, 18]. This is true for both IFN-γ and IFN-α; IFN-α acts in an autocrine or paracrine fashion in endotoxin activated macrophages [19].

Increased NOS2 transcription and increased NOS2 expression induced by IFN-γ/LPS and TNF is mediated in part by members of the MAP kinase family. For example, engagement of the IFN-γ/ receptor activates protein tyrosine kinases (such and the Janus kinases Jak1 and Jak2) which phosphorylate and activate STAT1α. The activated STAT1α translocates into the nucleus and induces transcription of IFN-γ-regulated genes by binding the consensus sequences in gene promoters. The p38 MAP kinase, extracellular signal-regulated kinase (ERK1/2), STAT1α, Janus kinases, and NF-κB have all been shown to be important in activation of NOS2 transcription by different stimuli [11,16,20–22].

Sequences in the 3′ untranslated region in NOS3 may determine mRNA stability [23], but this has not been demonstrated for NOS2. At the protein level, NOS may be regulated in many ways: calmodulin binding, dimer formation (the enzyme requires dimerization for function), substrate (L-arginine) depletion, substrate recycling (L-citrulline to L-arginine), tetrahydrobiopterin (BH_4) availability, end product inhibition (NO interaction with NOS heme), phosphorylation, and subcellular localization. Important NOS co-factors include FAD, FMN, NADPH, tetrahydro-biopterin, and calmodulin-calcium. For NOS2, calmodulin is tightly bound to protein, making it relatively resistant to inhibition by calcium chelators. Activities of NOS can be markedly influenced by levels of tetrahydrobiopterin—depleting cellular tetrahydrobiopterin by inhibitors of GTP cyclohydrolase I, sepiapterin reductase, and dihydrofolate reductase reduces NOS activity [24]. Cytokines and LPS can enhance tetrahydrobiopterin production by induction of GTP cyclohy-drolase, the rate limiting enzyme for tetrahydrobiopterin synthesis. NOS2 mRNA translation to protein is dependent on adequate levels of arginine [25]. Reduced levels of arginine cause decreased NOS2 protein even though NOS2 mRNA levels are unchanged. Arginine apparently negatively regulates the phosphorylation status of the eukaryotic initiation factor (eIF2 alpha), which, in turn, regulates translation of iNOS mRNA [25].

3.   ARGININE

Arginine is the substrate for NOS and the precursor of NO. Arginine is generally considered an essential amino acid in newborns and infants and a non-essential amino acid in adults [26]. This amino acid serves as a critical precursor for synthesis of proteins, NO, creatine, proline, citrulline, polyamines, urea, agmatine, and glutamate. As such, it is very important in eventual signal transduction, connective tissue physiology, cell proliferation, and general cellular function. In vivo, arginine derives from exogenous (diet) and endogenous (whole-body protein degradation plus endogenous synthesis from citrulline) sources [26]. In adults, de novo arginine synthesis accounts for only 5–15% of endogenous arginine flux. Whole-body protein turnover probably contributes the most to endogenous arginine flux. The intestine is the net site of citrulline synthesis from which the amino acid enters the circulation to be taken up by the kidneys. In the kidney, citrulline is converted to arginine almost exclusively in the proximal convoluted tubule via actions of the cytosolic enzymes ASS and ASL. Thus, the kidneys are considered to be the main organ site for net de novo arginine synthesis [26]. Arginine can also be synthesized in cells actively producing NO via the citrulline/NO cycle. As NOS2 is induced by inflammatory mediators, so are the enzymes that convert citrulline to arginine (ASS and ASL) [26].

Arginine can be catabolized through multiple pathways by a variety of enzymes. Some of these enzymes can be expressed within the same cells. For example, macrophages may express arginase and arginine decarboxylase, as well as NOS. The complex interactions noted in macrophages (especially those involving arginase) are likely balanced by the presence of NOS and the NOS intermediate molecule N^G-OH-arginine, a very potent arginase inhibitor in these cells.

Arginine transport is very important because it can regulate substrate availability and thus control production of NO by NOS [26, 27]. The cationic amino acid transporters (termed CAT-1 and CAT-2) serve to transport arginine, lysine, and ornithine across membranes in human cells (the system Y^+ amino acid transporters) [26, 28, 29]. CAT expression is regulated transcriptionally, and is co-induced with NOS2 in response to inflammatory stimuli [30]. As noted earlier, cellular production of NO by NOS is dependent on *extracellular* concentrations of arginine (and sufficient CAT to transport the arginine inside). Cells with apparent adequate intracellular levels of arginine (0.1 to 1 mM) for NO synthesis still require extra-cellular concentrations of arginine in the 75–150 uM range [26]. This "arginine paradox" (dependence of cellular NO production on exogenous L-arginine concentration despite the theoretical saturation of NOS enzymes with intracellular arginine) may be explained by the recent findings that arginine depletion suppresses translation of NOS2 [25]. The arginine controls NOS2 activity by regulating NOS2 expression through translational control pathways involving the amino acid control kinase GCN2 and eukaryotic initiation factor eIF2 alpha phosphorylation. Increasing intracellular arginine concentrations by increasing expression of CAT corrects the problem and allows adequate NOS2 translation and NO production [25]. The newly transported arginine not only increases arginine concentrations, it also increases the amount of NOS2 by a mechanism of translation.

Arginine has been safely administered to humans for decades [31, 32], and it is a component of the normal human diet. Orally supplemented arginine is well absorbed, with absorption varying from 30 to 70%. Peak plasma concentrations appear at 2 hours after oral ingestion on an empty stomach. Intravenous arginine is well tolerated. It is to given to children and adults at doses up to 30 grams by intra-venous bolus administration in studies of induction of growth hormone secretion [33, 34], an NO-mediated process. Arginine is well tolerated when given short term (6–30 g IV or orally) and long term (6–12 g/day orally) in healthy subjects, and subjects with severe cardiovascular disease and cystic fibrosis with minimal toxicity [31,32,35–38]. In these diseases, arginine increases NO metabolites and exhaled NO, with improvements in endothelial function, perfusion, symptom scores and exercise tolerance [31,32,35–37]. Arginine therapy corrects the hypoargininemia and impaired NO production found in patients with sickle cell vaso-occlusive syndrome (SCD VOCS) [39], a syndrome with endothelial dysfunction and impaired NO production and low plasma arginine levels similar to malaria [40]. Trials are also underway for treatment of pulmonary hypertension associated with SCD and in idiopathic pulmonary hypertension, conditions characterized by functional lack of NO, perhaps because of cell-free hemoglobin and elevated arginase from hemolysis.

4.   ARGINASES

Arginases are important enzymes that control availability of arginine for synthesis of NO, polyamines, agmatine, proline, and glutamate [41]. There are two distinct isozymes of arginase encoded by separate genes. Arginase I, a cytosolic enzyme, is very high in hepatocytes and a few other cells. Inherited deficiency of arginase I results in argininemia [42]. Arginase II, a mitochondrial enzyme is expressed at low levels, primarily in macrophages, kidney, brain, small intestine, and mammary gland [43]. There are no cases of inherited abnormalities in arginase II. Certain cells such as endothelial cells and macrophages may express both types I and II. Presence of arginase with consequent consumption of arginine can limit production of NO even when high levels of NOS are present [44–46]. Also, as noted above, specifics of arginine transport by CAT and regulation of NOS2 translation by levels of arginine may serve to further limit NO formation.

Arginase, through generation of polyamines, regulates cell proliferation and differentiation [26]. Inhibitors of arginase (e.g., N^G-OH-arginine) have been used to modulate the arginase influence on proliferation and differentiation [47]. Ornithine derived from arginase action may lead to proline synthesis which in turn is important for collagen synthesis and connective tissue physiology, and mammary gland function [26]. Arginase is important for synthesis of glutamate which plays important roles in neuronal signaling.

The arginase I gene is highly conserved among all mammalian species. Murine arginase I and II genes have eight exons, and their 5′-flanking sequences are 84% homologous [43]. The promoter region of arginase II is quite different than that of the arginase I gene, containing numerous potential binding sites for enhancer and promoter elements, including AP1, NF-kB, and CRE-BP2. However, arginase II does not contain a TATA box [43].

Arginase expression is increased by IL-4, IL-10, or IL-13 [44, 45, 48]. Macrophages induced to express arginase produce less NO [44–46, 49] and are termed "alternatively activated" macrophages [50, 51]. The alternatively activated macrophages also display other unique proteins such as FIZZ1 and YM1 [52]. Arginase may modulate resistance to parasitic diseases such as shistosomiasis, trypanosomiasis, and leishmaniasis [53]. These effects likely result from depletion of arginine and limitation of NO production and by increasing polyamines that enhance parasite growth and differentiation [29].

Arginase II is increased in synovial fluid macrophages from patients with RA [54]. Production by these macrophages could be increased by incubation in vitro with dibutyryl cyclic AMP, PGE_2, or endotoxin, while these factors reduced NO production by the synovial membrane cells. The researchers speculated that reciprocal regulation of arginase and NOS would NO production [54].

5. CYCLOOXYGENASES AND PROSTAGLANDINS

Cyclooxygenases (prostaglandin endoperoxide H synthases) catalyze conversion of arachidonic acid and oxygen to PGH_2, the committed step in prostanoid biosynthesis (Figure 2). COX enzymes catalyze both a *cyclooxygenase* reaction in which arachidonic acid is converted to PGG_2 and a *peroxidase* reaction in which PGG_2 is reduced to PGH_2 [55, 56]. PGH_2 can then be processed into various classes of bioactive lipids including thromboxanes, $PGF_{2\alpha}$, PGD_2, PGI_2, and PGE_2. NSAIDs (nonsteroidal anti-inflammatory drugs) compete directly with arachidonic acid binding to the cyclooxygenase site and inhibit cyclooxygenase activity. The two main isoforms of COX (COX1 and COX2) are 60% homologous, and are encoded by separate genes [56]. COX1 function is especially important for platelet, renal, and gastrointestinal mucosa function. COX2 mRNA is undetectable in most normal tissues. However, COX2 in increased in most inflammatory states. COX2 is inducible by a number of factors including IL-1, TNF, LPS, IL-2, GM-CSF, G-CSF, and TGF-β. COX2 is co-induced with NOS2 by many of the same stimulants (e.g., bacterial endotoxin and cytokines such as IFN-gamma and TNF). Several agents including glucocorticoids and IL-10 inhibit COX2 expression. Most evidence suggests that COX2 is the primary isoform involved in inflammation. However, animal studies with specific inhibitors and with COX2 gene knockout mice suggest that COX1 is also important [57], and COX2 may be involved in the resolution of inflammation [58]. There is some evidence that

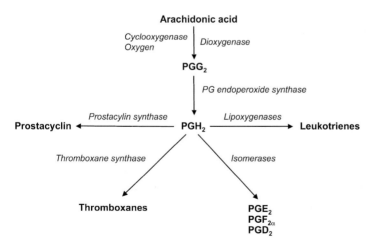

Figure 2. Arachidonic acid metabolism pathways. Simplified version of these pathways with several intermediates and enzymes omitted

COX3 is a COX expressed in the brain and heart that is inhibited by acetaminophen, an agent that can modify pain and fever but not inflammation [59].

Increased prostaglandin synthesis is a cellular response to activation by pro-inflammatory stimuli [60] and an important component in the pathogenesis of arthritis. Increased prostanoid release and COX2 expression are seen in arthritic compared with non-arthritic cartilage [61]. PGE_2 is a pleiotropic bioregulator with the ability to alter the expression of an increasing list of target genes involved in the pathophysiology of arthritic diseases. Since cartilage is avascular it is likely that effects are via paracrine and autocrine mechanisms. Cytokine stimulation of articular cartilage leads to PGE_2 release due to increased COX2 activity [62, 63]. PGE_2 plays a role in the regulation of chondrocyte proliferation and synthesis of extracellular components [64]. Low concentrations of PGE_2 increase collagen synthesis, while high doses decrease collagen synthesis [65]. Similarly, prostaglandins stimulate type II collagen gene (COL2A1) expression [66]. Addition of PGE_2 to chondrocytes can activate both the cAMP-protein kinase A and the Ca^{2+} and protein kinase C second messenger systems [67] which may account for the biphasic effect of PGE_2 on cartilage. PGE_2 upregulates the expression of IGF-1 and IGFBP-3 in chondrocytes by a cAMP independent pathway probably involving Ca^{2+}/calmodulin activated signaling systems [68]. Furthermore, IL-1 induced PGE_2 production by chondrocytes seems to involve protein tyrosine kinase pathway [62].

PGE_2 can also exert anti-catabolic and anti-inflammatory effects and can potently downregulate the expression and synthesis of inflammatory cytokines IL-1 and TNF, as well as NOS2, MMP1, MMP3 [69–72]. The pro-anabolic effects of PGE_2 on cartilage have been identified by increased proteoglycan synthesis and DNA synthesis [67] and increased collagen synthesis via an effector autocrine loop involving insulin-like growth factor 1 (IGF1) [65]. The onset of arthritis can be blocked *in vivo* using NOS inhibitors [73, 74 for review], but the mechanism likely involves an increase in PGE_2 in the presence of IL-1 *in vitro* [75]. IL-1 is prevalent in arthritic cartilage and induces chondrocyte catabolism [76]. Very little is known concerning the pathways involved in the stimulation of PGE_2 production under physiologic biomechanical conditions in the joint.

COX2 inhibitors have provided an alternative to non-specific NSAIDs in the treatment of arthritis. They are effective therapeutic agents for both OA and RA and also attenuate inflammation and hyperalgesia in several animal models of arthritis [60, 77]. COX2 expression is upregulated in a variety of cell types by pro-inflammatory cytokines and downregulated by anti-inflammatory cytokines and glucocorticoid hormones. COX2 is expressed in inflamed synovial tissue [78–80]. Certain drugs that have high selectivity against COX2 such as NS398, celocoxib, or rofecoxib have proven potent anti-inflammatory compounds with reduced side effects [81, 82]. However, the given the potential influence of prostaglandins on cartilage matrix turnover, the effect of COX inhibition on chondrocyte activity is unclear, particular with respect to mechanical stress. Because of important cardio-vascular side effects, their overall safety has been questioned [83].

6. NOS/NO – COX/PG INTERACTIONS

Products of NOS and COX can potently modulate functions of different cells and enzymes, and NO and PG can cross-regulate COX and NOS (Figure 1). Arachidonic acid metabolites play important roles in inflammation, and cyclooxygenase inhibitors are drugs useful in the management of inflammatory disease. Eicosanoids can reduce NOS2 expression and NO production [72, 84, 85], and NO modulates PGE_2 formation [86–88]. Stimuli that enhance NOS2 and NO formation also may induce COX2 expression, but the time course for induction differs. Arginine analogues such as N^G-monomethyl L-arginine (NMMA) may be anti-inflammatory by inhibiting both COX2 and NOS [89]. Furthermore, aspirin (in high doses) inhibits both cyclooxygenase and NOS2 [90]. Various researchers report different results. These divergent results may in part be related to use of different cells and experimental conditions, but some cannot be easily explained. PGE_2 has been reported to decrease NOS2 expression in mouse macrophages [72, 91, 92], or to increase NO production in rat liver macrophages (Kupffer cells) [93]. Some investigators reported that modulating NO levels by use NO donors, activation of cells, or inhibition of NO synthesis by arginine depletion or NOS inhibition either stimulated or inhibited PG synthesis [86,94–96]. These modulating effects were felt to be the result of altered transcription of COX genes, modulation of COX activity, or modification of PG metabolizing enzymes. The NO derivatives peroxynitrite or S-nitrosothiols may participate in these actions. NO enhances COX1 while inhibiting COX2 in mouse J774 macrophages [75]. We have consistently noted that NO apparently inhibits PG production by mouse J774 macrophages and pig cartilage cells [97, 98].

Marnett et al studied regulation of PG synthesis in mice with genetically disrupted NOS2 [57]. PGE_2 production was decreased in cells from the NOS2 knockout mice, but that COX2 protein was not different in cells from the wild type and NOS2 knockout mice. Urinary PGE_2 was lower and F_2-isoprostanes (an index of endogenous oxidant stress) were less in NOS2 knockout mice. Thromboxane B_2 from COX1 of platelets aggregating in vitro was higher in wildtype mice in the knockout mice. They concluded that NO or NO-related molecules modulate COX activity and eicosanoid production [57]. Experiments using purified COX showed that NO could bind to the iron in COX heme, but that in "physiologic" conditions, there was no evidence that it changed COX enzyme activity [99].

Kim et al [100] recently demonstrated that NOS2 binds and nitrosylates COX2 with resultant increased enzymatic activity of COX2. In experiments with mouse macrophage cell line cells, induced mouse peritoneal macrophages, and human embryonic kidney cells transfected with COX2 and NOS2, there NOS2 and COX2 co-immunoprecipitated after treatment with IFN-gamma and endotoxin indicating that COX2 and NOS2 were bound together. This was specific for COX2 since COX1 did not co-localize. The binding took place between the oxygenase domain (N terminus) of NOS2 and the C terminus of COX2. The interaction was accompanied and dependent on locally generated NO-induced S-nitrosylation of cysteine 526 of COX2. The authors calculated that about 50% of induced COX2 activity is determined by S-nitrosylation. The COX2-NOS2 physical proximity facilitates

COX2 S-nitrosylation [100]. These findings suggest that NOS2 and COX2 physical and biochemical interactions are key to functional modulation of COX2 activity and suggest that this NOS2/COX2/nitrosylation may be a target for therapy.

7.   CARTILAGE AND MENISCUS

Articular cartilage is a specialized connective tissue covering weight-bearing surfaces of diarthrodial joints (Figure 3). The cartilage layers covering bone ends function primarily to permit low-friction movement between bones, to distribute the trans-mitted forces, and they are responsible for synthesizing an array of molecules. Chondrocytes are the sole cell present in cartilage, but they synthesize the array of cartilage molecules. Under normal physiologic circumstances, articular cartilage functions as a nearly frictionless surface in diarthrodial joints while exposed to loads of several times body weight for decades. This remarkable function is attributed to the unique structure and composition that determine the mechanical properties of the cartilage extracellular matrix. The extracellular matrix of articular cartilage is primarily water, making up 60–85% of the tissue's wet weight. The remaining solid matrix is composed of a crosslinked network of type II collagen (15–22% by wet wt.), proteoglycan (4–7% by wet wt.), and lesser amounts of other collagen types (e.g., VI, IX, X) and non-collagenous proteins. The aggregating proteoglycan, or aggrecan, in cartilage is composed of a hyaluronic acid backbone to which numerous chondroitin and keratan sulfate chains are attached by a link protein. The constituents of articular cartilage are organized in a stratified structure that contributes the unique

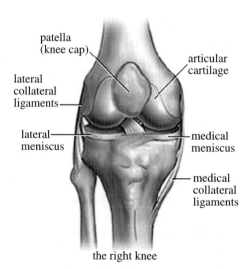

Figure 3. Anatomic relationships of the knee bones, cartilage, ligaments, and meniscus. From aclsolutions.com

mechanical behavior of the ECM. The cartilage ECM is maintained by the metabolic activity of a sparse population of cells (chondrocytes) embedded within the tissue.

The meniscus was originally believed to be a useless structure, but we now know that it is a critical component of the function of the knee joint. In the past, menisci have been primarily considered as anatomic structures that provide these mechanical functions. However, our recent work documents that the fibrochondrocyte cells in the menisci play an important role in modulating the biochemical environment of the knee joint through the synthesis and release of cytokines and inflammatory mediators such as PGE_2, NO, TNF, IL-1, and IFN-γ. In this regard, alterations in the mechanical loading history of the meniscus may have an important influence on the overall health and function of the knee joint. The menisci serve crucial biomechanical roles in load transmission, shock absorption, and joint stability [101, 102]. However, excluding ligament strains, the meniscus is the most frequently injured structure in the knee [103], and meniscal injuries are treated with either partial or total meniscectomy in up to 61 per 100,000 cases resulting in over 35,000 procedures per year in the US alone [104]. Treatment of meniscal tears usually involves partial meniscectomy, but specific conditions such as bucket handle tears or other severe injuries may necessitate total meniscectomy. Injury or removal of the meniscus eventually leads to progressive osteoarthritic degeneration of the human [105, 106].

The unique geometry and biomechanical properties of the menisci allow for their critical biomechanical roles within the knee (Figure 3). These include the transmission of load across the knee [107], increased joint congruence [101], distribution of stresses across the tibia [108], and stabilization of the knee [102]. Biomechanically, the meniscus (and other soft hydrated tissues such as articular cartilage) can be described as composite materials consisting of two separate phases (fluid and solid). The fluid phase is composed of water and dissolved electrolytes, comprising 63–75% of the tissue weight. The solid phase can be described as a porous, permeable, fiber-reinforced matrix consisting principally of type I collagen, with proteoglycans (primarily aggrecan, biglycan, and decorin), and other proteins, including collagen types II, III, V, and VI [109]. The mechanical behavior of the meniscus and articular cartilage can be described by a model that incorporates the fluid and solid phases. The elastic response of the tissue is governed by the properties of the solid matrix (shear, compressive and tensile moduli), while the time-dependent (viscoelastic) behavior is controlled by frictional interactions between the two phases (represented by the hydraulic permeability of the tissue). Fluid flow and pressurization are believed to be important factors in the load support and energy dissipation mechanisms of both meniscus and articular cartilage [110, 111].

The meniscus and osteoarthritis. Overwhelming evidence indicates that the presence of functional menisci is critical to the health of the knee. Degenerative changes resulting from meniscectomy were first noted by King [112] who observed lesions in the articular cartilage of dogs and rabbits following meniscectomy. In a later study, Fairbank [105] described radiographic changes after meniscectomy in the human knee, including narrowing of the joint space, ridge formation, and flattening of the femoral condyles. Since that time, these pathological findings have been reproduced in laboratory studies of partial or complete meniscectomy numerous animal models. Importantly, clinical studies have demonstrated that damage to or excision of the menisci results in accelerated osteoarthritis (OA) of the knee [106,113–115]. These changes include the onset of gross morphologic alterations such as joint space narrowing, cartilage fibrillation, erosion, osteophyte formation, and subchondral bone remodeling. Mechanical properties and structure of articular cartilage are significantly altered after meniscectomy [116]. The mechanism responsible for these degenerative changes is not known, but is believed to involve alterations in the normal biomechanics of the knee (e.g., increased contact stresses or alterations in the normal contact areas). This hypothesis is supported by the findings that meniscectomy results in a 50–60% reduction in femoral contact area and a seven-fold increase in stress on the tibial plateau [101, 107, 108]. However, little is known regarding the influence of the menisci on the biochemical milieu of the synovial joint. In particular, it is not clear whether the menisci are in part responsible for the production of inflammatory mediators that contribute to the pathogenesis of OA.

Mechanical stress and meniscus metabolism. Under normal physiological conditions, the components of the meniscus extracellular matrix are in a state of slow turnover, retained in a homeostatic balance between the catabolic and anabolic events of the fibrochondrocytes [109]. Meniscal fibrochondrocytes are sparsely distributed throughout the matrix and occupy only a small volume ($< 10\%$) of the total tissue. We and others have hypothesized that, despite this relatively low cell density, these cells have a large effect on the metabolism of not only the meniscus, but also adjacent cartilage and synovial tissue. The activities of meniscal fibrochondrocytes are controlled through the processing of both genetic and environmental information, which includes the action of soluble mediators (e.g., growth factors and cytokines), and extracellular matrix composition [107, 117, 118]. In other cartilaginous tissues such as articular cartilage, many studies have shown that the mechanical stress environment of the joint is an important factor which influences (and presumably regulates) the activity of articular cartilage chondrocytes [119]. However, little if any information is available on the response of meniscal fibrochondrocytes to mechanical stress. Recent evidence from *in vivo* studies suggests that mechanical stress also plays a role in regulating the metabolic activity of the meniscus. For example, treadmill exercise increases collagen and proteoglycan contents in rat menisci [120], while joint immobilization leads to a decrease in aggrecan gene expression [121]. Of particular interest is the finding that immobilization of the chick embryo prevents the formation of the knee menisci [122]. *In vivo* studies are limited, however, because of difficulties in determining the precise loading history of the meniscus. Further, such studies may be complicated by the effect of systemic factors or local soluble mediators (e.g., hormones, cytokines, enzymes) that are difficult to control *in vivo*. These confounding effects make it difficult to relate specific mechanical stimuli directly to the biological response of the meniscal fibrochondrocytes.

In vitro studies of the effects of mechanical loading on cartilage and meniscus metabolism. The sequence of biomechanical and biochemical events through which fibrochondrocytes perceive and respond to their mechanical environment are not fully understood. Much of the information available on the response of cartilaginous tissues to mechanical stress comes from the study of articular cartilage, the tissue lining the ends of bones in the diarthrodial joints. Previous studies have shown that mechanobiological factors may play a critical role in the development of the diarthrodial joint as well as in the etiopathogenesis of OA [123]. Clarification of the specific mechanisms of mechanical signaling in normal and inflamed tissues would not only provide a better understanding of the processes which regulate the physiology of meniscus and cartilage, but should also yield new insights on the pathogenesis of arthritis. In this respect, *in vitro* explant models of mechanical loading have provided a model system in which the biomechanical and biochemical environments can be more carefully controlled, as compared with the *in vivo* situation. Explant models of cartilage loading have been used in a number of different loading configurations, including unconfined compression, indentation, tension, and osmotic and hydrostatic pressure. The general consensus of these studies of articular cartilage is that static compression suppresses matrix biosynthesis, and cyclic and intermittent loading stimulate chondrocyte metabolism [124–129]. These responses have been reported over a wide range of loading magnitudes, and exhibit a stress-dose dependency [130 for review]. Excessive loading (e.g., high magnitude, long duration) seems to have a deleterious effect, resulting in cell death, tissue disruption and swelling [131]. Other studies showed that fluid shear stress increases proteoglycan synthesis by articular chondrocytes in monolayer through an NO-dependent pathway [132]. Other than our own previous work (detailed below), there is little information on the effects of mechanical stress on the meniscus *in vitro*. Imler et. al. [133] observed a decrease in protein synthesis in immature bovine meniscus explants subjected to static compression. Dynamic compression at 0.1 and 1.0 Hz increased protein synthesis rates relative to statically compressed samples, but not in comparison to free-swelling controls. There were no effects of compression on the rate of proteoglycan synthesis.

The synthesis and activity of cytokines can be influenced by mechanical stress. Physical therapy is important in mediating reparative and anabolic effects on diseased or inflamed synovial joints but its mechanism of intracellular action is largely unknown [134]. Continuous passive motion induces rapid recovery of inflamed joints and leads to increased proteoglycan synthesis in articular cartilage [135]. This has been mainly attributed to increased circulation and dissemination of inflammatory mediators from the inflamed joint. Cyclic tension has been proposed as an antagonist of IL-1 actions in chondrocyte monolayers and exerts its effects via transcriptional regulation of IL-1 response elements [136, 137]. In these studies, cyclic tension suppresses IL-1 dependent transcription of multiple genes involved in the initiation, of catabolic responses in chondrocytes such as NOS2, COX2 and matrix metalloproteinase I (MMP-I). Conversely, cyclic tension suppresses collagen degradation by abrogating IL-1-induced inhibition MMP-II and collagen type II expression. Cyclic tension also counteracts IL-1-dependent inhibition of aggrecan mRNA expression through hyper-induction of aggrecan, a prominent component of cartilage proteoglycans. To date, however, these relationships have only been studied in articular cartilage, without much work in meniscal fibrochondrocytes. We have been recently studying these relationships in meniscal explants (see below) [138].

Cytokines and arthritis. The disease pathogeneses of OA as well as rheumatoid arthritis (RA) have been associated with the presence of pro-inflammatory cytokines such as interleukin 1 (IL-1) and tumor necrosis factor alpha (TNF) [139]. Various cytokines can induce production and release of the mediators NO and PGE_2 in joint tissues [140–142]. These mediators are elevated in the articular cartilage, synovium, and synovial fluid of OA and RA joints [140,141,143–147]. IL-1 and TNF have been associated with matrix degradation, and more recently interleukin 17 (IL-17) has also been implicated in cartilage degradation and inflammation [148]. Importantly, there is significant evidence for potential synergy in the inter-action of these cytokines in the stimulation of NO production in other cells types [149], although their effects on meniscal fibrochondrocytes are unknown. We have evidence that TNF and IL-1 markedly interfere with the repair of torn/damaged menisci [150].

TNF and IL-1 play important roles in several human inflammatory diseases including rheumatoid arthritis, juvenile RA, Still's disease, inflammatory bowel disease, psoriasis, and inflammation associated with hereditary periodic fever syndromes [151–155]. A variety of antagonists against TNF and IL-1 are known to markedly improve all of these severe problems, and they are clinically approved and in clinical use. These include anti-TNF antibody (both humanized mouse anti-TNF antibody, and fully human anti-TNF antibody), soluble TNF receptor, and the IL-1 receptor antagonist [154]. In earlier work, our group demonstrated that the beneficial effects of the anti-TNF antibody infliximab in humans with RA is linked to NOS2. We demonstrated conclusively that the effectiveness of this anti-TNF therapy correlated closely with the degree of reduction in the overexpression of NOS2 in blood monocytes-lymphocytes from RA patients [155]. We proposed that some or all of the antibody's beneficial effects in RA are related to reducing the overproduction of NO in RA [155, 156]. The agents have been given successfully to many patients with RA, inflammatory bowel disease, and psoriasis. It is very important to note that the agents could be given locally (not systemically) to achieve benefit and to avoid any potential systemic side effects. Chevalier and co-workers have recently reported the safe use of intra-articular injection (up to 150 mg) in OA patients [157], but rigorous efficacy studies have not been done. We are not aware of any experimental or clinical use of the anti-cytokine treatments to enhance speed and effectiveness of meniscal repair.

NO and arthritis. NO has many actions including serving as a proinflammatory agent [158]. Several lines of evidence implicate NO in the pathogenesis of joint inflammation. Rodents in animal models of arthritis generate abundant quantities of NO as reflected by high levels of serum and urinary NOx that develop in association with disease manifestations [159–163]. Treatment of these animals with NOS inhibitors or NO quenchers suppresses NO production and effectively abrogates joint inflammation. These findings prompted studies in humans to determine if patients with RA, like the rodents with arthritis, also have heightened NO production. Some investigators analyzed NO production and NOS in human synovial tissue. For example, Sakurai et al [164] showed that macrophages and endothelial cells from synovial tissue of RA patients express NOS2 mRNA and protein, and generate NO in vitro. We noted that circulating mononuclear cells from patients with RA are activated to express NOS2 and overproduce NO [156]. Grabowski and colleagues [165] showed that patients with RA have 3-fold higher urinary nitrate/creatinine ratios than controls, implying that urinary NOx can be used in this clinical setting as a reliable index of excessive NO production. Farrell et al found that patients with RA or OA had higher serum nitrite (not nitrite + nitrate) levels than normal controls (with RA being higher than OA) [166]. Likewise, Euki and colleagues found that serum nitrite was higher in RA patients compared to normal controls and OA patients, and that nitrite levels correlated with clinical parameters of RA activity, C reactive protein, serum TNF, and serum IL-6 [167]. Onur and co-workers showed that patients with RA had higher serum NOx levels than controls, and that NOx correlated significantly C reactive protein and clinical disease activity [168]. Pham et al showed that RA patients had significantly higher serum NOx levels in comparison to normal control individuals and patients with OA [169].

We studied in detail a strain of mice (MRL-*lpr/lpr*) that spontaneously develop an autoimmune disease comparable to human RA and SLE [170, 171]. We discovered that these mice spontaneously overexpress NOS2 and overproduce NO and superoxide, and that blockage of NO production with an NOS inhibitor prevents the inflammatory disease and death. We have documented that the mice have high levels of nitrosohemoglobin and presence of a renal non-heme nitrosoprotein [172], and elevated levels of nitrated proteins in kidneys (evidence of in vivo peroxynitrite formation) [173].

We postulated that cells from patients with inflammation or infections would produce higher levels of NO. We have found that blood mononuclear cells (MNC) or monocytes from patients with inflammation or infection express more NOS2 and are more responsive to in vitro "activation" [156]. RA patients' monocytes had increased NOS activity, NOS2 antigen expression, NO production in vitro, increased NOS2 mRNA expression, and increased responsiveness to activation with IFN-gamma ± endotoxin [156]. There was a significant correlation between NOS activity and RA disease activity. This was the first demonstration of systemic activation of monocytes for NOS2 expression and NO production in RA. As noted above, we also found that patients treated with humanized, monoclonal anti-TNF antibody for RA had reduction of the overexpression of NOS activity and NOS2 antigen, and that the reduction in NOS correlated extremely closely with the degree of clinical improvement [155].

8.   OUR STUDIES OF CARTILAGE AND MENISCUS

We have been studying the interactions and influences of mechanical stress, cytokines, NO, and PG in normal and diseased/damaged cartilage and meniscus for the last several years. In these studies, we have used acutely isolated tissue explants of articular cartilage and meniscus from the knee joints of normal pigs and from human with RA or OA. The tissues are removed, and the cartilage and meniscus are carefully dissected and prepared for sterile culture and testing. Using this model system, we can examine the interactions of cytokines with controlled mechanical stresses relative to biochemistry, gene expression, and metabolic activity of these tissues. Figure 4. shows experimental methods for applying defined (mechanical stress quantity and desired stress regimen [static or dynamic]).

Mechanical stress induces NOS, COX, and LOX expression in cartilage. Using explants of porcine articular cartilage, we showed that static (0.1 MPa for 24 h) and intermittent (0.5 to 1.0 MPa at 0.5 Hz for 6 h-24 h) compression increased cartilage NO production and induced expression of NOS2 (but not NOS1 or NOS3) protein determined by immunoblot [174]. The increased NO production was inhibited by 1400W, a specific NOS2 inhibitor. In other studies, we showed that intermittent mechanical compression of cartilage induced not only NOS2 expression and NO production, but also COX2 expression and PGE_2 production [98] (Figure 5). PG production was fully inhibited the COX2-specific inhibitor NS398, and this drug also blocked NO production. On the other hand, compression in the presence of the NOS2-specific inhibitor 1400W markedly increased PGE_2 production (10 fold compared to uncompressed explants with 1400W and 40 fold compared to uncompressed explants without 1400W). These results suggest that PGE_2 production by chondrocytes in vivo may be regulated in part by mechanical stress through an NO-dependent pathway.

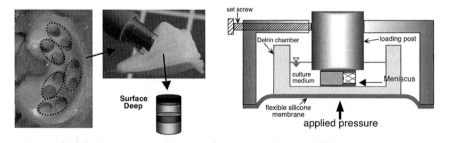

Figure 4. Experimental configuration for dynamic compression of tissue explants. Cartilage or meniscus (shown here) is manually dissected from the bone in a sterile fashion. Matched pairs of cylindrical discs 5 mm diameter and from 2 to 4 mm thick are harvested using a biopsy punch (left panel). Explants (either freshly-isolated or cultured as described) are subjected to precise compressive stresses in individual loading chambers using a computer-controlled instrument (Flexcell International, Hillsborough, NC). See references 98, 138, and 178 for further details

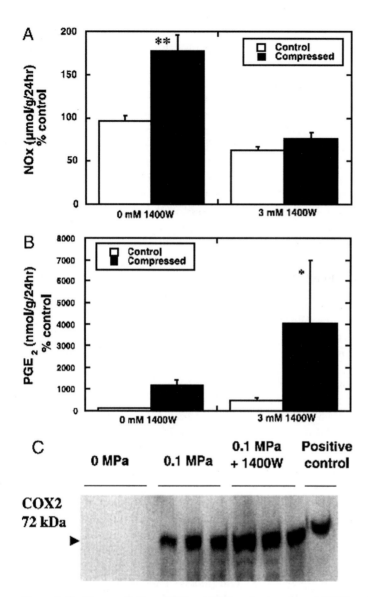

Figure 5. Cartilage production of NO and PGE$_2$ and expression of COX2 protein after mechanical compression and treatment with the NOS2 inhibitor 1400W. "A" shows the production of NO and "B" PGE$_2$ by articular cartilage explants intermittently compressed at 0.5 Hz at 0.1 MPa for 24 h in the presence of 1400W. Results are normalized to mean control value for each animal and are presented as mean ± SEM (n = 48, with * signifying p < 0.05 and ** signifying p < 0.01). "C" shows immunoblot analysis for COX2 (approximately 72 kD). Each lane represents a separate explant that was not compressed (lanes 1–3), compressed (lanes 4–6), or compressed in the presence of 1400W (lanes 7–9). The final lane is a positive control for COX2. From reference 98; see the text and reference 98 for more details

To determine if cartilage could express other enzymes in the arachidonate metabolism pathway, we examined the effects of mechanical stress on porcine production of leukotriene B_4(LTB_4) [175]. Application of dynamic compression for 1 hour in vitro followed by 23 hours of recovered resulted in appearance of 5-lipoxygenase (LOX) protein (by immunoblot) but no detectable of LTB_4. However, if the explants were cultured with the NOS2 inhibitor 1400W, there was more compression-induced LOX protein expression and markedly high LTB_4 production (Figure 6). The LTB_4 was functional as evidenced by the presence of chemotactic activity of the LTB_4-containing medium for rat basophilic leukemia (RBL) cells. RBL cells without LTB_4 receptor had minimal chemotaxis toward the medium from cartilage compressed in the presence of 1400W [175]. Thus, compression of cartilage induces production of both COX2 and LOX and PGE_2 and LTB_4 production in vitro. Furthermore, inhibition of NOS2 appears to superinduce PGE_2 and LTB_4 production by the chondrocytes in vitro. Leukotrienes, like certain prostaglandins, are proinflammatory, and LTB_4 antagonists can block experimental arthritis in mice [176].

Articular cartilage is an avascular tissue that functions at an oxygen tension that is lower than that of most tissues (6% oxygen in superficial zones and 1% in deep zones). Also, with mobilization and weight bearing, joints may undergo cycles of hypoxia and reoxygenation. We studied porcine cartilage explants to determine the effects of hypoxia and reoxygenation on cytokine-induced NO and PGE_2 production [177]. IL-1 and TNF induced increased NO and PGE_2 production in both hypoxic (1% oxygen) and normoxic (20% oxygen) conditions, but NO production was significantly lower in hypoxia. Explants cultured for 72 hours in 1% oxygen followed by 24 hours in 20% oxygen had sustained NO production with IL-1 or TNF, and this was significantly higher that tissues that had been cultured in only normoxic conditions. While IL-1 did not significantly increase PGE_2 production, co-culture with the NOS2 inhibitor 1400W resulted in a "superinduction" of PGE_2 [177].

Mechanical stress induces NOS and COX expression in meniscus. Like cartilage, the meniscus undergoes much mechanical compressive stress with normal function. We studied porcine meniscus to determine details of stress-induced meniscus NO and PG production in vitro [178]. Dynamic compression of medial or lateral meniscus significantly increased NO production. Compressed menisci contained NOS2 by immunoblot analysis, but those not compressed did not. There were some zonal differences in NO production (both basal and compression-induced), with surface zones producing more NO [178]. Our findings provide direct evidence that dynamic mechanical stress influences the biological activity of fibrochondrocytes. These results suggest that NO production in vivo may be in part regulated by mechanical stress acting upon the menisci.

We next examined menisci from patients with OA undergoing total knee replacement to determine production of basal and cytokine-stimulated PG and NO production [138]. All menisci constitutively produced NO, and significant increases in NO production were observed in the presence of IL-1, TNF, or IL-17. The combination of IL-17 and TNF significantly increased NO production compared to any

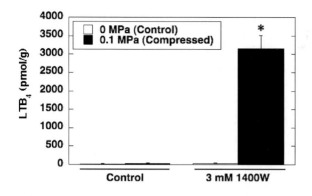

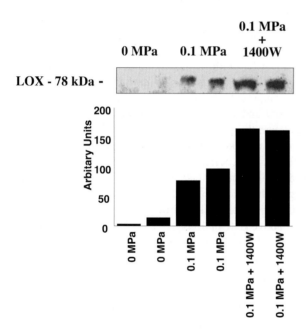

Figure 6. Cartilage production of leukotriene B_4 and expression of 5-lipoxygenase protein after mechanical compression and treatment with the NOS2 inhibitor 1400W. The upper panel shows LTB_4 production by porcine cartilage after application of compression at 0.1 MPa, 0.5 Hz for 1 h followed by 23 h recovery (with n = 24 and * signifying p < 0.001). The lower panel shows immunoblot analysis with an anti-5-LOX antibody demonstrating 5-LOX at approximately 78 kD. From reference 175; see the text and reference 175 for more details

cytokine alone. Basal and cytokine-stimulated NO synthesis was inhibited by the NOS inhibitors NMMA or 1400W. IL-1 significantly increased PGE_2 production. Combining IL-1 and TNF had an additive effect on PGE_2 production, while addition of IL-17 to TNF or IL-1 synergistically enhanced PGE_2 production. Inhibition of

NO production by 1400W significantly increased IL-1-stimulated PGE_2 production, and inhibition of PGE_2 production by the COX2 inhibitor NS398 significantly increased IL-17-stimulated NO production [138] (Figure 7). These results document that freshly isolated menisci from OA patients constitutively produce NO and PG, and that there is a complex interplay of the COX2 and NOS2 pathways in human arthritis.

Regulation of meniscus matrix turnover by IL-1, mechanical stress, and NO. We studied the influences of mechanical stress and IL-1 on porcine meniscal protein synthesis, proteoglycan synthesis and release, and NO production [179]. Mechanical stress (dynamic compression of approximate amplitude and frequency encountered physiologically) increased protein and proteoglycan synthesis and NO production as compared to uncompressed explants. IL-1 prevented compression-induced increases, and the NOS2 inhibitor 1400W blocked the IL-1 effect. IL-1 and compression increased release of proteoglycan from meniscus, and 1400W prevented the proteoglycan release. These findings suggest that IL-1 modulation of meniscus extracellular matrix turnover is dependent on NO [179].

Effects of mechanical tensile strain on meniscus NO and PG production. The meniscus repeatedly undergoes compressive forces, but the wedge-like cross-section of the meniscus also causes radial transmission of axial loads across the knee joint, producing tension in the radial periphery and circumferentially-oriented collagen fibers. This radial transmission of compressive forces causes cells to experience tension as well as compression in situ. This stretch of meniscal cells initiates signaling pathways in meniscal cells and brings about biological changes [180, 181]. Tensile forces can abrogate the effects of IL-1 on proteoglycan synthesis in temporomandibular joint fibrochondrocytes by inhibiting both the NOS2 and COX2 pathways [180], while as noted above IL-1 inhibits the anabolic effects of dynamic compression in meniscus explants through an NO mediated pathway [179]. We worked to determine if cyclic mechanical tensile strain of meniscal cells modulates the biosynthesis of matrix macromolecules and pro-inflammatory mediators, and to determine if this response is altered by TNF [182]. Cells were isolated from the inner two-thirds of porcine medial menisci and subjected to biaxial tensile strain of 5–15% at a frequency of 0.5 Hz. Cyclic tensile strain increased production of NO through the upregulation of NOS2 and also increased synthesis rates of PGE_2, proteoglycan, and total protein in a manner that depended on strain magnitude. TNF increased the production of NO and total protein, but inhibited proteoglycan synthesis rates. TNF prevented the mechanical stimulation of proteoglycan synthesis, and this effect was not dependent on NOS2. These findings indicate that pro-inflammatory cytokines can modulate the responses of meniscal cells to mechanical signals, and suggest that both biomechanical and inflammatory factors could contribute to the progression of joint disease as a consequence of altered loading of the meniscus.

    In separate recent work, we tested for intrinsic differences in the responsiveness of isolated meniscal cells from the inner and outer regions of porcine meniscus to

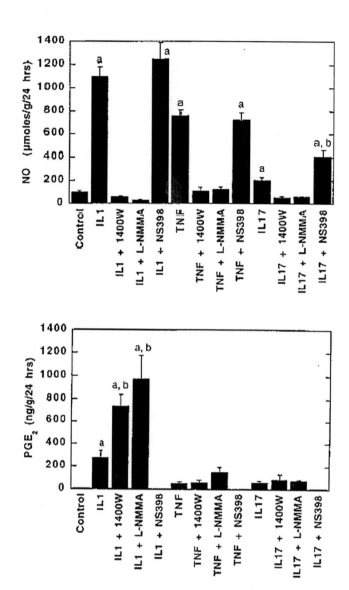

Figure 7. Modulation of human meniscus NO and prostaglandin production by IL-1, IL-17, TNF, and NOS inhibitors. Osteoarthritic human meniscus tissues from 17 patients were examined after they had received total knee replacements. Tissues were cultured for 24 hours with 0.1 ng/ml IL-1, 1 ng/ml TNF, or to 50 ng/ml IL-17, with or without the NOS inhibitors 1400W or NMMA (2 mM) or the COX inhibitor NS398. The upper panel shows results from NO production measurement (where "a" signifies $p < 0.05$ vs. control; "b" that $p < 0.01$ vs. IL-17), and the lower panel measures PGE_2 production (with "a" signifying $p < 0.05$ vs. control and "b" signifying $p < 0.01$ vs. IL-1). From reference 133; see the text and reference 133 for details

equivalent levels of biaxial stretch [183]. Results showed that inner meniscal cells have a more chondrocytic phenotype, as evidenced by the combination of higher levels of proteoglycan synthesis, increased gene expression for aggrecan, type II collagen, and NOS2, and decreased gene expression for type I collagen). Gene expression patterns for key extracellular matrix components differed in meniscus cells from the inner and outer regions during *in vitro* culture regardless of stretching condition. Cells from the inner meniscus expressed higher mRNA levels for type II collagen and lower mRNA levels for type I collagen as compared to outer meniscus cells. Inner cells expressed mRNA for aggrecan at significantly higher levels than that of outer meniscus cells. In contrast, meniscus cells from both regions expressed similar mRNA levels for the small proteoglycans decorin and biglycan. In addition to differences in gene expression for extracellular matrix proteins, inner and outer meniscus cells expressed significantly different mRNA levels for NOS2. Cyclic tensile biaxial stretch at a magnitude of 5% induced increases in protein synthesis and NOS2 mRNA expression in both inner and outer region cells [183].

Effects of mechanical force, IL-1, and NO on meniscus matrix turnover. We examined the influence of mechanical stress on matrix turnover in the meniscus in the presence of IL-1 and determined the role of NO in these processes [179]. Explants of porcine menisci were subjected to dynamic compressive stresses at 0.1 MPa for 24 h at 0.5 Hz with 1 ng/ml IL-1, and the synthesis of total protein, proteoglycan, and NO was measured. Dynamic compression significantly increased protein and proteoglycan synthesis by 68 and 58%, respectively, compared with uncompressed explants. This stimulatory effect of mechanical stress was prevented by the presence of IL-1 but was restored by specifically inhibiting NOS2 with 1400W. Release of proteoglycans into the medium was increased by IL-1 or mechanical compression and further enhanced by IL-1 and compression together. Stimulation of proteoglycan release in response to compression was dependent on NOS2 regardless of the presence of IL-1. These finding suggest that IL-1 may modulate the effects of mechanical stress on extracellular matrix turnover through a pathway that is dependent on NO [179].

9.   SUMMARY AND CONCLUSIONS

NO and PG play critical roles in the pathophysiology of inflammation. COX-nonspecific and COX2-specific inhibitors are used clinically to treat a variety of conditions. While NOS inhibitors are not now clinically approved for treatment of human disease, investigators and pharmaceutical companies are attempting to use these drugs for a variety of diseases including cardiovascular diseases, headache, inflammatory bowel disease, RA, and OA. Mechanical stress interacts with NO, NOS, PG, and COX to contribute to inflammation and tissue damage in arthritis. There are complex relationships of these enzymes and mediators relative to cartilage and meniscus. Our findings of overexpression of COX2 and 5-LOX and overproduction of PGE_2 and LTB_4 after treatment with NOS inhibitors indicates that treatment of inflammation with NOS alone could result in submaximal benefit or actual worsening of inflammation because of the induction of PGE_2 and LTB_4. Development of agents that simultaneously inhibit these multiple inflammation pathways will likely be the most beneficial.

ACKNOWLEDGEMENTS

The authors' research is supported in part by the Rehabilitation Research and Development Service of the Department of Veterans Affairs, and NIH grants AR48182, AR49790, AG15768, and AR50245.

REFERENCES

1. Amin AR, Dave M, Attur M, Abramson SB. COX-2, NO, and cartilage damage and repair. Curr Rheumatol Rep 2: 447–453, 2000.
2. Fernandes JC, Martel-Pelletier J, Pelletier JP. The role of cytokines in osteoarthritis pathophysiology. Biorheology 39: 237–246, 2002.
3. Goldring MB. Osteoarthritis and cartilage: the role of cytokines. Curr Rheumatol Rep 2: 459–465, 2000.
4. Guilak F, Fermor B, Keefe FJ, Kraus VB, Olson SA, Pisetsky DS, Setton LA, Weinberg JB. The role of biomechanics and inflammation in cartilage injury and repair. Clin Orthop Relat Res: 17–26, 2004.
5. Mollace V, Muscoli C, Masini E, Cuzzocrea S, Salvemini D. Modulation of prostaglandin biosynthesis by nitric oxide and nitric oxide donors. Pharmacol Rev 57: 217–252, 2005.
6. Moncada S, Higgs A. The L-arginine-nitric oxide pathway. New England Journal of Medicine 329: 2002–2012, 1993.
7. Magrinat G, Mason SN, Shami PJ, Weinberg JB. Nitric oxide modulation of human leukemia cell differentiation and gene expression. Blood 80: 1880–1884, 1992.
8. Stamler JS, Singel DJ, Loscalzo J. Biochemistry of nitric oxide and its redox-activated forms. [Review]. Science 258: 1898–1902, 1992.
9. Hess DT, Matsumoto A, Kim SO, Marshall HE, Stamler JS. Protein S-nitrosylation: purview and parameters. Nat Rev Mol Cell Biol 6: 150–166, 2005.
10. Palmer RM, Hickery MS, Charles IG, Moncada S, Bayliss MT. Induction of nitric oxide synthase in human chondrocytes. BBRC 193: 398–405, 1993.
11. Nathan C, Xie Q-W. Regulation of biosynthesis of nitric oxide. JBC 269: 13725–13728, 1994.
12. Spitsin SV, Koprowski H, Michaels FH. Characterization and functional analysis of the human inducible nitric oxide synthase gene promoter. Molecular Medicine 2: 226–235, 1996.
13. Devera ME, Shapiro RA, Nussler AK, Mudgett JS, Simmons RL, Morris SM, Billiar TR, Geller DA. Transcriptional regulation of human inducible nitric oxide synthase (NOS2) gene by cytokines - initial analysis of the human NOS2 promoter. Proceedings of the National Academy of Sciences of the United States of America 93: 1054–1059, 1996.
14. Taylor BS, Devera ME, Ganster RW, Wang Q, Shapiro RA, Morris SM, Billiar TR, Geller DA. Multiple NF-kappa-B enhancer elements regulate cytokine induction of the human inducible nitric oxide synthase gene. Journal of Biological Chemistry 273: 15148–15156, 1998.
15. Chartrain NA, Geller DA, Koty PP, Sitrin NF, Nussler AK, Hoffman EP, Billiar TR, Hutchinson NI, Mudgett JS. Molecular cloning, structure, and chromosomal localization of the human inducible nitric oxide synthase gene. J Biol Chem 269: 6765–6772, 1994.
16. Kleinert H, Wallerath T, Fritz G, Ihrig-Biedert I, Rodriguez-Pascual F, Geller DA, Forstermann U. Cytokine induction of NO synthase II in human DLD-1 cells: roles of the JAK-STAT, AP-1 and NF-kappaB-signaling pathways. Br J Pharmacol 125: 193–201, 1998.

17. Kamijo R, Harada H, Matsuyama T, Bosland M, Gerecitano J, Shapiro D, Le J, Koh SI, Kimura T, Green SJ, Mak TW, Taniguchi T, Vilcek J. Requirement for trnascription factor IRF-1 in NO synthase induction in macrophages. Science 263: 1612–1615, 1994.

18. Gao JJ, Morrison DC, Parmely TJ, Russell SW, Murphy WJ. An Interferon-Gamma-Activated Site (GAS) Is Necessary For Full Expression Of the Mouse Inos Gene In Response to Interferon-Gamma and Lipopolysaccharide. Journal of Biological Chemistry 272: 1226–1230, 1997.

19. Gao JJ, Filla MB, Fultz MJ, Vogel SN, Russell SW, Murphy WJ. Autocrine/paracrine IFN-alpha/beta mediates the lipopolysaccharide-induced activation of transcription factor Stat1alpha in mouse macrophages: pivotal role of Stat1alpha in induction of the inducible nitric oxide synthase gene. J Immunol 161: 4803–4810, 1998.

20. Chan ED, Winston BW, Uh ST, Wynes MW, Rose DM, Riches DWH. Evaluation of the role of mitogen-activated protein kinases in the expression of inducible nitric oxide synthase by IFN-gamma and TNF-alpha in mouse macrophages. J Immunol 162: 415–422, 1999.

21. Chen BC, Chen YH, Lin WW. Involvement of p38 mitogen-activated protein kinase in lipopolysaccharide-induced iNOS and COX-2 expression in J774 macrophages. Immunology 97: 124–129, 1999.

22. Singh K, Balligand JL, Fischer TA, Smith TW, Kelly RA. Regulation Of Cytokine-Inducible Nitric Oxide Synthase In Cardiac Myocytes and Microvascular Endothelial Cells - Role Of Extracellular Signal-Regulated Kinases 1 and 2 (Erk1/Erk2) and Stat1-Alpha. Journal of Biological Chemistry 271: 1111–1117, 1996.

23. Searles CD, Miwa Y, Harrison DG, Ramasamy S. Posttranscriptional regulation of endothelial nitric oxide synthase during cell growth. Circulation Research 85: 588–595, 1999.

24. Gross SS, Levi R. Tetrahydrobiopterin synthesis. An absolute requirement for cytokine-induced nitric oxide generation by vascular smooth muscle. Journal of Biological Chemistry 267: 25722–25729, 1992.

25. Lee J, Ryu H, Ferrante RJ, Morris SM Jr, Ratan RR. Translational control of inducible nitric oxide synthase expression by arginine can explain the arginine paradox. Proc Natl Acad Sci USA 100: 4843–4848, 2003.

26. Wu G, Morris SM Jr. Arginine metabolism: nitric oxide and beyond. Biochem J 336 (Pt 1): 1–17, 1998.

27. Nicholson B, Manner CK, Kleeman J, MacLeod CL. Sustained nitric oxide production in macrophages requires the arginine transporter CAT2. Journal of Biological Chemistry 276: 15881–15885, 2001.

28. Verrey F, Closs EI, Wagner CA, Palacin M, Endou H, Kanai Y. CATs and HATs: the SLC7 family of amino acid transporters. Pflugers Arch 447: 532–542, 2004.

29. Mori M, Gotoh T. Regulation of nitric oxide production by arginine metabolic enzymes. Biochem Biophys Res Commun 275: 715–719, 2000.

30. Hammermann R, Dreiig MDM, Dreissig MDM, Mossner J, Fuhrmann M, Berrino L, Gothert M, Racke K. Nuclear factor-kappa B mediates simultaneous induction of inducible nitric-oxide synthase and up-regulation of the cationic amino acid transporter CAT-2B in rat alveolar macrophages. Mol Pharmacol 58: 1294–1302, 2000.

31. Barbul A. Arginine: biochemistry, physiology, and therapeutic implications. JPEN J Parenter Enteral Nutr 10: 227–238, 1986.

32. Boger RH, Bode-Boger SM. The clinical pharmacology of L-arginine. Annu Rev Pharmacol Toxicol 41: 79–99, 2001.

33. Merimee TJ, Rabinowtitz D, Fineberg SE. Arginine-initiated release of human growth hormone. Factors modifying the response in normal man. N Engl J Med 280: 1434–1438, 1969.

34. Merimee TJ, Rabinowitz D, Riggs L, Burgess JA, Rimoin DL, McKusick VA. Plasma growth hormone after arginine infusion. Clinical experiences. N Engl J Med 276: 434–439, 1967.

35. Boger RH, Bode-Boger SM, Thiele W, Creutzig A, Alexander K, Frolich JC. Restoring vascular nitric oxide formation by L-arginine improves the symptoms of intermittent claudication in patients with peripheral arterial occlusive disease. J Am Coll Cardiol 32: 1336–1344, 1998.

36. Ceremuzynski L, Chamiec T, Herbaczynska-Cedro K. Effect of supplemental oral L-arginine on exercise capacity in patients with stable angina pectoris. Am J Cardiol 80: 331–333, 1997.

37. Lerman A, Burnett JC Jr, Higano ST, McKinley LJ, Holmes DR Jr. Long-term L-arginine supplementation improves small-vessel coronary endothelial function in humans. Circulation 97: 2123–2128, 1998.

38. Grasemann H, Gartig SS, Wiesemann HG, Teschler H, Konietzko N, Ratjen F. Effect of L-arginine infusion on airway NO in cystic fibrosis and primary ciliary dyskinesia syndrome. Eur Respir J 13: 114–118, 1999.

39. Morris CR, Kuypers FA, Larkin S, Sweeters N, Simon J, Vichinsky EP, Styles LA. Arginine therapy: a novel strategy to induce nitric oxide production in sickle cell disease. Br J Haematol 111: 498–500, 2000.

40. Morris CR, Kuypers FA, Larkin S, Vichinsky EP, Styles LA. Patterns of arginine and nitric oxide in patients with sickle cell disease with vaso-occlusive crisis and acute chest syndrome. Journal of Pediatric Hematology Oncology 22: 515–520, 2000.

41. Iyer R, Jenkinson CP, Vockley JG, Kern RM, Grody WW, Cederbaum S. The human arginases and arginase deficiency. J Inherit Metab Dis 21 Suppl 1: 86–100, 1998.

42. Jenkinson CP, Grody WW, Cederbaum SD. Comparative properties of arginases. Comp Biochem Physiol B Biochem Mol Biol 114: 107–132, 1996.

43. Shi O, Kepka-Lenhart D, Morris SM Jr, O'Brien WE. Structure of the murine arginase II gene. Mamm Genome 9: 822–824, 1998.

44. Munder M, Eichmann K, Moran JM, Centeno F, Soler G, Modolell M. Th1/Th2-regulated expression of arginase isoforms in murine macrophages and dendritic cells. J Immunol 163: 3771–3777, 1999.

45. Hesse M, Modolell M, La Flamme AC, Schito M, Fuentes JM, Cheever AW, Pearce EJ, Wynn TA. Differential regulation of nitric oxide synthase-2 and arginase-1 by type 1/type 2 cytokines in vivo: Granulomatous pathology is shaped by the pattern of L-arginine metabolism. J Immunol 167: 6533–6544, 2001.

46. Munder M, Eichmann K, Modolell M. Alternative metabolic states in murine macrophages reflected by the nitric oxide synthase/arginase balance: competitive regulation by CD4+ T cells correlates with Th1/Th2 phenotype. J Immunol 160: 5347–5354, 1998.

47. Wei LH, Wu G, Morris SM Jr, Ignarro LJ. Elevated arginase I expression in rat aortic smooth muscle cells increases cell proliferation. Proc Natl Acad Sci USA 98: 9260–9264, 2001.

48. Wei LH, Jacobs AT, Morris SM, Ignarro LJ. IL-4 and IL-13 upregulate arginase I expression by cAMP and JAK/STAT6 pathways in vascular smooth muscle cells. American Journal of Physiology - Cell Physiology 279: C248-C256, 2000.

49. Modolell M, Corraliza IM, Link F, Soler G, Eichmann K. Reciprocal regulation of the nitric oxide synthase/arginase balance in mouse bone marrow-derived macrophages by TH1 and TH2 cytokines. Eur J Immunol 25: 1101–1104, 1995.

50. Dal-Pizzol F. Alternative activated macrophage: A new key for systemic inflammatory response syndrome and sepsis treatment? Crit Care Med 32: 1971–1972, 2004.

51. Gordon S. Alternative activation of macrophages. Nat Rev Immunol 3: 23–35, 2003.

52. Raes G, De Baetselier P, Noel W, Beschin A, Brombacher F, Hassanzadeh Gh G. Differential expression of FIZZ1 and Ym1 in alternatively versus classically activated macrophages. J Leukoc Biol 71: 597–602, 2002.

53. Vincendeau P, Gobert AP, Daulouede S, Moynet D, Mossalayi MD. Arginases in parasitic diseases. Trends Parasitol 19: 9–12, 2003.

54. Corraliza I, Moncada S. Increased expression of arginase II in patients with different forms of arthritis. Implications of the regulation of nitric oxide. J Rheumatol 29: 2261–2265, 2002.

55. Appleton I, Tomlinson A, Willoughby DA. Induction of cyclo-oxygenase and nitric oxide synthase in inflammation. Adv Pharmacol 35: 27–78, 1996.

56. Smith WL, Garavito RM, DeWitt DL. Prostaglandin endoperoxide H synthases (cyclooxygenases)-1 and -2. Journal of Biological Chemistry 271: 33157–33160, 1996.

57. Marnett LJ, Wright TL, Crews BC, Tannenbaum SR, Marrow JD. Regulation of prostaglandin biosynthesis by nitric oxide is revealed by targeted deletion of inducible nitric-oxide synthase. Journal of Biological Chemistry 275: 13427–13430, 2000.

58. Gilroy DW, Colville-Nash PR. New insights into the role of COX 2 in inflammation. Journal of Molecular Medicine-Jmm 78: 121–129, 2000.

59. Chandrasekharan NV, Dai H, Roos KL, Evanson NK, Tomsik J, Elton TS, Simmons DL. COX-3, a cyclooxygenase-1 variant inhibited by acetaminophen and other analgesic/antipyretic drugs: cloning, structure, and expression. Proc Natl Acad Sci USA 99: 13926–13931, 2002.

60. Vane JR, Botting RM. Mechanism of action of antiinflammatory drugs. Int J Tissue React 20: 3–15, 1998.

61. Abramson SB. The role of COX-2 produced by cartilage in arthritis. Osteoarthritis & Cartilage 7: 380–381, 1999.

62. Geng Y, Blanco FJ, Cornelisson M, Lotz M. Regulation of cyclooxygenase-2 expression in normal human articular chondrocytes. J Immunol 155: 796–801, 1995.

63. Lyons-Giordana B, Pratta M, Galbraith W, Davis G, Arner E. Interleukin-1 differentially modulates chondrocyte expression of cyclooxygenase-2 and phospholipase A2. Exp Cell Res 206: 58, 1993.

64. Dingle J. Cartilage maintenance in osteoarthritis: interaction of cytokines, NSAID and prostaglandins in articular cartilage damage and repair. J Rheumatol Suppl 28: 30, 1991.

65. Di Battista JA, Dore S, Martel-Pelletier J, Pelletier JP. Prostaglandin E2 stimulates incorporation of proline into collagenase digestible proteins in human articular chondrocytes: identification of an effector autocrine loop involving insulin-like growth factor I. Mol Cell Endocrinol 123: 27–35, 1996.

66. Goldring M, Suen L-F, Yamin R, Lai W-F. Regulation of collagen gene expression by prostaglandins and interleukin-1beta in cultured chondrocytes and fibroblasts. Am J Therapeutics 3: 9–16, 1996.

67. Lowe GN, Fu YH, McDougall S, Polendo R, Williams A, Benya PD, Hahn TJ. Effects of prostaglandins on deoxyribonucleic acid and aggrecan synthesis in the RCJ 3.1C5.18 chondrocyte cell line: role of second messengers. Endocrinology 137: 2208–2216, 1996.

68. Di Battista JA, Dore S, Morin N, He Y, Pelletier JP, Martel-Pelletier J. Prostaglandin E2 stimulates insulin-like growth factor binding protein-4 expression and synthesis in cultured human articular chondrocytes: possible mediation by Ca(++)-calmodulin regulated processes. J Cell Biochem 65: 408–419, 1997.

69. Di Battista JA, Martel-Pelletier J, Fujimoto N, Obata K, Zafarullah M, Pelletier JP. Prostaglandins E2 and E1 inhibit cytokine-induced metalloprotease expression in human synovial fibroblasts. Mediation by cyclic-AMP signalling pathway. Lab Invest 71: 270–278, 1994.

70. Blanco FJ, Lotz M. IL-1-induced nitric oxide inhibits chondrocyte proliferation via PGE2. Exp Cell Res 218: 319–325, 1995.

71. Knudsen PJ, Dinarello CA, Strom TB. Prostaglandins posttranscriptionally inhibit monocyte expression of interleukin 1 activity by increasing intracellular cyclic adenosine monophosphate. Journal of Immunology 137: 3189–3194, 1986.

72. Milano S, Arcoleo F, Dieli M, D'Agostino R, D'Agostino P, De Nucci G, Cillari E. Prostaglandin E2 regulates inducible nitric oxide synthase in the murine macrophage cell line J774. Prostaglandins 49: 105–115, 1995.

73. Studer R, Jaffurs D, Stefanovic-Racic M, Robbins PD, Evans CH. Nitric oxide in osteoarthritis. Osteoarthritis & Cartilage 7: 377–379, 1999.

74. Clancy RM, Abramson SB. Nitric oxide: A novel mediator of inflammation. Proceedings of the Society of Experimental Biology and Medicine 210: 93–101, 1995.

75. Clancy R, Varenika B, Huang WQ, Ballou L, Attur M, Amin AR, Abramson SB. Nitric oxide synthase/COX cross-talk: Nitric oxide activates COX-1 but inhibits COX-2-derived prostaglandin production. J Immunol 165: 1582–1587, 2000.

76. Benton H, Tyler J. Inhibition of cartilage proteoglycan synthesis by interleukin-1. Biochem Biophys Res Comm 145: 421–428, 1988.

77. Anderson GD, Hauser SD, McGarity KL, Bremer ME, Isakson PC, Gregory SA. Selective inhibition of cyclooxygenase (COX)-2 reverses inflammation and expression of COX-2 and interleukin-6 in rat adjuvant arthritis. Journal of Clinical Investigation 97: 2672–2679, 1996.

78. Bombardieri S, Cattani P, Giabattoni G, Di Munno O, Paero G, Patrono C, Pinca E, Pugliese F. The synovial prostaglandin system in chronic inflammatory arthritis: differential effects of steroidal and non-steroidal antiinflammatory drugs. Br J Pharmacol 73: 893–901, 1981.

79. Crofford LJ, Wilder RL, Ristimaki AP, Sano H, Remmers EF, Epps HR, Hla T. Cyclooxygenase-1 and -2 expression in rheumatoid synovial tissues: effects of interleukin-1beta, phorbol ester, and corticosteroids. J Clin Inv 93: 1095–1101, 1994.

80. Davies P, Bailey PJ, Goldenberg MM, Ford-Hutchinson AW. The role of arachidonic acid oxygenation products in pain and inflammation. Annu Rev Immunol 2: 335–357, 1984.

81. Engelhardt G, Homma D, Schlegel K, Utzmann R, Schnitzler C. Anti-inflammatory, analgesic, antipyretic and related properties of meloxicam, a new non-steroidal anti-inflammatory agent with favourable gastrointestinal tolerance. Inflamm Res 44: 423–433, 1995.

82. Penning TD, Talley JJ, Bertenshaw SR, Carter JS, Collins PW, Docter S, Graneto MJ, Lee LF, Malecha JW, Miyashiro JM, Rogers RS, Rogier DJ, Yu SS, AndersonGd, Burton EG, Cogburn JN, Gregory SA, Koboldt CM, Perkins WE, Seibert K, Veenhuizen AW, Zhang YY, Isakson PC. Synthesis and biological evaluation of the 1,5-diarylpyrazole class of cyclooxygenase-2 inhibitors: identification of 4-[5-(4-methylphenyl)-3-(trifluoromethyl)-1H-pyrazol-1-yl]benze nesulfonamide (SC-58635, celecoxib). J Med Chem 40: 1347–1365, 1997.

83. Topol EJ. Arthritis medicines and cardiovascular events–"house of coxibs". JAMA 293: 366–368, 2005.

84. Tetsuka T, Daphna-Iken D, Srivastava SK, Baier LD, DuMaine J, Morrison AR. Cross-talk between cyclooxygenase and nitric oxide pathways: prostaglandin E2 negatively modulates induction of nitric oxide synthase by interleukin 1. Proc Natl Acad Sci USA 91: 12168–12172, 1994.

85. Weinberg JB. Nitric oxide synthase 2 and cyclooxygenase 2 interactions in inflammation. Immunol Res 22: 319–341, 2000.

86. Salvemini D, Misko TP, Masferrer JL, Seibert K, Currie MG, Needleman P. Nitric oxide activates cyclooxygenase enzymes. Proc Natl Acad Sci USA 90: 7240–7244, 1993.

87. Swierkosz TA, Mitchell JA, Warner TD, Botting RM, Vane JR. Co-induction of nitric oxide synthase and cyclo-oxygenase: interactions between nitric oxide and prostanoids. Br J Pharmacol 114: 1335–1342, 1995.

88. Vane JR, Mitchell JA, Appleton I, Tomlinson A, Bishop-Bailey D, Croxtall J, Willoughby DA. Inducible isoforms of cyclooxygenase and nitric-oxide synthase in inflammation. Proc Natl Acad Sci USA 91: 2046–2050, 1994.

89. Salvemini D, Manning PT, Zweifel BS, Seibert K, Connor J, Currie MG, Needleman P, Masferrer JL. Dual inhibition of nitric oxide and prostaglandin production contributes to the anti-inflammatory properties of nitric oxide synthase inhibitors. Journal of Clinical Investigation 96: 301–308, 1995.

90. Amin AR, Vyas P, Attur M, Leszczynska-Piziak J, Patel IR, Weissmann G, Abramson SB. The mode of action of aspirin-like drugs: effect on inducible nitric oxide synthase. Proc Natl Acad Sci USA 92: 7926–7930, 1995.

91. Pang L, Hoult JR. Repression of inducible nitric oxide synthase and cyclooxygenase-2 by prostaglandin E2 and other cyclic AMP stimulants in J774 macrophages [published erratum appears in Biochem Pharmacol 1997 Jun 15;53(12):1945]. Biochem Pharmacol 53: 493–500, 1997.

92. Marotta P, Sautebin L, Di Rosa M. Modulation of the induction of nitric oxide synthase by eicosanoids in the murine macrophage cell line J774. Br J Pharmacol 107: 640–641, 1992.

93. Stadler J, Stefanovic-Racic M, Billiar TR, Curran RD, McIntyre LA, Georgescu HI, Simmons RL, Evans CH. Articular chondrocytes synthesize nitric oxide in response to cytokines and lipopolysaccharide. J Immunol 147: 3915–3920, 1991.

94. Salvemini D, Masferrer JL. Interactions of nitric oxide with cyclooxygenase: in vitro, ex vivo, and in vivo studies. Methods Enzymol 269: 12–25, 1996.

95. Salvemini D, Manning PT, Zweifel BS, Seibert K, Connor J, Currie MG, Needleman P, Masferrer JL. Dual inhibition of nitric oxide and prostaglandin production contributes to the antiinflammatory properties of nitric oxide synthase inhibitors. J Clin Invest 96: 301–308, 1995.

96. Lianos EA, Guglielmi K, Sharma M. Regulatory interactions between inducible nitric oxide synthase and eicosanoids in glomerular immune injury. Kidney Int 53: 645–653, 1998.

97. Ghosh DK, Misukonis MA, Reich C, Pisetsky DS, Weinberg JB. Host response to infection: the role of CpG DNA in induction of cyclooxygenase 2 and nitric oxide synthase 2 in murine macrophages. Infect Immun 69: 7703–7710, 2001.

98. Fermor B, Weinberg JB, Pisetsky DS, Misukonis MA, Fink C, Guilak F. Induction of cyclooxygenase-2 by mechanical stress through a nitric oxide-regulated pathway. Osteoarthritis Cartilage 10: 792–798, 2002.

99. Tsai AL, Wei C, Kulmacz RJ. Interaction between nitric oxide and prostaglandin H synthase. Arch Biochem Biophys 313: 367–372, 1994.

100. Kim SF, Huri DA, Snyder SH. Inducible nitric oxide synthase binds, S-nitrosylates, and activates cyclooxygenase-2. Science 310: 1966–1970, 2005.

101. Kurosawa H, Fukubayashi T, Nakajuma H. Load-bearing mode of the knee joint: physical behavior of the knee joint with or without menisci. Clinical Orthopaedics & Related Research 149: 283–290, 1980.

102. Levy IM, Torzilli PA, Fisch ID. The contribution of the menisci to the stability of the knee. In: Mow VC, Jackson DW, Arnoczky SP, eds. Knee Meniscus: Basic and Clinical Foundations. New York: Raven Press; 1992:107–115.

103. Baker BE, Peckham AC, Pupparo F, Sanborn JC. Review of meniscal injury and associated sports. Am J Sports Med 13: 1–4, 1985.

104. Praemer A, Furner S, Rice DP. Musculoskeletal Conditions in the United States. Rosement, IL: American Academy of Orthopaedic Surgeons; 1999.

105. Fairbank TJ. Knee joint changes after meniscectomy. Journal of Bone and Joint Surgery 30B: 664–670, 1948.

106. Roos H, Lauren M, Adalberth T, Roos EM, Jonsson K, Lohmander LS. Knee osteoarthritis after meniscectomy: prevalence of radiographic changes after twenty-one years, compared with matched controls. Arthritis & Rheumatism 41: 687–693, 1998.

107. Walker PS, Erkman MJ. The role of the menisci in force transmission across the knee. Clinical Orthopaedics & Related Research: 184–192, 1975.

108. Radin EL, de Lamotte F, Maquet P. Role of the menisci in the distribution of stress in the knee. Clinical Orthopaedics & Related Research: 290–294, 1984.

109. McDevitt CA, Webber RJ. The ultrastructure and biochemistry of meniscal cartilage. Clinical Orthopaedics & Related Research: 8–18, 1990.

110. Fithian DC, Kelly MA, Mow VC. Material properties and structure-function relationships in the menisci. Clinical Orthopaedics & Related Research: 19–31, 1990.

111. Mow VC, Kuei SC, Lai WM, Armstrong CG. Biphasic creep and stress relaxation of articular cartilage in compression: Theory and experiments. Journal of Biomechanical Engineering 102: 73–84, 1980.

112. King D. The healing of semilunar cartilages. J Bone Joint Surg Am 54A: 349, 1936.

113. Aagaard H, Verdonk R. Function of the normal meniscus and consequences of meniscal resection. Scand J Med Sci Sports 9: 134–140, 1999.

114. Fairbank TJ. Knee joint changes after meniscectomy. J Bone Joint Surg 30B: 664–670, 1948.

115. McNicholas MJ, Rowley DI, McGurty D, Adalberth T, Abdon P, Lindstrand A, Lohmander LS. Total meniscectomy in adolescence. A thirty-year follow-up. J Bone Joint Surg Br 82: 217–221, 2000.

116. Elliott DM, Guilak F, Vail TP, Wang JY, Setton LA. Tensile properties of articular cartilage are altered by meniscectomy in a canine model of osteoarthritis. Journal of Orthopaedic Research 17: 503–508, 1999.

117. Bhargava MM, Attia ET, Murrell GA, Dolan MM, Warren RF, Hannafin JA. The effect of cytokines on the proliferation and migration of bovine meniscal cells. American Journal of Sports Medicine 27: 636–643, 1999.

118. Collier S, Ghosh P. Effects of transforming growth factor beta on proteoglycan synthesis by cell and explant cultures derived from the knee joint meniscus. Osteoarthritis & Cartilage 3: 127–138, 1995.

119. Guilak F, Ratcliffe A, Lane N, Rosenwasser MP, Mow VC. Mechanical and biochemical changes in the superficial zone of articular cartilage in canine experimental osteoarthritis. Journal of Orthopaedic Research 12: 474–484, 1994.

120. Vailas AC, Zernicke RF, Matsuda J, Curwin S, Durivage J. Adaptation of rat knee meniscus to prolonged exercise. Journal of Applied Physiology 60: 1031–1034, 1986.

121. Djurasovic M, Aldridge JW, Grumbles R, Rosenwasser MP, Howell D, Ratcliffe A. Knee joint immobilization decreases aggrecan gene expression in the meniscus. American Journal of Sports Medicine 26: 460–466, 1998.

122. Mikic B, Johnson TL, Chhabra AB, Schalet BJ, Wong M, Hunziker EB. Differential effects of embryonic immobilization on the development of fibrocartilaginous skeletal elements. Journal of Rehabilitation Research & Development 37: 127–133, 2000.

123. Beaupre GS, Stevens SS, Carter DR. Mechanobiology in the development, maintenance, and degeneration of articular cartilage. J Rehabil Res Dev 37: 145–151, 2000.

124. Burton-Wurster N, Vernier-Singer M, Farquhar T, Lust G. Effect of compressive loading and unloading on the synthesis of total protein, proteoglycan, and fibronectin by canine cartilage explants. J Orthop Res 11: 717–729, 1993.

125. Gray ML, Pizzanelli AM, Grodzinsky AJ, Lee RC. Mechanical and physiochemical determinants of the chondrocyte biosynthetic response. J Orthop Res 6: 777–792, 1988.

126. Palmoski MJ, Brandt KD. Effects of static and cyclic compressive loading on articular cartilage plugs in vitro. Arthritis Rheum 27: 675–681, 1984.

127. Sah RL, Kim YJ, Doong JY, Grodzinsky AJ, Plaas AH, Sandy JD. Biosynthetic response of cartilage explants to dynamic compression. J Orthop Res 7: 619–636, 1989.

128. Torzilli PA, Grigiene R. Continuous cyclic load reduces proteoglycan release from articular cartilage. Osteoarthritis Cartilage 6: 260–268, 1998.

129. Guilak F, Meyer BC, Ratcliffe A, Mow VC. The effects of matrix compression on proteoglycan metabolism in articular cartilage explants. Osteoarthritis & Cartilage 2: 91–101, 1994.

130. Guilak F, Sah RL, Setton LA. Physical regulation of cartilage metabolism. In: Mow VC, Hayes WC, eds. Basic Orthopaedic Biomechanics (2nd ed). Philadelphia: Lippincott-Raven; 1997:179–207.

131. Farquhar T, Xia Y, Mann K, Bertram J, Burton-Wurster N, Jelinski L, Lust G. Swelling and fibronectin accumulation in articular cartilage explants after cyclical impact. J Orthop Res 14: 417–423, 1996.

132. Das P, Schurman DJ, Smith RL. Nitric oxide and G proteins mediate the response of bovine articular chondrocytes to fluid-induced shear. J Orthop Res 15: 87–93, 1997.

133. Imler SM, Vanderploeg EJ, Hunter CJ, Levenston ME. Static and oscillatory compression modulate protein and proteoglycan synthesis by meniscal fibrochondrocytes. Transactions of the Orthopaedic Research Society 26: 552, 2001.

134. Kim H, Kerr R, Cruz T, Salter R. Effects of continuous motion and immobilization on synovitis and cartilage degradation in an antigen induced arthritis. J Rheumatology 22: 1714, 1995.

135. Salter R. THe physiologic basis of continuous passive motion for articular cartilage healing and regeneration. Hand Clin 10: 211, 1994.

136. Gassner R, Buckley M, Georgescu R, Studer M, Stefanovich-Racic M, Piesco N, Evans C, Agarwal S. Cyclic tensile stress exerts anti-inflammatory actions on chondrocytes by inhibiting inducible nitric oxide synthase. J Immunol 163: 2187, 1999.

137. Xu Z, Buckley M, Evans C, Agarwal S. Cyclic tensile strain acts as an antagonist of IL1beta actions in chondrocytes. The Journal of Imunology 165: 453–460, 2000.

138. LeGrand A, Fermor B, Fink C, Pisetsky DS, Vail TP, Weinberg JB, Guilak F. IL-1, TNF-a and IL-17 induction of inflammatory mediator production by human osteoarthritic knee menisci. Arthritis Rheum 44: 2078–2083, 2001.

139. Harris ED Jr. Textbook of rheumatology (4th edn). Philadelphia: W.B. Saunders Company; 1993.

140. Hashimoto S, Takahashi K, Ochs RL, Coutts RD, Amiel D, Lotz M. Nitric oxide production and apoptosis in cells of the meniscus during experimental osteoarthritis. Arthritis Rheum 42: 2123–2131, 1999.

141. Hughes FJ, Buttery LD, Hukkanen MV, O'Donnell A, Maclouf J, Polak JM. Cytokine-induced prostaglandin E2 synthesis and cyclooxygenase-2 activity are regulated both by a nitric oxide-dependent and -independent mechanism in rat osteoblasts in vitro. Journal of Biological Chemistry 274: 1776–1782, 1999.

142. Jang D, Murrell GAC. NITRIC OXIDE IN ARTHRITIS [Review]. Free Radical Biology & Medicine 24: 1511–1519, 1998.

143. Amin AR, Di Cesare PE, Vyas P, Attur M, Tzeng E, Billiar TR, Stuchin SA, Abramson SB. The expression and regulation of nitric oxide synthase in human osteoarthritis-affected chondrocytes: evidence for up-regulated neuronal nitric oxide synthase. J Exp Med 182: 2097–2102, 1995.

144. Amin AR, Attur M, Patel RN, Thakker GD, Marshall PJ, Rediske J, Stuchin SA, Patel IR, Abramson SB. Superinduction Of Cyclooxygenase-2 Activity In Human Osteoarthritis-Affected Cartilage - Influence Of Nitric Oxide. Journal of Clinical Investigation 99: 1231–1237, 1997.

145. Clancy RM, Amin AR, Abramson SB. The role of nitric oxide in inflammation and immunity [Review]. Arthritis & Rheumatism 41: 1141–1151, 1998.

146. Evans CH, Stefanovic-Racic M, Lancaster JR Jr. Nitric oxide and its role in orthopaedic disease [Review]. Clinical Orthopaedics & Related Research 312: 275–294, 1995.

147. Grabowski PS, Wright PK, Vanthof RJ, Helfrich MH, Ohshima H, Ralston SH. Immunolocalization Of Inducible Nitric Oxide Synthase In Synovium and Cartilage In Rheumatoid Arthritis and Osteoarthritis. British Journal of Rheumatology 36: 651–655, 1997.

148. Shalom-Barak T, Quach J, Lotz M. Interleukin-17-induced gene expression in articular chondrocytes is associated with activation of mitogen-activated protein kinases and NF-kappaB. J Biol Chem 273: 27467–27473, 1998.

149. Kwon S, George SC. Synergistic cytokine-induced nitric oxide production in human alveolar epithelial cells. Nitric Oxide 3: 348–357, 1999.

150. Hennerbichler A, Moutos FT, Hennerbichler D, Weinberg JB, Guilak F. Integrative repair of the inner and outer regions of the meniscus in vitro. Am J Sports Med, in Press, 2006.

151. Dinarello CA. The many worlds of reducing interleukin-1. Arthritis Rheum 52: 1960–1967, 2005.

152. Kastner DL. Hereditary periodic fever syndromes. Hematology 2005—American Society of Hematology Education Book: 74–81, 2005.

153. Reich K, Nestle FO, Papp K, Ortonne JP, Evans R, Guzzo C, Li S, Dooley LT, Griffiths CE. Infliximab induction and maintenance therapy for moderate-to-severe psoriasis: a phase III, multicentre, double-blind trial. Lancet 366: 1367–1374, 2005.

154. Weaver AL. The impact of new biologicals in the treatment of rheumatoid arthritis. Rheumatology (Oxford) 43 Suppl 3: iii17-iii23, 2004.

155. Perkins DJ, St Clair EW, Misukonis MA, Weinberg JB. Reduction of NOS2 overexpression in rheumatoid arthritis patients treated with anti-tumor necrosis factor alpha monoclonal antibody (cA2). Arthritis Rheum 41: 2205–2210, 1998.

156. St. Clair EW, Wilkinson WE, Lang T, Sanders L, Misukonis MA, Gilkeson GS, Pisetsky DS, Granger DL, Weinberg JB. Increased expression of blood mononuclear cell nitric oxide synthase type 2 in rheumatoid arthritis patients. Journal of Experimental Medicine 184: 1173–1178, 1996.

157. Chevalier X, Giraudeau B, Conrozier T, Marliere J, Kiefer P, Goupille P. Safety study of intraarticular injection of interleukin 1 receptor antagonist in patients with painful knee osteoarthritis: a multicenter study. J Rheumatol 32: 1317–1323, 2005.

158. Clancy RM, Abramson SB. Nitric oxide—a novel mediator of inflammation [Review]. Proceedings of the Society of Experimental Biology and Medicine 210: 93–101, 1995.

159. Ialenti A, Moncada S, Di Rosa M. Modulation of adjuvant arthritis by endogenous nitric oxide. Br J Pharmacol 110: 701–706, 1993.

160. Stefanovic-Racic M, Meyers K, Meschter C, Coffey JW, Hoffman RA, Evans CH. N-monomethyl arginine, an inhibitor of nitric oxide synthase, suppresses the development of adjuvant arthritis in rats. Arthritis Rheum 37: 1062–1069, 1994.

161. McCartney-Francis N, Allen JB, Mizel DE, Albina JE, Xie QW, Nathan CF, Wahl SM. Suppression of arthritis by an inhibitor of nitric oxide synthase. J Exp Med 178: 749–754, 1993.

162. Connor JR, Manning PT, Settle SL, Moore WM, Jerome GM, Webber RK, Tjoeng FS, Currie MG. Suppression Of Adjuvant-Induced Arthritis By Selective Inhibition Of Inducible Nitric Oxide Synthase. European Journal of Pharmacology 273: 15–24, 1995.

163. Weinberg JB. Nitric oxide as an inflammatory mediator in autoimmune MRL-lpr/lpr mice. Environ Health Perspect 106: 1131–1137, 1998.

164. Sakurai H, Kohsaka H, Liu MF, Higashiyama H, Hirata Y, Kanno K, Saito I, Miyasaka N. Nitric oxide production and inducible nitric oxide synthase expression in inflammatory arthritides. Journal of Clinical Investigation 96: 2357–2363, 1995.

165. Grabowski PS, England AJ, Dykhuizen R, Copland M, Benjamin N, Reid DM, Ralston SH. Elevated Nitric Oxide Production In Rheumatoid Arthritis – Detection Using the Fasting Urinary Nitrate/Creatinine Ratio. Arthritis & Rheumatism 39: 643–647, 1996.

166. Farrell AJ, Blake DR, Palmer RM, Moncada S. Increased concentrations of nitrite in synovial fluid and serum samples suggest increased nitric oxide synthesis in rheumatic diseases. Annals of the Rheumatic Diseases 51: 1219–1222, 1992.

167. Ueki Y, Miyake S, Tominaga Y, Eguchi K. Increased nitric oxide levels in patients with rheumatoid arthritis. Journal of Rheumatology 23: 230–236, 1996.

168. Onur O, Akinci AS, Akbiyik F, Unsal I. Elevated levels of nitrate in rheumatoid arthritis. Rheumatol Int 20: 154–158, 2001.

169. Pham TN, Rahman P, Tobin YM, Khraishi MM, Hamilton SF, Alderdice C, Richardson VJ. Elevated serum nitric oxide levels in patients with inflammatory arthritis associated with co-expression of inducible nitric oxide synthase and protein kinase C-eta in peripheral blood monocyte-derived macrophages. J Rheumatol 30: 2529–2534, 2003.

170. Weinberg JB, Granger DL, Pisetsky DS, Seldin MF, Misukonis MA, Mason SN, Pippen AM, Ruiz P, Wood ER, Gilkeson GS. The role of nitric oxide in the pathogenesis of spontaneous murine autoimmune disease: increased nitric oxide production and nitric oxide synthase expression in MRL-lpr/lpr mice, and reduction of spontaneous glomerulonephritis and arthritis by orally administered NG-monomethyl-L-arginine. J Exp Med 179: 651–660, 1994.

171. Dang-Vu AP, Pisetsky DS, Weinberg JB. Functional alterations of macrophages in autoimmune MRL-lpr/lpr mice. J Immunol 138: 1757–1761, 1987.

172. Weinberg JB, Gilkeson GS, Mason RP, Chamulitrat W. Nitrosylation of blood hemoglobin and renal nonheme proteins in autoimmune MRL-lpr/lpr mice. Free Radical Biology & Medicine 24: 191–196, 1998.

173. Keng T, Privalle CT, Gilkeson GS, Weinberg JB. Peroxynitrite formation and decreased catalase activity in autoimmune MRL-lpr/lpr mice. Mol Med 6: 779–792, 2000.

174. Fermor B, Weinberg JB, Pisetsky DS, Misukonis MA, Banes AJ, Guilak F. The effects of static and intermittent compression on nitric oxide production in articular cartilage explants. J Orthop Res 19: 729–737, 2001.

175. Fermor B, Haribabu B, Weinberg JB, Pisetsky DS, Guilak F. Mechanical stress and nitric oxide influence leukotriene production in cartilage. Biochem Biophys Res Commun 285: 806–810, 2001.

176. Griffiths RJ, Pettipher ER, Koch K, Farrell CA, Breslow R, Conklyn MJ, Smith MA, Hackman BC, Wimberly DJ, Milici AJ, et al. Leukotriene B4 plays a critical role in the progression of collagen-induced arthritis. Proc Natl Acad Sci U S A 92: 517–521, 1995.

177. Cernanec J, Guilak F, Weinberg JB, Pisetsky DS, Fermor B. Influence of hypoxia and reoxygenation on cytokine-induced production of proinflammatory mediators in articular cartilage. Arthritis Rheum 46: 968–975, 2002.

178. Fink C, Fermor B, Weinberg JB, Pisetsky DS, Misukonis MA, Guilak F. The effect of dynamic mechanical compression on nitric oxide production in the meniscus. Osteoarthritis Cartilage 9: 481–487, 2001.

179. Shin SJ, Fermor B, Weinberg JB, Pisetsky DS, Guilak F. Regulation of matrix turnover in meniscal explants: role of mechanical stress, interleukin-1, and nitric oxide. J Appl Physiol 95: 308–313, 2003.

180. Agarwal S, Long P, Gassner R, Piesco NP, Buckley MJ. Cyclic tensile strain suppresses catabolic effects of interleukin-1beta in fibrochondrocytes from the temporomandibular joint. Arthritis Rheum 44: 608–617, 2001.
181. Agarwal S, Long P, Seyedain A, Piesco N, Shree A, Gassner R. A central role for the nuclear factor-kappaB pathway in anti-inflammatory and proinflammatory actions of mechanical strain. Faseb J 17: 899–901, 2003.
182. Fermor B, Jeffcoat D, Hennerbichler A, Pisetsky DS, Weinberg JB, Guilak F. The effects of cyclic mechanical strain and tumor necrosis factor alpha on the response of cells of the meniscus. Osteoarthritis Cartilage 12: 956–962, 2004.
183. Upton ML, Hennerbichler A, Fermor B, Guilak F, Weinberg JB, Setton LA. Biaxial strain effects on cells from the inner and outer regions of the meniscus. Collagen Tissue Research Connect Tissue Res 47: 207–214, 2006.

CHAPTER 3

OBESITY, INFLAMMATION, AND VASCULAR DISEASE
The role of the adipose tissue as an endocrine organ

PAOLO CALABRO'[*,1,2] AND EDWARD T. H. YEH[2,3]

[1]*Division of Cardiology, Department of Cardiothoracic Sciences, Second University of Naples, Italy,*
[2]*The Brown Foundation Institute of Molecular Medicine for the Prevention of Human Diseases,*
The University of Texas-Houston Health Science Center, and
[3]*The Department of Cardiology, The University of Texas-M.D. Anderson Cancer Center,*
Houston, Texas

Abstract: Insulin resistance, both in nondiabetic and diabetic subjects, is frequently associated with obesity, particularly with an excess of central fat. With the growing prevalence of obesity, scientific interest in the biology of adipose tissue has been extended to the secretory products of adipocytes, since they are increasingly shown to influence several aspects in the pathogenesis of obesity-related diseases

Until relatively recently, the role of fat itself in the development of obesity and its consequences was considered to be a passive one; adipocytes were considered to be little

[*]E-mail: paolo.calabro@unina2.it and etyeh@mdanderson.org

R. E. Harris (ed.), Inflammation in the Pathogenesis of Chronic Diseases, 63–91.

more than storage cells for fat. It is now clear that, in addition to storing calories as triglycerides, they also secrete a large variety of proteins, including cytokines, chemokines and hormone-like factors, such as leptin, adiponectin and resistin. This production of pro-atherogenic chemokines by adipose tissue is of particular interest since their local secretion, e.g. by perivascular adipose depots, may provide a novel mechanistic link between obesity and the associated vascular complications.

Recent research has revealed many functions of adipocytokines extending far beyond metabolism, such as immunity, cancer and bone formation. This remarkable understanding is allowing us to more clearly define the role that adipocytes play in health and in obesity and how inflammatory mediators act as signaling molecules in this process.

Moreover, on a molecular level, we are beginning to comprehend how such variables as hormonal control, exercise, food intake, and genetic variation interact and result in a given phenotype, and how pharmacological intervention may modulate adipose tissue biology

1.   INTRODUCTION

The metabolic syndrome is a constellation of abnormalities—generally considered to include abdominal obesity, high blood glucose/impaired glucose tolerance, dyslip-idaemia, and high blood pressure—that together increase risk of overt diabetes mellitus and cardiovascular disease (CVD). A variety of data indicate that glucose intolerance plays a central role in coronary artery disease (CAD) risk.

Obesity, the most common nutritional disorder in industrial countries, is associated with increased cardiovascular mortality and morbidity. [1–3] Until recently, the adipocyte was largely thought to be an inert storage cell whose main function was to store excess energy in the form of triglycerides. It is now apparent that adipocytes have a more complex role in the organism. [4] For example, adipocytes produce a large number of hormones, peptides, and smaller molecules that affect metabolism and cardiovascular function, not only in an endocrine manner, but also by autocrine and paracrine influences. [5–7]

One of the key vasoactive substances produced by adipocytes is leptin, which is an important regulator of food intake. [8] Other adipocyte-derived molecules, including prostaglandins, adiponectin and the more recently discovered resistin, affect metabolic function and might play a role in causing cardiovascular end-organ damage. [9, 10] In addition, obese individuals have high circulating levels of a range of inflammatory markers produced by adipose tissue, including Tumor Necrosis Factor alpha (TNF-alpha), interleukin-1 (IL-1), and IL-6. [11, 12] These factors, whose levels can be reduced by weight loss, are likely to contribute to vascular damage in obese individuals.

2.   THE IMPORTANT ROLE OF FAT TISSUE
FOR HUMAN HEALTH

The adipose organ consists of two distinct tissues, namely brown (BAT) and white adipose tissue (WAT), and there is continuing debate on the extent to which there is inter-convertibility between them. [13] BAT is specialized for heat production by non-shivering thermogenesis through the presence of the tissue-specific uncoupling protein-1 (UCP1) located in the inner mitochondrial membrane. [14] In brown fat, the lipid droplets (normally multiple within each brown adipocyte), are considered to serve primarily as a fuel for thermogenesis. In WAT, on the other hand, the stored triacylglycerols provide a long-term fuel reserve for the organism as a whole. Indeed, white fat is the main energy reservoir in mammals and birds, triacylglycerols providing storage at a high energy density, both because of the considerable caloric value of lipid and because, in contrast to carbohydrate, triacylglycerols can be stored with little associated water.

Until relatively recently, the physiology of WAT centered on lipogenesis and lipolysis, and the regulation of these two opposing metabolic pathways. However, a revolution in our understanding of the biological role of white fat has occurred over the past decade; it is now recognized as a major endocrine and signaling tissue which interacts extensively with other organs in overall physiological and metabolic control.

The rapid escalation in the incidence of obesity, with its concomitant disorders, has been the major impetus behind much of the current work on WAT. Obesity is the most prevalent nutrition-related disorder in Westernized countries, and in the UK, for example, some 23% of adult males and 24% of adult females are now clinically obese (Body Mass Index, BMI > 30), [15] while a further one-third of the population are overweight (BMI 25–29.9). In contrast, in the early 1980s, just 6% of adult men and 8% of adult women in the UK were obese. [16] Obesity not only reduces life expectancy (by 8 years), but there is also an increased risk of developing several major diseases; these diseases include type 2 diabetes, coronary heart disease and certain cancers. In the case of diabetes, the risk increases approximately 10-fold once a BMI of 30 is reached and the more obese the greater the relative risk. Paradoxically, white fat has been something of a 'poor relation' in energy balance and obesity research, most attention having been directed towards the perceived more complex neuroendocrine pathways involved in the hypothalamic control of food intake, together with the peripheral mechanisms of adaptive thermogenesis.

The importance of adipocytes for health was shown very elegantly through the use of the mouse model of lipoatrophic diabetes. [17, 18] These mice were genetically altered so they had virtually no white fat tissue. They also had characteristics similar to those seen in humans with severe lipoatrophic diabetes: insulin resistance, hyperglycemia, hyperlipidemia, and fatty livers. Transplantation of adipose tissue from healthy mice into these lipoatrophic mice resulted in a dramatic reversal of the hyperglycemia, accompanied by lowered insulin concentrations and improved muscle insulin sensitivity, decreased serum triacylglycerols, decreased hepatic gluconeogenesis, and decreased amounts of fat deposited in muscle and liver. These beneficial effects were dependent on the presence of transplanted adipose tissue. In other words, the introduction of adipocytes into these mice completely reversed the characteristic phenotype. Thus, the absence of adipocytes is metabolically detrimental. These experiments provided an elegant platform for the argument that fat cells play a role in health. [17]

3.   INFLAMMATION AND OBESITY

An important recent development in our understanding of obesity is the emergence of the concept that, along with diabetes, it is characterized by a state of chronic low-grade inflammation.[19–21] The basis for this view is that increased circulating levels of several markers of inflammation, both pro-inflammatory cytokines and acute-phase proteins, are elevated in the obese; these markers include IL-6, the TNF-alpha system, C-reactive protein (CRP) and haptoglobin. [22, 23] The implications in terms of the site of inflammation itself, whether systemic or local, are unclear. Nevertheless, it is increasingly evident that the inflammatory state may be causal in the development of insulin resistance and the other disorders associated with obesity, such as hyperlipidemia and the metabolic syndrome. [24, 25] While the general assumption is that inflammation is consequent to obesity, it has been suggested that obesity is in fact a result of inflammatory disease. [23]

A central question is the origin of the inflammatory markers in obesity, and there are three possibilities. The first is that it reflects production and release from organs other than adipose tissue, primarily the liver (and immune cells). The second explanation is that WAT is secreting factors that stimulate the production of inflammatory markers from the liver and other organs; this may well be the case with CRP, where it is argued that hepatic and extra-hepatic production is stimulated by increased IL-6 from the expanded fat mass of the obese. [12, 25, 26] The third possibility is that adipocytes themselves are the immediate source of some, or most, of these inflammatory markers, with the raised circulating levels in obesity reflecting production from the increased WAT mass. [27] There is also, of course, the possibility of there being a combination of production in adipose tissue and other organs.

Given that adipocytes secrete a number of cytokines and acute phase proteins, the question arises as to the extent to which the expanded WAT mass contributes, either directly or indirectly, to the increased production and circulating levels of inflammation-related factors in obesity.

From the perspective of adipose tissue biology, a key question is whether adipocytes (or adipose tissue) directly contribute to the raised circulating levels of specific inflammatory markers and, if so, to what extent? Although obtaining quantitative information on the contribution from particular cells within adipose tissue is difficult, the issue that can be readily addressed is whether adipocytes express certain inflammatory genes and their encoded proteins secreted. Recent reports demonstrating that WAT is infiltrated by macrophages in obesity clearly suggest that the non-adipocyte fraction may be a significant component of the inflammatory state within adipose tissue. [28, 29]

However, we have recently demonstrated, using an in vitro model, that the mature adipocytes fraction isolated from human adipose tissue is directly involved in both CRP and serum amyloid A (SAA) release. [27, 30] Furthermore, close links between adipocytes and immune cells are increasingly apparent, and preadipocytes have been reported to act as 'macrophage-like' cells. [31]

Following from these observations is the growing view that the inflammatory state plays a causal role in the development of type 2 diabetes and the metabolic syndrome associated with obesity. In this context, the reduction in adiponectin in the obese [32, 33] is of particular interest in view of the anti-inflammatory effect of this adipokine. [9, 34]

As we have mentioned before, the inflammatory state of adipose tissue in obesity has been highlighted by recent reports demonstrating that there is extensive infiltration of the tissue by macrophages in the obese. [28, 29] The arrival of macrophages en masse is likely to lead to a considerable amplification of the inflammatory state in white fat, and TNF-alpha may play a pivotal role in this infiltration. Two key chemokines are released by adipocytes: monocyte chemotactic protein 1 (MCP-1) and monocyte inhibiting factor (MIF),, which are important in relation to attracting and preventing the exodus, respectively, of macrophages into tissue. [35–38] Expression and secretion of MCP-1 is strongly up-regulated by TNF-alpha. [35, 39]

An important issue is why adipose tissue should mount a strong inflammatory response as fat mass expands in obesity. One possibility is that WAT is providing inflammatory mediators for a site, or sites, elsewhere in the body, whether because of inflammation in another specific locus or more systemically. However, Trayhurn et al. have recently argued the parsimonious view that WAT is itself in a state of inflammation as a reflection of local events within the tissue, with raised circulating levels of inflammatory markers reflecting spillover. [40] We have further suggested that the inflammation may be a response to relative hypoxia in clusters of adipocytes distant from the capillary network as WAT mass expands, in advance of angiogenesis. Indeed, the proportion of cardiac output that goes to adipose tissue is decreased in obesity, and the obese do not show the postprandial increase in blood flow which occurs in lean individuals. [41]

Activation of a transcription factor, hypoxia inducible factor-1 (HIF-1), through the stimulation of the expression of the HIF-1alpha subunit – the molecular sensor of hypoxia [42–44]– may be the mechanism through which low oxygen tension links to inflammation. [40] The target genes for HIF-1 include vascular endothelial growth factor (VEGF) and leptin, and expression of both of these has been shown to be stimulated in 3T3-L1 adipocytes in response to hypoxia. [45]

4.   ADIPOSE TISSUE AS AN ENDOCRINE ORGAN

As briefly introduced before, increasing evidence indicates that adipose tissue is an important source of cytokines [46] and that adiposity contributes to a pro-inflammatory milieu. [21]

Fat is both a dynamic endocrine organ, as well a highly active metabolic tissue that produces and secretes inflammatory factors, which are well known to play important roles in the atherosclerotic process. Collectively, these factors are called adipocytokines or adipokines. These include TNF-alpha, leptin, adiponectin, resistin, plasminogen activator inhibitor-1 (PAI-1), IL-6, and angiotensinogen. [46] Serum adipokine levels are elevated in humans and animals with excess adiposity [21, 47–49], and visceral fat appears to produce several of these adipokines more actively than subcutaneous adipose tissue. [50–52] Reduction in fat mass correlates with decrease in the serum levels of many of these adipokines [53–55], implying that approaches designed to promote fat loss should be useful in attenuating the pro-inflammatory milieu associated with obesity. Some of these adipokines, in addition to their pro-inflammatory actions, also affect insulin action.

As individuals become obese and their adipocytes enlarge, adipose tissue undergoes molecular and cellular alterations affecting systemic metabolism. First, several pro-inflammatory factors are produced in adipose tissue with increasing obesity. Compared with that of lean individuals, adipose tissue in obese persons shows higher expression of pro-inflammatory proteins, including TNF-alpha, inter-leukin 6 (IL-6), MCP-1, inducible nitric oxide synthase (i-NOS), transforming growth factor beta 1 (TGF-beta 1), procoagulant proteins such as PAI-1, tissue factor (TF), and factor VII.[37, 48, 51, 56–62]

Macrophage numbers in adipose tissue also increase with obesity [28, 29], where they apparently function to scavenge moribund adipocytes, which increase dramatically with obesity. [63] Macrophages are thought to be responsible for most of the cytokine production in obese adipose tissue. [28, 29, 51] In fact, adipose tissue macrophages are responsible for almost all adipose tissue TNF-alpha expression and significant amounts of IL-6 and i-NOS expression. [28] Of particular note, Xu et al. [29] reported that the increased expression of inflammation-specific genes by macrophages in the adipose tissue of obese mice preceded a dramatic increase in insulin production. Furthermore, when those mice were treated with rosigli-tazone, an insulin-sensitizing drug, the expression of these genes declined. Thus, the chronological appearance of these inflammatory molecules before the development of insulin resistance, as well as their known ability to promote insulin resistance and other complications of obesity, strongly suggests adipose tissue inflammation as an important protagonist in the development of obesity-related complications.

Inflammation is thought to contribute also to the development of the sequelae of obesity. For example, adipose tissue TNF-alpha concentrations are correlated with obesity and insulin resistance in patients with and without type 2 diabetes. [64, 65] In obese women, TNF-alpha messenger RNA expression in adipose tissue is correlated with fasting plasma glucose, insulin, and triacylglycerol concentrations. [57] TNF-alpha may increase systemic insulin resistance by promoting the release of fatty acids from adipose tissue into the bloodstream to act on tissues such as muscle and liver. Thus, adipose tissue TNF-alpha can act locally in adipose tissue, which ultimately promotes insulin resistance in peripheral tissues.

Furthermore, IL-6 expression is also increased in obese adipose tissue; for example, its expression in adipose tissue from obese individuals is 10-fold that in adipose tissue from lean individuals if normalized for the number of adipocytes present. Also, IL-6 expression varies between adipose tissue sites: expression is higher in visceral than in peripheral adipocytes, and ±90% of IL-6 expressed in adipose tissue is produced by cells other than adipocytes. [51] Plasma concentrations of IL-6 increase with obesity, unlike those of TNF-alpha, which acts in an autocrine and paracrine fashion [66]; in obese individuals, adipose tissue is a major determinant of plasma IL-6 concentrations, contributing as much as 30% of total body production. [66] IL-6 increases lipolysis and fat oxidation in humans [67], and plasma IL-6 concentrations correlate with insulin resistance. [65] Recently, IL-6 was shown directly to cause insulin resistance in the liver. [68] Elevated IL-6 concentrations are a predictor for development of type 2 diabetes and for myocardial infarction. [69, 70]

Clearly, several inflammatory mediators are implicated in the development of obesity. Nevertheless, the precise mechanisms responsible for the development of the chronic diseases associated with obesity are still unclear. In the following sections, we analyze and discuss the main adipokines individually.

4.1.   Adiponectin

Adiponectin, a hormone also known as adipoQ or adipocyte complement-related protein, is an adipocyte-derived collagen-like protein identified through an extensive search of adipose tissue transcripts in the human genome project. Expression of adiponectin mRNA occurs exclusively in adipose tissue. The protein is composed of two structurally distinct domains: the C-terminal collagen-like fibrous domain and the complement C1q-like globular domain. Adiponectin is abundant in the circulating plasma, amounting to $5–20\,\mu g/mL$ in normal subjects in multimeric form.

This hormone enhances insulin sensitivity in muscle and liver and increases free fatty acid (FFA) oxidation in several tissues, including muscle fibers. [71–73] It also decreases serum FFA, glucose, and triacylglycerol concentrations: e.g., when normal, lean mice were given injections of adiponectin in conjunction with a meal high in fat and sugar, the normal postprandial increases in plasma glucose, FFA, and triacylglycerol concentrations were smaller as the result of an increased rate of clearance from the blood rather than a reduced rate of absorption from the gut. [71] In contrast, when insulin-resistant mice were treated with physiologic concentrations of adiponectin, glucose tolerance was improved and insulin resistance reduced. [73] In humans, plasma adiponectin concentrations fall with increasing obesity and visceral fat accumulation, and this effect is greater in men than in women. [32] A Japanese case–control study demonstrated that patients with hypoadiponecti-naemia (plasma level less than $4\mu g/mL$) together with multiple cardiovascular risk factors had an increased risk of coronary artery disease, indicating that hypoad-iponectinaemia may be a key factor in the metabolic syndrome. [74] A prospective study performed in the USA confirmed that high adiponectin concentrations are associated with a lower risk of myocardial infarction in men than women. [75] Interestingly there is a close negative correlation between the concentration of adiponectin and visceral adiposity determined by CT scan.

Reduced adiponectin concentrations correlate with insulin resistance and hyper-insulinaemia. [33, 76] In addition, several polymorphisms of the adiponectin gene (APM1, mapped to chromosome 3q27) have been identified that are associated with reduced plasma adiponectin concentration [77–79] and an increased risk of type 2 diabetes, insulin resistance, or the metabolic syndrome. [77, 78, 80] There is a genetic form of hypoadiponectinaemia caused by a missense mutation that exhibits the clinical phenotype of metabolic syndrome. [78]

Adiponectin appears to play a key role in opposing insulin resistance. [27] Plasma adiponectin concentrations are lower in subjects with type 2 diabetes mellitus than in controls matched for body mass index. Studies in Pima Indians and obese monkeys have shown that plasma concentrations have a strong positive correlation with insulin sensitivity, suggesting that low plasma concentrations are related to insulin resistance. [81]

Plasma levels of adiponectin are also decreased in hypertensive subjects. Endothelium-dependent vasoreactivity is impaired in subjects with hypoadiponecti-naemia, which is thought to be a cause of hypertension in obesity. [82] Most importantly, plasma concentrations of adiponectin are lower in subjects with coronary heart disease than controls, even when body mass index and age are matched. [9] Kaplan–Meyer analysis in Italian subjects with renal insufficiency demonstrated that the high adiponectin group had a lower mortality rate from cardiovascular disease than other groups. [83]

In mice deficient in apolipoprotein E (and thus susceptible to atherosclerosis), treatment with human adiponectin inhibits lesion formation in the aortic sinus by 30% compared with that in untreated control animals ($P < 0.05$). [84] Adiponectin knockout mice show more severe intimal thickening by endothelial injury than wild-type mice. In addition, over-expression of human adiponectin by adenovirus transfection attenuated plaque formation in apoE knockout mice. [84]

Adiponectin concentrations are reduced in patients with coronary artery disease [76], whereas high levels appear to block critical cellular phenomena in the development of atherosclerosis. [85, 86] When the endothelial barrier is injured by attacking factors such as oxidized low-density lipoprotein, chemical substances and mechanical stress, adiponectin accumulates in the sub-endothelial space of vascular walls by binding to sub-endothelial collagen (collagens I, III and V) where it inhibits key components of atherogenesis. For example, adiponectin suppresses monocyte attachment to vascular endothelial cells by inhibiting TNF-alpha-induced expression of adhesion molecules such as vascular cell adhesion molecule-1, ICAM-1 and E-selectin via the inhibition of NF-κB activation. Adiponectin also attenuates growth-factor-induced proliferation of vascular smooth muscle cells by inhibition of the MAPK process. Furthermore, adiponectin suppresses the transformation of macrophages to foam cells by inhibiting scavenger receptor class A. [9, 85]

The vulnerability of atherosclerotic plaque to rupture is considered to be the most important prognostic determinant of acute coronary syndrome (myocardial infarction and stroke) in cardiovascular disease. In this process, matrix metallopro-teinase (MMP) secreted from macrophages is considered to play an important role in plaque vulnerability, and the tissue inhibitor of metalloproteinase (TIMP) may protect against plaque rupture by inhibiting MMP. Adiponectin has been found to enhance the expression of mRNA and protein production of TIMP in macrophages via the induction of interleukin-10 (IL-10) synthesis, suggesting that adiponectin may prevent plaque rupture by the inhibition of MMP function through the induction of IL-10-dependent TIMP production. [86]

Adiponectin may also inhibit plaque development by stimulating production of NO [87] and decreasing cytokine production from macrophages by inhibiting NF-kB signaling through cyclic adenosine monophosphate (cAMP)-dependent pathways. [34, 88] Interleukin-6 inhibits adiponectin expression and secretion in 3T3-L1 adipocytes. [89] Thus, adiponectin might indirectly inhibit CRP and IL-6 expression through its ability to inhibit production of TNF-alpha. Furthermore, adiponectin directly stimulates production of NO in endothelial cells using phosphatidyli-nositol (PI) 3-kinase-dependent pathways involving phosphorylation of endothelial nitric oxide synthase (eNOS) by adenosine-monophosphate–activated protein kinase (AMPK). [90]

The clinical and experimental evidence presented above suggests that adiponectin may have therapeutic value for cardiovascular disease, diabetes mellitus, and metabolic syndrome. However, observed plasma levels are variable and often extremely high, and direct administration to diseased patients may not be practical because of the difficulty in achieving and maintaining optimum levels. A further complication is that adiponectin in its high-molecular weight form has the greatest anti-atherogenic activity, and molecular mechanisms of signal transduction may therefore be extremely complex. As discussed below, the search for enhancers of endogenous synthesis may be the most efficacious method to identify therapeutic applications related to adiponectin.

Lifestyle modification (primarily weight loss through exercise and diet) signifi-cantly increased adiponectin levels in diabetic or obese subjects. [55, 91] Treatment with temocapril and candesartan significantly increased adiponectin levels as well as insulin sensitivity without affecting degree of adiposity. [92] Recent clinical trials suggest that blockade of the renin-angiotensin system lowers the risk of development of type II diabetes. One possible mechanism for this effect is the correlated increase in adiponectin levels. In hypercholesterolemic, hypertensive patients, losartan alone or combined therapy with simvastatin and losartan significantly increased plasma adiponectin levels relative to baseline measurements, whereas simvastatin therapy alone did not. [93] Potential mechanisms by which losartan increases adiponectin levels include direct effects on insulin-stimulated glucose uptake, promotion of adipogenesis and induction of PPAR-alpha activity that promotes adipocyte differ-entiation. [94] Fenofibrate therapy significantly increased plasma adiponectin levels and insulin sensitivity in patients with primary hypertriglyceridemia. [95]

Thiazolidindione derivatives have also been shown to be potent enhancers of adiponectin synthesis. For example, troglitazone was reported to increase plasma levels of adiponectin three fold in subjects with visceral obesity. Administration of thiazolidinediones significantly increased plasma adiponectin concentrations in insulin-resistant humans and rodents without affecting body weight, and adiponectin messenger-RNA expression was normalized or increased by thiazolidinediones in the adipose tissues of obese mice. Nevertheless, since thiazolidindione may have unexpected effects as a PPAR-γ agonist, a search is underway for derivatives that can specifically enhance adiponectin without producing such effects. [96]

4.2.   Leptin

Leptin, the first adipocyte hormone identified, influences food intake through a direct effect on the hypothalamus. [97, 98] In humans and rodents, plasma leptin concentrations are highly correlated with BMI. [99] Mice lacking the gene coding for leptin (ob/ob mice) are very obese and diabetic, and if ob/ob mice are treated with regular injections of leptin, they reduce their food intake, increase their metabolic rate, and lose weight. [97, 100] Mice and rats with a genetic mutation affecting the leptin receptor in the hypothalamus exhibit a similar phenotype to ob/ob mice. [98, 101]

These functions seem to be mediated mainly by the central nervous system, because intracerebroventricular injection of leptin produces significant effects with much smaller amounts than those required by systemic injection, although application of anti-obese treatment using adipocytokines has been tried.

Signal transduction mediated by leptin has been clarified more precisely than that of adiponectin. Leptin receptors (OB-Rs) are single membrane-spanning receptors with homology to members of the cytokine receptor superfamily. Seven different leptin receptors, produced by alternative splicing, have been identified. The receptor-containing transmembrane domains can be divided into two groups: one group has a short amino acid residue intracellular domain (OB-Ra, OB-Rc, OB-Rd and OB-Rf), and the other group has a short amino acid residue intracellular domain (OB-Rb). OB-Rb is mainly expressed in the hypothalamus, whereas the short forms are expressed in a variety of tissues. The long form of the receptor has two Janus kinase sites in the intracellular domain and the short form has one. Only the long form can activate the signal transducers and activators of the transcription family (STAT). C57B1/Ks db/db mice that lack the long form of the receptor and have intact short forms exhibit a phenotype that is almost identical to ob/ob mice, which lack leptin.

As animals and humans become obese, the role of leptin in regulating body weight becomes more complex. There are rare cases where mutations affecting the genes coding for either leptin or its receptor have been found in families with a high prevalence of morbid obesity [102–104], and leptin therapy does have a beneficial effect in children with congenital leptin deficiency. [105, 106] However, in most obese individuals, leptin concentrations are already high because of the increased amount of leptin-secreting adipose tissue. [107] It appears that with increasing leptin concentrations, the hormone induces target cells to become resistant to its actions. In mice that became obese after being fed a high-fat diet, leptin concentrations increased accompanied by an increased expression of suppressor-of-cytokine-signaling 3 (SOCS-3), a potent inhibitor of leptin signaling. [108] Thus, the central effects of leptin are blocked by SOCS-3 produced as a result of the increasing concentrations of leptin found in obesity.

Leptin appears to have important effects on peripheral metabolism. In a mouse model of congenital lipodystrophy (little or no fat), insulin resistance, hyperinsulinaemia, hyperglycemia, and enlarged fatty liver, leptin therapy reversed the insulin resistance and diabetes. [18] Humans with a rare disorder called lipoatrophic diabetes have little or no fat mass, reduced serum adipokines such as leptin, and very elevated serum triacylglycerol concentrations. In fact, triacylglycerol concentrations tend to be so high that some individuals require regular plasmapheresis to reduce serum triacylglycerol. These elevated lipid concentrations lead to an enlarged fatty liver, which can lead to severe liver disease, and some individuals die secondary to liver complications.

In a pioneering study by Oral et al. [109], administration of exogenous leptin to individuals with lipoatrophic diabetes resulted in marked reductions in triacylglycerol concentrations, liver volume, and glycated hemoglobin, and discontinuation or a large reduction in antidiabetic therapy

Clearly, adiponectin and leptin are important hormones with central and peripheral effects on metabolism and energy balance. Recent data suggest that at least some of their actions that reduce circulating fatty acids and triacylglycerol are due to increased fat oxidation. The increase in fat oxidation is mediated by activating the enzyme AMP-activated protein kinase (AMPK), which also increases glucose transport in muscle. [110, 111] Interestingly, exercise activates AMPK, which also increases fat oxidation and reduces insulin resistance. [112] Thus, the adipocyte hormones and exercise act via a similar signal transduction pathway to increase fat oxidation and promote insulin sensitivity.

The potential effects of leptin in the pathophysiology of cardiovascular complications of obesity are still diverse, despite evidence of leptin resistance to metabolic actions. This protein may elevate blood pressure by stimulation of the autonomic nervous system. Recent reports suggest that leptin contributes to atherosclerosis and cardiovascular disease in obese subjects. [113] Further studies are necessary to verify the significance of therapeutic strategies using leptin.

4.3. Resistin

Resistin is the most recent example of an adipokine with contrasting roles in mouse and man. Resistin belongs to a family of cysteine rich secretory proteins known as resistin-like molecules or FIZZ (found in inflammatory zones) proteins.

This protein was initially shown to be released in large amounts from mouse adipocytes; its release was increased in obese mice and accompanied by insulin resistance. [114] The adverse effects of obesity were neutralised by antibodies against resistin, and rosiglitazone reduced resistin levels. Adipocyte-derived resistin was therefore thought to link obesity to diabetes. [114]

Further studies in rodents have suggested that resistin mRNA levels are higher in abdominal fat depots, compared with depots from the thigh [115], and that serum resistin levels are positively correlated with body mass index (BMI). [116]

Additionally, resistin has been found to modulate hepatic insulin action [117, 118] and possibly play a role in maintaining fasting blood glucose levels. [119]

Confirmation of these findings in human populations has been difficult and may be due to the fact that resistin appears to be derived from different sources in humans and rodents. Reports point to the adipocyte as the sole source of resistin in mice [114, 120], whereas investigations in humans suggest that very little resistin is expressed in adipocytes, but rather, monocytes and macrophages produce large quantities of resistin. [121, 122]

Studies determined the resistin gene, referred to as Retn, encoded a 114-amino acid polypeptide [114] secreted as a disulphide-linked homodimer. [123] Recent X-ray crystallographic studies of resistin [124] have determined its complex hexameric structure. Resistin was shown to circulate in two distinct assembly states; the more predominant HMM (high-molecular-mass) hexamer and the substantially more bioactive LMM (low-molecularmass) complex, which is unable to form intertrimer disulphide bonds. [124] This implies that regulated processing through disulphide cleavage is required to initiate bioactivity of the LMM form, and suggests a potential target site for receptor interaction. [124]

The lack of homology between the human and mouse resistin genes also suggests an interspecies divergence in function. [125] Although resistin appears to be involved in rodent metabolism, the data in humans are less clear. Rather, resistin may be an inflammatory marker in humans, because macrophages are known inflammatory modulators. In support of its possible inflammatory role in humans, recombinant resistin activates human endothelial cells, as measured by increased expression of endothelin-1 and various adhesion molecules and chemokines, while simultaneously increasing CD40 ligand signaling by down-regulating tumor necrosis factor receptor-associated factor-3. [126] Moreover, we have also recently shown that resistin promotes human coronary artery smooth muscle cell proliferation through activation of extracellular signal-regulated kinase 1/2 (ERK) and phosphatidylinositol 3-kinase (PI3K) pathways. [127]

These findings suggest a possible mechanistic link between resistin and cardio-vascular disease via proinflammatory pathways. Recently Burnet et al. [128] demonstrated that resistin mRNA and protein are present in atherosclerotic lesions in the aorta of apoE-deficient mice. In addition, they found elevated serum levels of resistin in apoE-deficient mice compared with wild type controls, and in patients with premature coronary artery disease compared with individuals with angiographically normal coronary arteries.

Most subsequent studies of resistin in mouse models support the notion that resistin is an adipokine regulator of insulin action. [129] In contrast, human studies reflect a different picture. Human fat cells, unlike those of mice, do not produce resistin, [130] although segments of human adipose tissue appear to support its release. [131] Resistin is therefore not a true adipokine in man, but is derived from as yet unidentified cells in the stromal compartment of human adipose tissue. To examine the influence of resistin on insulin sensitivity in man, Utzschneider et al. [132] measured plasma resistin in 177 non-diabetic individuals, and found no difference between those with a high or low body mass index (BMI), or high or low insulin sensitivity. Nor did resistin levels correlate with visceral fat accumulation, although visceral fat is a strong determinant of insulin sensitivity. In contrast, circulating levels of other adipose tissue derived factors such as adiponectin, plasminogen activator inhibitor-1 and leptin were markedly influenced by these parameters. These results demonstrate that the level of resistin does not provide a link between the adipocyte and insulin sensitivity in man but, as the authors point out, do not exclude other possible roles for resistin within human adipose tissue. [132]

Many recent observations do support a role for resistin in obesity. Studies by Lee et al. [133] using various murine models showed that obese mice had higher circulating resistin levels than their lean counterparts. These observations coincide with studies of rodents by Rajala and coworkers [134], showing that circulating resistin levels were significantly elevated and concordant with increasing levels of insulin, glucose and lipids; thus substantiating the initial evidence that linked increasing resistin and adiposity with the aetiology of these conditions. [114] Recently, Asensio et al. [135] determined that mice fed a high fat diet showed heightened adipocyte differentiation denoted by induction of fatty acid binding protein (AP-2) gene expression (a surrogate marker of differentiation) that was positively correlated with resistin gene expression. Subsequently, in view of this and previous studies [120, 134], it was suggested that elevated resistin expression was a result of adipocyte differentiation. [135] Moreover, the increase in adipocyte number may have caused a rise in local resistin production, inhibiting insulin action on glucose uptake in adipose tissue, and thus preventing further adipocyte differentiation. [135] Therefore, at least in rodents, a regulatory feedback mechanism for resistin in adipogenesis may exist, acting as an adipose sensor for nutritional status. In accordance with these observations, Kim et al. [136] generated transgenic mice overexpressing a dominant inhibitory form of resistin which functioned to reverse the inhibition of resistin-mediated adipocyte differentiation. These transgenic mice developed obesity, possibly owing to enhanced adipocyte differentiation and adipocyte hypertrophy, as indicated by increased circulating levels of adiponectin and leptin. [136]

In humans, serum resistin is elevated in obese subjects compared to lean subjects [116, 137, 138], and resistin levels are positively correlated with increased BMI (body mass index) and visceral fat area. [116, 139, 140] The implication that resistin is important in human adipose tissue has been corroborated by studies showing increased protein expression with obesity. [116] as well as protein secretion from isolated adipocytes. [141] These recent observations are concomitant with initial studies that showed increased serum resistin levels [142] and gene expression levels in abdominal depots [115, 143] in states of increased adiposity. Additional studies have shown significant reductions in circulating resistin levels following moderate weight loss [144] and post-gastric bypass. [138] Collectively, these observations suggest that resistin could be subjected to nutritional regulation in humans.

Contrary to the studies suggesting a role for resistin in obesity, Maebuchi et al. [145] reported that resistin was undetectable in the serum of obese mice, and in the same study, they observed reductions in resistin mRNA and protein expression with obesity. Other investigators have also reported no association of resistin expression with increased adiposity, despite observing elevated circulating levels.[133–135] It has been suggested that resistin mRNA expression may not necessarily correlate with protein expression. [134] Possible explanations for such diverse observations include variability in post-transcriptional and post-translational modifications that influence secretory rates of resistin.

Increased serum levels may enhance transcript degradation rates via negative feedback mechanisms, or the initiation and recruitment of inhibitors of translation. The secreted form of resistin is considered to have paracrine properties, and this may imply that the majority of regulation occurs at the protein level. Similarly, Rajala and co-workers [134] have suggested that binding of serum cofactors to the resistin protein may prolong its half-life, thereby reducing clearance; this hypothesis is supported by studies showing that protein interactions and tertiary alterations can influence adipocytokines, such as leptin and TNF-alpha. [146–148] Indeed, these studies demonstrate the limitations of attempting to derive all necessary information regarding resistin and obesity from gene expression studies. Further recent human studies have shown no correlation of serum [149] or plasma levels of resistin with any markers of adiposity. [150] Heilbronn et al. [151] reported no relationship between resistin serum levels and percentage body fat, visceral adiposity and BMI. However, the authors suggested that the lack of correlation of serum resistin and increased adiposity was partly due to the confounding variable of age, as non-obese subjects were significantly younger than obese subjects. [151] Another study showed similar levels of resistin expressed in gluteal femoral and subcutaneous abdominal depots in non-diabetic subjects. [152] However, no indication of the number of 'gluteal' subjects compared with 'abdominal' subjects was given. Moreover, the study used a high proportion of male subjects and, as previous studies had shown resistin to exhibit sexual dimorphism,with women having approx. 20% higher levels than men [140, 149, 150], this may explain these findings. Although a high degree of discrepancy has emerged from publications regarding the association of resistin with obesity in the context of mRNA and serum levels, it is worth highlighting the importance of developing highly accurate methods of determining serum resistin concentrations. Methodological limitations may result in variations among serum concentrations, mRNA and protein levels, or may simply indicate that resistin does not play a significant role in the pathophysiology of obesity mediated insulin resistance. However, with reference to the use of commercially available ELISAs, both rodent and human ELISAs have potential to cross-react with circulating RELMs. To date, not all studies using resistin ELISAs have assessed RELM cross-reactivity prior to analysis; therefore it may be that different ELISAs used may provide varying serum concentrations. [153–155] Similarly, assessment of serum resistin in rodents has proved contentious. [133, 134] Furthermore, due to recent advances in the understanding of the tertiary and quaternary structure of resistin [124], further studies are required to establish whether the complex distribution of the individual structural forms of resistin affect the validity of the currently available human and rodent assays.

4.4. Newly Emergent Adipokines

4.4.1. Acute phase protein

More than 20 prospective epidemiologic studies demonstrate that high-sensitivity CRP is an independent predictor of risk of myocardial infarction, stroke, peripheral arterial disease, and sudden cardiac death, even in apparently healthy individuals. [156] Esposito et al. [157], investigated effects of weight loss and lifestyle changes on vascular inflammatory markers in obese women. After two years, body mass index decreased more in the intervention group than in control subjects, as did serum concentrations of IL-6, IL-18, and CRP, whereas adiponectin levels increased significantly. Beneficial effects of a Mediterranean-style diet on endothelial function and vascular inflammatory markers were documented in patients with the metabolic syndrome. Compared with patients consuming the control diet, patients consuming a Mediterranean-style diet had significantly reduced serum concentrations of high-sensitivity CRP, IL-6, IL-7, and IL-18 as well as decreased insulin resistance. [158] In addition, two recent studies demonstrate that exercise training with weight reduction lowers CRP levels significantly. [159, 160] After supervised aerobic exercises, both weight and CRP levels were decreased; however, changes in CRP levels were not proportionally associated with the extent of weight reduction. In quartile analysis of percent weight reduction, the largest weight reduction quartile did not show significant decreases in CRP levels, whereas the middle quartiles showed remarkable CRP decreases. Considering inflammatory status, there might be an optimal pace of exercise combined with weight loss. [160] In another study, CRP levels decreased significantly with training, although none of the CRP variants were associated with training-induced CRP changes. C-reactive protein $+219G/A$ and $-732A/G$ genotypes and haplotypes and exercise training appear to modulate CRP levels; however, training-induced CRP reductions are independent of genotype at these loci. [159]

Ouchi et al. demonstrated CRP mRNA expression in human adipose tissue by using the quantitative real-time polymerase chain reaction method. [161] In the same article, the authors proposed that adipose tissue is an important source of circulating CRP. However, they made no attempt to investigate the stimuli able to induce CRP. [161] Accordingly, we have recently investigated whether CRP is produced by cells in adipose tissue in response to inflammatory stimuli in culture and we have demonstrated that human adipocytes, but not preadipocytes, cultured in vitro produced CRP following exposure to inflammatory cytokines such as IL-1beta, IL-6, TNF-alpha, LPS, and resistin. Moreover, the response to the different molecules was additive, peaking in adipocytes incubated with all the stimuli. Interestingly, resistin, the most recently identified adipocytokine that is proposed as an inflammatory marker for atherosclerosis, also induced an increase in CRP production by adipocytes. [27]

These data confirm that the adipocyte, largely thought to be an inert storage cell whose main function was to store excess energy in the form of triglycerides, has a more complex role in the organism, thus suggesting a new link between obesity, adipose tissue and vascular inflammation.

Furthermore, using the same *in vitro* model, we have recently demonstrated the production of serum amyloid A (SAA), another acute phase protein, by mature adipocytes isolated from human adipose tissue. [30] Elevated levels of SAA have been found in subjects at risk for developing future coronary heart disease, as well as in patients with coronary and peripheral vascular disease. [162–165]

PAI-1 is an inhibitor of plasminogen activators and fibrinolytic activity that is thought to be synthesized mainly in endothelial cells and the liver. Random sequence analysis demonstrated that adipose tissue expressed the PAI-1 gene, and mRNA expression was markedly enhanced, especially in visceral adipose tissue, during the development of obesity. [166] Plasma levels of PAI-1 are positively correlated with the amount of visceral fat determined by computer tomography (CT) scan in human subjects. It is well known that plasma levels of PAI-1 are elevated in subjects with type 2 diabetes and hypertriglyceridaemia, although the precise mechanism is unclear. Type 2 diabetes and hypertriglyceridaemia are often associated with visceral fat accumulation, so PAI-1 produced by accumulated visceral fat may explain the high plasma concentration of PAI-1 in these conditions. It is not yet known why adipocytes secrete a large amount of PAI-1. Adipocytes change their cell size dramatically in response to nutritional conditions. Plasmin may work to destroy the basement membrane to facilitate cell expansion, and PAI-1 may control the activity of plasminogen activators to prevent the overproduction of plasmin.

4.4.2.   Other adipokines

The number and range of adipocyte secretory proteins is continuing to expand rapidly. In the year 2005 alone, three major new adipokines were reported: apelin, visfatin and zinc-a2-glycoprotein (ZAG), production of each of which was originally described in other tissues. Apelin was first identified as the endogenous ligand of the orphan G protein-coupled receptor, APJ [167], and has now been found to be secreted from adipocytes. [168] It is synthesized as a 77 amino acid preproprotein, which is cleaved to a 55 amino acid product and then to further products, the biologically active form apparently being apelin-36. [167] Apelin expression and circulating levels are increased in hyperinsulinemia associated obesities, including in humans, and in cell culture its expression rises after adipocyte differentiation. Production of apelin is stimulated by insulin and it is suggested that this factor is a potential link with obesity-related changes in insulin sensitivity. [168]

A 'new' adipocytokine was isolated by Fukuhara et al in 2004. [169] This adipocytokine, named 'visfatin', was found to be highly enriched in the visceral adipose tissue of both humans and rodents. Visfatin was found to be identical to the previously known pre-B cell colony enhancing factor, a cytokine expressed by lymphocytes. Visfatin has a molecular weight of 52 kDa. The coding region of the gene encodes for 491 amino acids. When given to mice, visfatin lowers blood glucose, [169] resembling the effects of insulin. In vitro, it mimics insulin action as evidenced by phosphorylation of the insulin receptor, insulin receptor substrates (IRS-1 and IRS-2), and the binding of Leptin, resistin and adiponectin 537 phosphatidyl-inositol-3-kinase to IRS-1 and IRS-2. In 3T3-F442A adipocytes, visfatin leads to phosphorylation and activation of Akt and MAP kinases. Apparently, visfatin is able to directly interact with the insulin receptor, although the exact mechanisms of this interaction are not yet known. The binding equilibrium dissociation constant of visfatin to the insulin receptor in human embryonic kidney -293 cells (4.4 nM) is similar to that of insulin (6.1 nM). In contrast, visfatin does not bind to the insulin-like growth factor-1 receptor. Taking all the available data together, it seems that visfatin activates the insulin receptor signaling cascade but in a manner distinct from insulin. [169] Such an action is not only surprising in itself, but also in relation to the augmented expression in visceral adipose tissue given the particular association between this fat depot and the metabolic syndrome.

Zinc-alpha-2-glycoprotein, the third novel adipokine, is a 43 000 mol. wt glycoprotein which is synthesized by certain malignant tumors and which has been used as a marker for cancer. The protein stimulates lipid loss in cachexia, and this occurs through the activation of lipolysis [170, 171] via b3-adrenoceptors. [172] ZAG has recently been shown to be directly synthesized by white (and brown) adipocytes, there being a powerful upregulation at both the gene expression and protein levels in mice bearing the MAC16 tumor (a model for cachexia). [173] ZAG mRNA was increased 10-fold in the WAT of tumor bearing mice, while the level of leptin mRNA was reduced some 30-fold. [173] In studies using human SGBS (Simpson–Golabi–Behmel syndrome) adipocytes, ZAG has now been shown to be released from fat cells, indicating that it is an adipokine. [174] Expression of ZAG in human adipocytes is stimulated by the PPAR-gamma agonist rosiglitazone and suppressed by TNF-alpha and this is similar to adiponectin. [174] It has been proposed that ZAG may play a local role in modulating lipolysis in WAT, the selective increase in tumor bearing animals being responsible, at least in part, for fat depletion in cancer cachexia. [173] Intriguingly, overexpression of ZAG is also reported to lead to an increase in adiponectin mRNA level in 3T3-L1 adipocytes, consistent with a linkage between these two adipokines. [175]

Further study of this natural insulinmimetic should help to determine its role in maintaining normal glucose homeostasis in humans. This in itself may boost diabetes research and possibly offer new therapeutic options for people with diabetes. [176]

5. FUTURE DIRECTIONS

Obesity appears to be associated with a low-grade state of inflammation, probably as a consequence of the secretion of proinflammatory cytokines by adipocytes. These cytokines may underlie many of the components of the insulin resistance syndrome, as well as endothelial dysfunction and, potentially, cardiovascular risk.

From the wide range of protein signals and factors here discussed, it is evident that WAT is a secretory organ of considerable complexity which is highly integrated into the general homeostatic mechanisms of mammals. [40, 118, 177, 178] A corollary to the diversity of the adipokines is that WAT communicates extensively with other organs and is involved in multiple metabolic systems. Co-culture studies, for example, have indicated that adipocytes directly signal to other tissues, such as the adrenal cortex and skeletal muscle [179, 180], and there is a critical conversation between white adipocytes and the brain through leptin and the sympathetic system. [181] Extensive crosstalk between preadipocytes and adipocytes is likely, and between these cells and macrophages as part of the inflammatory response. The emergence of the adipocyte as a key endocrine and secretory cell has been a major development, not only in the sphere of energy balance and obesity, but more generally – with growing impact in areas such as inflammation and aging. The adipocyte is not, however, alone in its unexpected range of secreted factors; cells such as chondrocytes also release a wide range of protein signals, including many again linked to inflammation. [182] Even skeletal muscle is now recognized to release large quantities of IL-6 on exercise, raising the possibility that there may be a family of 'myokines', [183, 184] paralleling the recent evolution of the adipokines.

A question of great importance is: how can we avoid or reverse the deleterious effects of obesity? We know about diet and exercise, and that both leptin and adiponectin act through at least one common pathway, i.e., AMPK, as does exercise. In recent years, new and interesting pharmacotherapuetic findings have emerged. Members of the antidiabetic class of drugs, the thiazolidinediones (TZDs, e.g., rosiglitazone), activate peroxisome proliferator-activated receptor gamma (PPAR-gamma), a nuclear transcription factor that in turn activates many genes that are highly expressed in adipose tissue. [185] PPAR-gamma, once activated, reduces plasma FFA and glucose concentrations and improves insulin sensitivity, producing beneficial effects for persons with diabetes. In ob/ob mice, the TZDs inhibit leptin gene expression. [186] TZDs have also been shown to increase adiponectin, and decrease IL-6 and TNF-alpha. [187] Rosiglitazone treatment also has positive effects on markers of cardiovascular disease both in vitro and in patients with type 2 diabetes mellitus. [27, 188, 189] As we have discussed, all these effects are beneficial. Remarkably, the TZDs, have been shown to activate AMPK, similar to the effects of exercise, leptin, and adiponectin, [190] Metformin, another drug commonly used to treat diabetic patients also activates AMPK, although unlike the TZDs, it does not increase adiponectin concentrations. [191] Obviously, none of the available drugs provide a cure for diabetes and certainly not obesity. Further therapeutic options are needed, including pharmacotherapy, nutrients, and diets that enhance insulin action and regulate appetite. A combination of therapeutic agents may prove to be most efficacious.

In conclusion, it is now apparent that adipocytes are not simply a storage reservoir of fat but are active endocrine organs that play multiple roles in the body. Their metabolic role changes as they enlarge with increasing obesity. This increased understanding of the role of the adipocyte and its associated adipokines, such as leptin and adiponectin, is allowing us to dissect the all-too prevalent metabolic syndrome and perhaps affect its course for the better. We are also beginning to understand the interplay of inflammation and obesity, although our knowledge remains incomplete. Finally, the intracellular mechanisms by which these factors affect energy intake, utilization, and metabolism are being better understood, and we are developing therapies that manipulate these pathways.

REFERENCES

1. Eckel RH, Krauss RM. American Heart Association call to action: obesity as a major risk factor for coronary heart disease. AHA Nutrition Committee. Circulation 1998; 97:2099–2100.
2. Grundy SM. Obesity, metabolic syndrome, and coronary atherosclerosis. Circulation 2002; 105:2696–2698.
3. Sowers JR. Obesity as a cardiovascular risk factor. Am J Med 2003; 115 Suppl 8A:37S–41S.
4. Sharma AM. Adipose tissue: a mediator of cardiovascular risk. Int J Obes Relat Metab Disord 2002; 26 Suppl 4:S5–7.
5. Engeli S, Sharma AM. Role of adipose tissue for cardiovascular-renal regulation in health and disease. Horm Metab Res 2000; 32:485–499.
6. Guerre-Millo M. Adipose tissue and adipokines: for better or worse. Diabetes Metab 2004; 30:13–19.
7. Poirier P, Eckel RH. Obesity and cardiovascular disease. Curr Atheroscler Rep 2002; 4:448–453.
8. Peelman F, Waelput W, Iserentant H, Lavens D, Eyckerman S, Zabeau L, Tavernier J. Leptin: linking adipocyte metabolism with cardiovascular and autoimmune diseases. Prog Lipid Res 2004; 43:283–301.
9. Ouchi N, Kihara S, Arita Y, Maeda K, Kuriyama H, Okamoto Y, Hotta K, Nishida M, Takahashi M, Nakamura T, Yamashita S, Funahashi T, Matsuzawa Y. Novel modulator for endothelial adhesion molecules: adipocyte-derived plasma protein adiponectin. Circulation 1999; 100:2473–2476.
10. Shuldiner AR, Yang R, Gong DW. Resistin, obesity and insulin resistance–the emerging role of the adipocyte as an endocrine organ. N Engl J Med 2001; 345:1345–1346.
11. Bullo-Bonet M, Garcia-Lorda P, Lopez-Soriano FJ, Argiles JM, Salas-Salvado J. Tumour necrosis factor, a key role in obesity? FEBS Lett 1999; 451:215–219.
12. Yudkin JS, Kumari M, Humphries SE, Mohamed-Ali V. Inflammation, obesity, stress and coronary heart disease: is interleukin-6 the link? Atherosclerosis 2000; 148:209–214.
13. Cinti S. The adipose organ: morphological perspectives of adipose tissues. Proc Nutr Soc 2001; 60:319–328.
14. Cannon B, Nedergaard J. Brown adipose tissue: function and physiological significance. Physiol Rev 2004; 84:277–359.
15. Rennie KL, Jebb SA. Prevalence of obesity in Great Britain. Obes Rev 2005; 6:11–12.
16. Prentice AM, Jebb SA. Obesity in Britain: gluttony or sloth? Bmj 1995; 311:437–439.
17. Gavrilova O, Marcus-Samuels B, Graham D, Kim JK, Shulman GI, Castle AL, Vinson C, Eckhaus M, Reitman ML. Surgical implantation of adipose tissue reverses diabetes in lipoatrophic mice. J Clin Invest 2000; 105:271–278.
18. Shimomura I, Hammer RE, Ikemoto S, Brown MS, Goldstein JL. Leptin reverses insulin resistance and diabetes mellitus in mice with congenital lipodystrophy. Nature 1999; 401:73–76.
19. Engstrom G, Stavenow L, Hedblad B, Lind P, Eriksson KF, Janzon L, Lindgarde F. Inflammation-sensitive plasma proteins, diabetes, and mortality and incidence of myocardial infarction and stroke: a population-based study. Diabetes 2003; 52:442–447.
20. Festa A, D'Agostino R Jr, Williams K, Karter AJ, Mayer-Davis EJ, Tracy RP, Haffner SM. The relation of body fat mass and distribution to markers of chronic inflammation. Int J Obes Relat Metab Disord 2001; 25:1407–1415.

21. Yudkin JS, Stehouwer CD, Emeis JJ, Coppack SW. C-reactive protein in healthy subjects: associations with obesity, insulin resistance, and endothelial dysfunction: a potential role for cytokines originating from adipose tissue? Arterioscler Thromb Vasc Biol 1999; 19:972–978.
22. Bullo M, Garcia-Lorda P, Megias I, Salas-Salvado J. Systemic inflammation, adipose tissue tumor necrosis factor, and leptin expression. Obes Res 2003; 11:525–531.
23. Das UN. Is obesity an inflammatory condition? Nutrition 2001; 17:953–966.
24. Hotamisligil GS. Inflammatory pathways and insulin action. Int J Obes Relat Metab Disord 2003; 27 Suppl 3:S53–55.
25. Yudkin JS. Adipose tissue, insulin action and vascular disease: inflammatory signals. Int J Obes Relat Metab Disord 2003; 27 Suppl 3:S25–28.
26. Calabro P, Willerson JT, Yeh ET. Inflammatory cytokines stimulated C-reactive protein production by human coronary artery smooth muscle cells. Circulation 2003; 108:1930–1932.
27. Calabro P, Chang DW, Willerson JT, Yeh ET. Release of C-reactive protein in response to inflammatory cytokines by human adipocytes: linking obesity to vascular inflammation. J Am Coll Cardiol 2005; 46:1112–1113.
28. Weisberg SP, McCann D, Desai M, Rosenbaum M, Leibel RL, Ferrante AW Jr. Obesity is associated with macrophage accumulation in adipose tissue. J Clin Invest 2003; 112:1796–1808.
29. Xu H, Barnes GT, Yang Q, Tan G, Yang D, Chou CJ, Sole J, Nichols A, Ross JS, Tartaglia LA, Chen H. Chronic inflammation in fat plays a crucial role in the development of obesity-related insulin resistance. J Clin Invest 2003; 112:1821–1830.
30. Calabro P, Chang DW, Willerson JT, Yeh ET. Production of C-reactive protein and serum amyloid A in response to inflammatory cytokines by human adipocytes. Eur H Journal 2005; 26:334–335.
31. Cousin B, Munoz O, Andre M, Fontanilles AM, Dani C, Cousin JL, Laharrague P, Casteilla L, Penicaud L. A role for preadipocytes as macrophage-like cells. Faseb J 1999; 13:305–312.
32. Arita Y, Kihara S, Ouchi N, Takahashi M, Maeda K, Miyagawa J, Hotta K, Shimomura I, Nakamura T, Miyaoka K, Kuriyama H, Nishida M, Yamashita S, Okubo K, Matsubara K, Muraguchi M, Ohmoto Y, Funahashi T, Matsuzawa Y. Paradoxical decrease of an adipose-specific protein, adiponectin, in obesity. Biochem Biophys Res Commun 1999; 257:79–83.
33. Hotta K, Funahashi T, Arita Y, Takahashi M, Matsuda M, Okamoto Y, Iwahashi H, Kuriyama H, Ouchi N, Maeda K, Nishida M, Kihara S, Sakai N, Nakajima T, Hasegawa K, Muraguchi M, Ohmoto Y, Nakamura T, Yamashita S, Hanafusa T, Matsuzawa Y. Plasma concentrations of a novel, adipose-specific protein, adiponectin, in type 2 diabetic patients. Arterioscler Thromb Vasc Biol 2000; 20:1595–1599.
34. Ouchi N, Kihara S, Arita Y, Okamoto Y, Maeda K, Kuriyama H, Hotta K, Nishida M, Takahashi M, Muraguchi M, Ohmoto Y, Nakamura T, Yamashita S, Funahashi T, Matsuzawa Y. Adiponectin, an adipocyte-derived plasma protein, inhibits endothelial NF-kappaB signaling through a cAMP-dependent pathway. Circulation 2000; 102:1296–1301.
35. Gerhardt CC, Romero IA, Cancello R, Camoin L, Strosberg AD. Chemokines control fat accumulation and leptin secretion by cultured human adipocytes. Mol Cell Endocrinol 2001; 175:81–92.
36. Hirokawa J, Sakaue S, Tagami S, Kawakami Y, Sakai M, Nishi S, Nishihira J. Identification of macrophage migration inhibitory factor in adipose tissue and its induction by tumor necrosis factor-alpha. Biochem Biophys Res Commun 1997; 235:94–98.
37. Sartipy P, Loskutoff DJ. Monocyte chemoattractant protein 1 in obesity and insulin resistance. Proc Natl Acad Sci USA 2003; 100:7265–7270.
38. Skurk T, Herder C, Kraft I, Muller-Scholze S, Hauner H, Kolb H. Production and release of macrophage migration inhibitory factor from human adipocytes. Endocrinology 2005; 146:1006–1011.
39. Wang B, Jenkins JR, Trayhurn P. Expression and secretion of inflammation-related adipokines by human adipocytes differentiated in culture: integrated response to TNF-alpha. Am J Physiol Endocrinol Metab 2005; 288:E731–740.
40. Trayhurn P, Wood IS. Adipokines: inflammation and the pleiotropic role of white adipose tissue. Br J Nutr 2004; 92:347–355.

41. Karpe F, Fielding BA, Ilic V, Macdonald IA, Summers LK, Frayn KN. Impaired postprandial adipose tissue blood flow response is related to aspects of insulin sensitivity. Diabetes 2002; 51:2467–2473.

42. Hopfl G, Ogunshola O, Gassmann M. HIFs and tumors–causes and consequences. Am J Physiol Regul Integr Comp Physiol 2004; 286:R608–623.

43. Semenza GL. HIF-1 and mechanisms of hypoxia sensing. Curr Opin Cell Biol 2001; 13:167–171.

44. Wenger RH. Cellular adaptation to hypoxia: O2-sensing protein hydroxylases, hypoxia-inducible transcription factors, and O2-regulated gene expression. Faseb J 2002; 16:1151–1162.

45. Lolmede K, Durand de Saint Front V, Galitzky J, Lafontan M, Bouloumie A. Effects of hypoxia on the expression of proangiogenic factors in differentiated 3T3-F442A adipocytes. Int J Obes Relat Metab Disord 2003; 27:1187–1195.

46. Ahima RS, Flier JS. Adipose tissue as an endocrine organ. Trends Endocrinol Metab 2000; 11:327–332.

47. Samad F, Loskutoff DJ. Tissue distribution and regulation of plasminogen activator inhibitor-1 in obese mice. Mol Med 1996; 2:568–582.

48. Samad F, Yamamoto K, Pandey M, Loskutoff DJ. Elevated expression of transforming growth factor-beta in adipose tissue from obese mice. Mol Med 1997; 3:37–48.

49. Zhang B, Graziano MP, Doebber TW, Leibowitz MD, White-Carrington S, Szalkowski DM, Hey PJ, Wu M, Cullinan CA, Bailey P, Lollmann B, Frederich R, Flier JS, Strader CD, Smith RG. Down-regulation of the expression of the obese gene by an antidiabetic thiazolidinedione in Zucker diabetic fatty rats and db/db mice. J Biol Chem 1996; 271:9455–9459.

50. Eriksson P, Van Harmelen V, Hoffstedt J, Lundquist P, Vidal H, Stemme V, Hamsten A, Arner P, Reynisdottir S. Regional variation in plasminogen activator inhibitor-1 expression in adipose tissue from obese individuals. Thromb Haemost 2000; 83:545–548.

51. Fried SK, Bunkin DA, Greenberg AS. Omental and subcutaneous adipose tissues of obese subjects release interleukin-6: depot difference and regulation by glucocorticoid. J Clin Endocrinol Metab 1998; 83:847–850.

52. Giacchetti G, Faloia E, Mariniello B, Sardu C, Gatti C, Camilloni MA, Guerrieri M, Mantero F. Overexpression of the renin-angiotensin system in human visceral adipose tissue in normal and overweight subjects. Am J Hypertens 2002; 15:381–388.

53. Dandona P, Weinstock R, Thusu K, Abdel-Rahman E, Aljada A, Wadden T. Tumor necrosis factor-alpha in sera of obese patients: fall with weight loss. J Clin Endocrinol Metab 1998; 83:2907–2910.

54. Itoh K, Imai K, Masuda T, Abe S, Tanaka M, Koga R, Itoh H, Matsuyama T, Nakamura M. Relationship between changes in serum leptin levels and blood pressure after weight loss. Hypertens Res 2002; 25:881–886.

55. Ziccardi P, Nappo F, Giugliano G, Esposito K, Marfella R, Cioffi M, D'Andrea F, Molinari AM, Giugliano D. Reduction of inflammatory cytokine concentrations and improvement of endothelial functions in obese women after weight loss over one year. Circulation 2002; 105:804–809.

56. De Pergola G, Pannacciulli N. Coagulation and fibrinolysis abnormalities in obesity. J Endocrinol Invest 2002; 25:899–904.

57. Hotamisligil GS, Shargill NS, Spiegelman BM. Adipose expression of tumor necrosis factor-alpha: direct role in obesity-linked insulin resistance. Science 1993; 259:87–91.

58. Perreault M, Marette A. Targeted disruption of inducible nitric oxide synthase protects against obesity-linked insulin resistance in muscle. Nat Med 2001; 7:1138–1143.

59. Samad F, Pandey M, Loskutoff DJ. Tissue factor gene expression in the adipose tissues of obese mice. Proc Natl Acad Sci USA 1998; 95:7591–7596.

60. Vgontzas AN, Papanicolaou DA, Bixler EO, Kales A, Tyson K, Chrousos GP. Elevation of plasma cytokines in disorders of excessive daytime sleepiness: role of sleep disturbance and obesity. J Clin Endocrinol Metab 1997; 82:1313–1316.

61. Visser M, Bouter LM, McQuillan GM, Wener MH, Harris TB. Elevated C-reactive protein levels in overweight and obese adults. Jama 1999; 282:2131–2135.

62. Weyer C, Yudkin JS, Stehouwer CD, Schalkwijk CG, Pratley RE, Tataranni PA. Humoral markers of inflammation and endothelial dysfunction in relation to adiposity and in vivo insulin action in Pima Indians. Atherosclerosis 2002; 161:233–242.

63. Cinti S, Mitchell G, Barbatelli G, Murano I, Ceresi E, Faloia E, Wang S, Fortier M, Greenberg AS, Obin MS. Adipocyte death defines macrophage localization and function in adipose tissue of obese mice and humans. J Lipid Res 2005; 46:2347–2355.

64. Hotamisligil GS, Spiegelman BM. Tumor necrosis factor alpha: a key component of the obesity-diabetes link. Diabetes 1994; 43:1271–1278.

65. Kern PA, Ranganathan S, Li C, Wood L, Ranganathan G. Adipose tissue tumor necrosis factor and interleukin-6 expression in human obesity and insulin resistance. Am J Physiol Endocrinol Metab 2001; 280:E745–751.

66. Mohamed-Ali V, Goodrick S, Rawesh A, Katz DR, Miles JM, Yudkin JS, Klein S, Coppack SW. Subcutaneous adipose tissue releases interleukin-6, but not tumor necrosis factor-alpha, in vivo. J Clin Endocrinol Metab 1997; 82:4196–4200.

67. van Hall G, Steensberg A, Sacchetti M, Fischer C, Keller C, Schjerling P, Hiscock N, Moller K, Saltin B, Febbraio MA, Pedersen BK. Interleukin-6 stimulates lipolysis and fat oxidation in humans. J Clin Endocrinol Metab 2003; 88:3005–3010.

68. Klover PJ, Zimmers TA, Koniaris LG, Mooney RA. Chronic exposure to interleukin-6 causes hepatic insulin resistance in mice. Diabetes 2003; 52:2784–2789.

69. Pradhan AD, Manson JE, Rifai N, Buring JE, Ridker PM. C-reactive protein, interleukin 6, and risk of developing type 2 diabetes mellitus. Jama 2001; 286:327–334.

70. Ridker PM, Rifai N, Stampfer MJ, Hennekens CH. Plasma concentration of interleukin-6 and the risk of future myocardial infarction among apparently healthy men. Circulation 2000; 101:1767–1772.

71. Fruebis J, Tsao TS, Javorschi S, Ebbets-Reed D, Erickson MR, Yen FT, Bihain BE, Lodish HF. Proteolytic cleavage product of 30-kDa adipocyte complement-related protein increases fatty acid oxidation in muscle and causes weight loss in mice. Proc Natl Acad Sci USA 2001; 98:2005–2010.

72. Scherer PE, Williams S, Fogliano M, Baldini G, Lodish HF. A novel serum protein similar to C1q, produced exclusively in adipocytes. J Biol Chem 1995; 270:26746–26749.

73. Yamauchi T, Kamon J, Waki H, Terauchi Y, Kubota N, Hara K, Mori Y, Ide T, Murakami K, Tsuboyama-Kasaoka N, Ezaki O, Akanuma Y, Gavrilova O, Vinson C, Reitman ML, Kagechika H, Shudo K, Yoda M, Nakano Y, Tobe K, Nagai R, Kimura S, Tomita M, Froguel P, Kadowaki T. The fat-derived hormone adiponectin reverses insulin resistance associated with both lipoatrophy and obesity. Nat Med 2001; 7:941–946.

74. Kumada M, Kihara S, Sumitsuji S, Kawamoto T, Matsumoto S, Ouchi N, Arita Y, Okamoto Y, Shimomura I, Hiraoka H, Nakamura T, Funahashi T, Matsuzawa Y. Association of hypoad-iponectinemia with coronary artery disease in men. Arterioscler Thromb Vasc Biol 2003; 23:85–89.

75. Pischon T, Girman CJ, Hotamisligil GS, Rifai N, Hu FB, Rimm EB. Plasma adiponectin levels and risk of myocardial infarction in men. Jama 2004; 291:1730–1737.

76. Hotta K, Funahashi T, Bodkin NL, Ortmeyer HK, Arita Y, Hansen BC, Matsuzawa Y. Circulating concentrations of the adipocyte protein adiponectin are decreased in parallel with reduced insulin sensitivity during the progression to type 2 diabetes in rhesus monkeys. Diabetes 2001; 50:1126–1133.

77. Hara K, Boutin P, Mori Y, Tobe K, Dina C, Yasuda K, Yamauchi T, Otabe S, Okada T, Eto K, Kadowaki H, Hagura R, Akanuma Y, Yazaki Y, Nagai R, Taniyama M, Matsubara K, Yoda M, Nakano Y, Tomita M, Kimura S, Ito C, Froguel P, Kadowaki T. Genetic variation in the gene encoding adiponectin is associated with an increased risk of type 2 diabetes in the Japanese population. Diabetes 2002; 51:536–540.

78. Kondo H, Shimomura I, Matsukawa Y, Kumada M, Takahashi M, Matsuda M, Ouchi N, Kihara S, Kawamoto T, Sumitsuji S, Funahashi T, Matsuzawa Y. Association of adiponectin mutation with type 2 diabetes: a candidate gene for the insulin resistance syndrome. Diabetes 2002; 51:2325–2328.

79. Takahashi M, Arita Y, Yamagata K, Matsukawa Y, Okutomi K, Horie M, Shimomura I, Hotta K, Kuriyama H, Kihara S, Nakamura T, Yamashita S, Funahashi T, Matsuzawa Y. Genomic structure and mutations in adipose-specific gene, adiponectin. Int J Obes Relat Metab Disord 2000; 24:861–868.

80. Kissebah AH, Sonnenberg GE, Myklebust J, Goldstein M, Broman K, James RG, Marks JA, Krakower GR, Jacob HJ, Weber J, Martin L, Blangero J, Comuzzie AG. Quantitative trait loci on chromosomes 3 and 17 influence phenotypes of the metabolic syndrome. Proc Natl Acad Sci USA 2000; 97:14478–14483.

81. Lindsay RS, Funahashi T, Hanson RL, Matsuzawa Y, Tanaka S, Tataranni PA, Knowler WC, Krakoff J. Adiponectin and development of type 2 diabetes in the Pima Indian population. Lancet 2002; 360:57–58.

82. Adamczak M, Wiecek A, Funahashi T, Chudek J, Kokot F, Matsuzawa Y. Decreased plasma adiponectin concentration in patients with essential hypertension. Am J Hypertens 2003; 16:72–75.

83. Zoccali C, Mallamaci F, Tripepi G, Benedetto FA, Cutrupi S, Parlongo S, Malatino LS, Bonanno G, Seminara G, Rapisarda F, Fatuzzo P, Buemi M, Nicocia G, Tanaka S, Ouchi N, Kihara S, Funahashi T, Matsuzawa Y. Adiponectin, metabolic risk factors, and cardiovascular events among patients with end-stage renal disease. J Am Soc Nephrol 2002; 13:134–141.

84. Okamoto Y, Kihara S, Ouchi N, Nishida M, Arita Y, Kumada M, Ohashi K, Sakai N, Shimomura I, Kobayashi H, Terasaka N, Inaba T, Funahashi T, Matsuzawa Y. Adiponectin reduces atherosclerosis in apolipoprotein E-deficient mice. Circulation 2002; 106:2767–2770.

85. Ouchi N, Kihara S, Arita Y, Nishida M, Matsuyama A, Okamoto Y, Ishigami M, Kuriyama H, Kishida K, Nishizawa H, Hotta K, Muraguchi M, Ohmoto Y, Yamashita S, Funahashi T, Matsuzawa Y. Adipocyte-derived plasma protein, adiponectin, suppresses lipid accumulation and class A scavenger receptor expression in human monocyte-derived macrophages. Circulation 2001; 103:1057–1063.

86. Kumada M, Kihara S, Ouchi N, Kobayashi H, Okamoto Y, Ohashi K, Maeda K, Nagaretani H, Kishida K, Maeda N, Nagasawa A, Funahashi T, Matsuzawa Y. Adiponectin specifically increased tissue inhibitor of metalloproteinase-1 through interleukin-10 expression in human macrophages. Circulation 2004; 109:2046–2049.

87. Chen H, Montagnani M, Funahashi T, Shimomura I, Quon MJ. Adiponectin stimulates production of nitric oxide in vascular endothelial cells. J Biol Chem 2003; 278:45021–45026.

88. Kawanami D, Maemura K, Takeda N, Harada T, Nojiri T, Imai Y, Manabe I, Utsunomiya K, Nagai R. Direct reciprocal effects of resistin and adiponectin on vascular endothelial cells: a new insight into adipocytokine-endothelial cell interactions. Biochem Biophys Res Commun 2004; 314:415–419.

89. Fasshauer M, Kralisch S, Klier M, Lossner U, Bluher M, Klein J, Paschke R. Adiponectin gene expression and secretion is inhibited by interleukin-6 in 3T3-L1 adipocytes. Biochem Biophys Res Commun 2003; 301:1045–1050.

90. Ouchi N, Kobayashi H, Kihara S, Kumada M, Sato K, Inoue T, Funahashi T, Walsh K. Adiponectin stimulates angiogenesis by promoting cross-talk between AMP-activated protein kinase and Akt signaling in endothelial cells. J Biol Chem 2004; 279:1304–1309.

91. Brekke HK, Lenner RA, Taskinen MR, Mansson JE, Funahashi T, Matsuzawa Y, Jansson PA. Lifestyle modification improves risk factors in type 2 diabetes relatives. Diabetes Res Clin Pract 2005; 68:18–28.

92. Furuhashi M, Ura N, Higashiura K, Murakami H, Tanaka M, Moniwa N, Yoshida D, Shimamoto K. Blockade of the renin-angiotensin system increases adiponectin concentrations in patients with essential hypertension. Hypertension 2003; 42:76–81.

93. Koh KK, Quon MJ, Han SH, Chung WJ, Ahn JY, Seo YH, Kang MH, Ahn TH, Choi IS, Shin EK. Additive beneficial effects of losartan combined with simvastatin in the treatment of hypercholesterolemic, hypertensive patients. Circulation 2004; 110:3687–3692.

94. Nielsen S, Lihn AS, Ostergaard T, Mogensen CE, Schmitz O. Increased plasma adiponectin in losartan-treated type 1 diabetic patients. a mediator of improved insulin sensitivity? Horm Metab Res 2004; 36:194–196.

95. Koh KK, Han SH, Quon MJ, Yeal Ahn J, Shin EK. Beneficial effects of fenofibrate to improve endothelial dysfunction and raise adiponectin levels in patients with primary hypertriglyceridemia. Diabetes Care 2005; 28:1419–1424.

96. Maeda N, Takahashi M, Funahashi T, Kihara S, Nishizawa H, Kishida K, Nagaretani H, Matsuda M, Komuro R, Ouchi N, Kuriyama H, Hotta K, Nakamura T, Shimomura I, Matsuzawa Y. PPARgamma ligands increase expression and plasma concentrations of adiponectin, an adipose-derived protein. Diabetes 2001; 50:2094–2099.

97. Halaas JL, Gajiwala KS, Maffei M, Cohen SL, Chait BT, Rabinowitz D, Lallone RL, Burley SK, Friedman JM. Weight-reducing effects of the plasma protein encoded by the obese gene. Science 1995; 269:543–546.

98. Lee GH, Proenca R, Montez JM, Carroll KM, Darvishzadeh JG, Lee JI, Friedman JM. Abnormal splicing of the leptin receptor in diabetic mice. Nature 1996; 379:632–635.

99. Maffei M, Halaas J, Ravussin E, Pratley RE, Lee GH, Zhang Y, Fei H, Kim S, Lallone R, Ranganathan S, et al. Leptin levels in human and rodent: measurement of plasma leptin and ob RNA in obese and weight-reduced subjects. Nat Med 1995; 1:1155–1161.

100. Pelleymounter MA, Cullen MJ, Baker MB, Hecht R, Winters D, Boone T, Collins F. Effects of the obese gene product on body weight regulation in ob/ob mice. Science 1995; 269:540–543.

101. Chua SC Jr, Chung WK, Wu-Peng XS, Zhang Y, Liu SM, Tartaglia L, Leibel RL. Phenotypes of mouse diabetes and rat fatty due to mutations in the OB (leptin) receptor. Science 1996; 271:994–996.

102. Clement K, Vaisse C, Lahlou N, Cabrol S, Pelloux V, Cassuto D, Gourmelen M, Dina C, Chambaz J, Lacorte JM, Basdevant A, Bougneres P, Lebouc Y, Froguel P, Guy-Grand B. A mutation in the human leptin receptor gene causes obesity and pituitary dysfunction. Nature 1998; 392:398–401.

103. Farooqi IS, Keogh JM, Kamath S, Jones S, Gibson WT, Trussell R, Jebb SA, Lip GY, O'Rahilly S. Partial leptin deficiency and human adiposity. Nature 2001; 414:34–35.

104. Montague CT, Farooqi IS, Whitehead JP, Soos MA, Rau H, Wareham NJ, Sewter CP, Digby JE, Mohammed SN, Hurst JA, Cheetham CH, Earley AR, Barnett AH, Prins JB, O'Rahilly S. Congenital leptin deficiency is associated with severe early-onset obesity in humans. Nature 1997; 387:903–908.

105. Farooqi IS, Jebb SA, Langmack G, Lawrence E, Cheetham CH, Prentice AM, Hughes IA, McCamish MA, O'Rahilly S. Effects of recombinant leptin therapy in a child with congenital leptin deficiency. N Engl J Med 1999; 341:879–884.

106. Farooqi IS, Matarese G, Lord GM, Keogh JM, Lawrence E, Agwu C, Sanna V, Jebb SA, Perna F, Fontana S, Lechler RI, DePaoli AM, O'Rahilly S. Beneficial effects of leptin on obesity, T cell hyporesponsiveness, and neuroendocrine/metabolic dysfunction of human congenital leptin deficiency. J Clin Invest 2002; 110:1093–1103.

107. Considine RV, Sinha MK, Heiman ML, Kriauciunas A, Stephens TW, Nyce MR, Ohannesian JP, Marco CC, McKee LJ, Bauer TL, et al. Serum immunoreactive-leptin concentrations in normal-weight and obese humans. N Engl J Med 1996; 334:292–295.

108. Munzberg H, Flier JS, Bjorbaek C. Region-specific leptin resistance within the hypothalamus of diet-induced obese mice. Endocrinology 2004; 145:4880–4889.

109. Oral EA, Simha V, Ruiz E, Andewelt A, Premkumar A, Snell P, Wagner AJ, DePaoli AM, Reitman ML, Taylor SI, Gorden P, Garg A. Leptin-replacement therapy for lipodystrophy. N Engl J Med 2002; 346:570–578.

110. Minokoshi Y, Kahn BB. Role of AMP-activated protein kinase in leptin-induced fatty acid oxidation in muscle. Biochem Soc Trans 2003; 31:196–201.

111. Yamauchi T, Kamon J, Minokoshi Y, Ito Y, Waki H, Uchida S, Yamashita S, Noda M, Kita S, Ueki K, Eto K, Akanuma Y, Froguel P, Foufelle F, Ferre P, Carling D, Kimura S, Nagai R, Kahn BB, Kadowaki T. Adiponectin stimulates glucose utilization and fatty-acid oxidation by activating AMP-activated protein kinase. Nat Med 2002; 8:1288–1295.

112. Ruderman N, Prentki M. AMP kinase and malonyl-CoA: targets for therapy of the metabolic syndrome. Nat Rev Drug Discov 2004; 3:340–351.

113. Luo JD, Zhang GS, Chen MS. Leptin and cardiovascular diseases. Timely Top Med Cardiovasc Dis 2005; 9:E34.

114. Steppan CM, Bailey ST, Bhat S, Brown EJ, Banerjee RR, Wright CM, Patel HR, Ahima RS, Lazar MA. The hormone resistin links obesity to diabetes. Nature 2001; 409:307–312.

115. McTernan CL, McTernan PG, Harte AL, Levick PL, Barnett AH, Kumar S. Resistin, central obesity, and type 2 diabetes. Lancet 2002; 359:46–47.

116. Degawa-Yamauchi M, Bovenkerk JE, Juliar BE, Watson W, Kerr K, Jones R, Zhu Q, Considine RV. Serum resistin (FIZZ3) protein is increased in obese humans. J Clin Endocrinol Metab 2003; 88:5452–5455.

117. Muse ED, Obici S, Bhanot S, Monia BP, McKay RA, Rajala MW, Scherer PE, Rossetti L. Role of resistin in diet-induced hepatic insulin resistance. J Clin Invest 2004; 114:232–239.

118. Rajala MW, Obici S, Scherer PE, Rossetti L. Adipose-derived resistin and gut-derived resistin-like molecule-beta selectively impair insulin action on glucose production. J Clin Invest 2003; 111:225–230.

119. Banerjee RR, Rangwala SM, Shapiro JS, Rich AS, Rhoades B, Qi Y, Wang J, Rajala MW, Pocai A, Scherer PE, Steppan CM, Ahima RS, Obici S, Rossetti L, Lazar MA. Regulation of fasted blood glucose by resistin. Science 2004; 303:1195–1198.

120. Kim KH, Lee K, Moon YS, Sul HS. A cysteine-rich adipose tissue-specific secretory factor inhibits adipocyte differentiation. J Biol Chem 2001; 276:11252–11256.

121. Patel L, Buckels AC, Kinghorn IJ, Murdock PR, Holbrook JD, Plumpton C, Macphee CH, Smith SA. Resistin is expressed in human macrophages and directly regulated by PPAR gamma activators. Biochem Biophys Res Commun 2003; 300:472–476.

122. Savage DB, Sewter CP, Klenk ES, Segal DG, Vidal-Puig A, Considine RV, O'Rahilly S. Resistin/Fizz3 expression in relation to obesity and peroxisome proliferator-activated receptor-gamma action in humans. Diabetes 2001; 50:2199–2202.

123. Banerjee RR, Lazar MA. Dimerization of resistin and resistin-like molecules is determined by a single cysteine. J Biol Chem 2001; 276:25970–25973.

124. Patel SD, Rajala MW, Rossetti L, Scherer PE, Shapiro L. Disulfide-dependent multimeric assembly of resistin family hormones. Science 2004; 304:1154–1158.

125. Yang RZ, Huang Q, Xu A, McLenithan JC, Eisen JA, Shuldiner AR, Alkan S, Gong DW. Comparative studies of resistin expression and phylogenomics in human and mouse. Biochem Biophys Res Commun 2003; 310:927–935.

126. Verma S, Li SH, Wang CH, Fedak PW, Li RK, Weisel RD, Mickle DA. Resistin promotes endothelial cell activation: further evidence of adipokine-endothelial interaction. Circulation 2003; 108:736–740.

127. Calabro P, Samudio I, Willerson JT, Yeh ET. Resistin promotes smooth muscle cell proliferation through activation of extracellular signal-regulated kinase 1/2 and phosphatidylinositol 3-kinase pathways. Circulation 2004; 110:3335–3340.

128. Burnett MS, Lee CW, Kinnaird TD, Stabile E, Durrani S, Dullum MK, Devaney JM, Fishman C, Stamou S, Canos D, Zbinden S, Clavijo LC, Jang GJ, Andrews JA, Zhu J, Epstein SE. The potential role of resistin in atherogenesis. Atherosclerosis 2005; 182:241–248.

129. Adeghate E. An update on the biology and physiology of resistin. Cell Mol Life Sci 2004; 61:2485–2496.

130. Nagaev I, Smith U. Insulin resistance and type 2 diabetes are not related to resistin expression in human fat cells or skeletal muscle. Biochem Biophys Res Commun 2001; 285:561–564.

131. Fain JN, Cheema PS, Bahouth SW, Lloyd Hiler M. Resistin release by human adipose tissue explants in primary culture. Biochem Biophys Res Commun 2003; 300:674–678.

132. Utzschneider KM, Carr DB, Tong J, Wallace TM, Hull RL, Zraika S, Xiao Q, Mistry JS, Retzlaff BM, Knopp RH, Kahn SE. Resistin is not associated with insulin sensitivity or the metabolic syndrome in humans. Diabetologia 2005; 48:2330–2333.

133. Lee JH, Bullen JW Jr, Stoyneva VL, Mantzoros CS. Circulating resistin in lean, obese, and insulin-resistant mouse models: lack of association with insulinemia and glycemia. Am J Physiol Endocrinol Metab 2005; 288:E625–632.

134. Rajala MW, Qi Y, Patel HR, Takahashi N, Banerjee R, Pajvani UB, Sinha MK, Gingerich RL, Scherer PE, Ahima RS. Regulation of resistin expression and circulating levels in obesity, diabetes, and fasting. Diabetes 2004; 53:1671–1679.

135. Asensio C, Cettour-Rose P, Theander-Carrillo C, Rohner-Jeanrenaud F, Muzzin P. Changes in glycemia by leptin administration or high- fat feeding in rodent models of obesity/type 2 diabetes suggest a link between resistin expression and control of glucose homeostasis. Endocrinology 2004; 145:2206–2213.

136. Kim KH, Zhao L, Moon Y, Kang C, Sul HS. Dominant inhibitory adipocyte-specific secretory factor (ADSF)/resistin enhances adipogenesis and improves insulin sensitivity. Proc Natl Acad Sci USA 2004; 101:6780–6785.

137. Schaffler A, Buchler C, Muller-Ladner U, Herfarth H, Ehling A, Paul G, Scholmerich J, Zietz B. Identification of variables influencing resistin serum levels in patients with type 1 and type 2 diabetes mellitus. Horm Metab Res 2004; 36:702–707.

138. Vendrell J, Broch M, Vilarrasa N, Molina A, Gomez JM, Gutierrez C, Simon I, Soler J, Richart C. Resistin, adiponectin, ghrelin, leptin, and proinflammatory cytokines: relationships in obesity. Obes Res 2004; 12:962–971.

139. Azuma K, Katsukawa F, Oguchi S, Murata M, Yamazaki H, Shimada A, Saruta T. Correlation between serum resistin level and adiposity in obese individuals. Obes Res 2003; 11:997–1001.

140. Yannakoulia M, Yiannakouris N, Bluher S, Matalas AL, Klimis-Zacas D, Mantzoros CS. Body fat mass and macronutrient intake in relation to circulating soluble leptin receptor, free leptin index, adiponectin, and resistin concentrations in healthy humans. J Clin Endocrinol Metab 2003; 88:1730–1736.

141. McTernan PG, Fisher FM, Valsamakis G, Chetty R, Harte A, McTernan CL, Clark PM, Smith SA, Barnett AH, Kumar S. Resistin and type 2 diabetes: regulation of resistin expression by insulin and rosiglitazone and the effects of recombinant resistin on lipid and glucose metabolism in human differentiated adipocytes. J Clin Endocrinol Metab 2003; 88:6098–6106.

142. Zhang J, Qin Y, Zheng X, Qiu J, Gong L, Mao H, Jia W, Guo J. [The relationship between human serum resistin level and body fat content, plasma glucose as well as blood pressure]. Zhonghua Yi Xue Za Zhi 2002; 82:1609–1612.

143. McTernan PG, McTernan CL, Chetty R, Jenner K, Fisher FM, Lauer MN, Crocker J, Barnett AH, Kumar S. Increased resistin gene and protein expression in human abdominal adipose tissue. J Clin Endocrinol Metab 2002; 87:2407.

144. Valsamakis G, McTernan PG, Chetty R, Al Daghri N, Field A, Hanif W, Barnett AH, Kumar S. Modest weight loss and reduction in waist circumference after medical treatment are associated with favorable changes in serum adipocytokines. Metabolism 2004; 53:430–434.

145. Maebuchi M, Machidori M, Urade R, Ogawa T, Moriyama T. Low resistin levels in adipose tissues and serum in high-fat fed mice and genetically obese mice: development of an ELISA system for quantification of resistin. Arch Biochem Biophys 2003; 416:164–170.

146. Huang L, Wang Z, Li C. Modulation of circulating leptin levels by its soluble receptor. J Biol Chem 2001; 276:6343–6349.

147. Lahlou N, Clement K, Carel JC, Vaisse C, Lotton C, Le Bihan Y, Basdevant A, Lebouc Y, Froguel P, Roger M, Guy-Grand B. Soluble leptin receptor in serum of subjects with complete resistance to leptin: relation to fat mass. Diabetes 2000; 49:1347–1352.

148. Winkler G, Kiss S, Keszthelyi L, Sapi Z, Ory I, Salamon F, Kovacs M, Vargha P, Szekeres O, Speer G, Karadi I, Sikter M, Kaszas E, Dworak O, Gero G, Cseh K. Expression of tumor necrosis factor (TNF)-alpha protein in the subcutaneous and visceral adipose tissue in correlation with adipocyte cell volume, serum TNF-alpha, soluble serum TNF-receptor-2 concentrations and C-peptide level. Eur J Endocrinol 2003; 149:129–135.

149. Lee JH, Chan JL, Yiannakouris N, Kontogianni M, Estrada E, Seip R, Orlova C, Mantzoros CS. Circulating resistin levels are not associated with obesity or insulin resistance in humans and are not regulated by fasting or leptin administration: cross-sectional and interventional studies in normal, insulin-resistant, and diabetic subjects. J Clin Endocrinol Metab 2003; 88:4848–4856.

150. Silha JV, Krsek M, Skrha JV, Sucharda P, Nyomba BL, Murphy LJ. Plasma resistin, adiponectin and leptin levels in lean and obese subjects: correlations with insulin resistance. Eur J Endocrinol 2003; 149:331–335.

151. Heilbronn LK, Rood J, Janderova L, Albu JB, Kelley DE, Ravussin E, Smith SR. Relationship between serum resistin concentrations and insulin resistance in nonobese, obese, and obese diabetic subjects. J Clin Endocrinol Metab 2004; 89:1844–1848.

152. Smith SR, Bai F, Charbonneau C, Janderova L, Argyropoulos G. A promoter genotype and oxidative stress potentially link resistin to human insulin resistance. Diabetes 2003; 52:1611–1618.

153. Fujinami A, Obayashi H, Ohta K, Ichimura T, Nishimura M, Matsui H, Kawahara Y, Yamazaki M, Ogata M, Hasegawa G, Nakamura N, Yoshikawa T, Nakano K, Ohta M. Enzyme-linked immunosorbent assay for circulating human resistin: resistin concentrations in normal subjects and patients with type 2 diabetes. Clin Chim Acta 2004; 339:57–63.

154. Pfutzner A, Langenfeld M, Kunt T, Lobig M, Forst T. Evaluation of human resistin assays with serum from patients with type 2 diabetes and different degrees of insulin resistance. Clin Lab 2003; 49:571–576.

155. Youn BS, Yu KY, Park HJ, Lee NS, Min SS, Youn MY, Cho YM, Park YJ, Kim SY, Lee HK, Park KS. Plasma resistin concentrations measured by enzyme-linked immunosorbent assay using a newly developed monoclonal antibody are elevated in individuals with type 2 diabetes mellitus. J Clin Endocrinol Metab 2004; 89:150–156.

156. Ridker PM, Koenig W, Fuster V. C-reactive protein and coronary heart disease. N Engl J Med 2004; 351:295–298; author reply 295–298.

157. Esposito K, Pontillo A, Di Palo C, Giugliano G, Masella M, Marfella R, Giugliano D. Effect of weight loss and lifestyle changes on vascular inflammatory markers in obese women: a randomized trial. Jama 2003; 289:1799–1804.

158. Esposito K, Marfella R, Ciotola M, Di Palo C, Giugliano F, Giugliano G, D'Armiento M,D' Andrea F, Giugliano D. Effect of a mediterranean-style diet on endothelial dysfunction and markers of vascular inflammation in the metabolic syndrome: a randomized trial. Jama 2004; 292:1440–1446.

159. Obisesan TO, Leeuwenburgh C, Phillips T, Ferrell RE, Phares DA, Prior SJ, Hagberg JM. C-reactive protein genotypes affect baseline, but not exercise training-induced changes, in C-reactive protein levels. Arterioscler Thromb Vasc Biol 2004; 24:1874–1879.

160. Okita K, Nishijima H, Murakami T, Nagai T, Morita N, Yonezawa K, Iizuka K, Kawaguchi H, Kitabatake A. Can exercise training with weight loss lower serum C-reactive protein levels? Arterioscler Thromb Vasc Biol 2004; 24:1868–1873.

161. Ouchi N, Kihara S, Funahashi T, Nakamura T, Nishida M, Kumada M, Okamoto Y, Ohashi K, Nagaretani H, Kishida K, Nishizawa H, Maeda N, Kobayashi H, Hiraoka H, Matsuzawa Y. Reciprocal association of C-reactive protein with adiponectin in blood stream and adipose tissue. Circulation 2003; 107:671–674.

162. Erren M, Reinecke H, Junker R, Fobker M, Schulte H, Schurek JO, Kropf J, Kerber S, Breithardt G, Assmann G, Cullen P. Systemic inflammatory parameters in patients with atherosclerosis of the coronary and peripheral arteries. Arterioscler Thromb Vasc Biol 1999; 19:2355–2363.

163. Fyfe AI, Rothenberg LS, DeBeer FC, Cantor RM, Rotter JI, Lusis AJ. Association between serum amyloid A proteins and coronary artery disease: evidence from two distinct arteriosclerotic processes. Circulation 1997; 96:2914–2919.

164. Ridker PM, Hennekens CH, Buring JE, Rifai N. C-reactive protein and other markers of inflammation in the prediction of cardiovascular disease in women. N Engl J Med 2000; 342:836–843.

165. Ridker PM, Rifai N, Pfeffer MA, Sacks FM, Moye LA, Goldman S, Flaker GC, Braunwald E. Inflammation, pravastatin, and the risk of coronary events after myocardial infarction in patients with average cholesterol levels. Cholesterol and Recurrent Events (CARE) Investigators. Circulation 1998; 98:839–844.

166. Shimomura I, Funahashi T, Takahashi M, Maeda K, Kotani K, Nakamura T, Yamashita S, Miura M, Fukuda Y, Takemura K, Tokunaga K, Matsuzawa Y. Enhanced expression of PAI-1 in visceral fat: possible contributor to vascular disease in obesity. Nat Med 1996; 2:800–803.

167. Tatemoto K, Hosoya M, Habata Y, Fujii R, Kakegawa T, Zou MX, Kawamata Y, Fukusumi S, Hinuma S, Kitada C, Kurokawa T, Onda H, Fujino M. Isolation and characterization of a novel endogenous peptide ligand for the human APJ receptor. Biochem Biophys Res Commun 1998; 251:471–476.

168. Boucher J, Masri B, Daviaud D, Gesta S, Guigne C, Mazzucotelli A, Castan-Laurell I, Tack I, Knibiehler B, Carpene C, Audigier Y, Saulnier-Blache JS, Valet P. Apelin, a newly identified adipokine up-regulated by insulin and obesity. Endocrinology 2005; 146:1764–1771.

169. Fukuhara A, Matsuda M, Nishizawa M, Segawa K, Tanaka M, Kishimoto K, Matsuki Y, Murakami M, Ichisaka T, Murakami H, Watanabe E, Takagi T, Akiyoshi M, Ohtsubo T, Kihara S, Yamashita S, Makishima M, Funahashi T, Yamanaka S, Hiramatsu R, Matsuzawa Y, Shimomura I. Visfatin: a protein secreted by visceral fat that mimics the effects of insulin. Science 2005; 307:426–430.

170. Hirai K, Hussey HJ, Barber MD, Price SA, Tisdale MJ. Biological evaluation of a lipid-mobilizing factor isolated from the urine of cancer patients. Cancer Res 1998; 58:2359–2365.

171. Todorov PT, McDevitt TM, Meyer DJ, Ueyama H, Ohkubo I, Tisdale MJ. Purification and characterization of a tumor lipid-mobilizing factor. Cancer Res 1998; 58:2353–2358.

172. Russell ST, Hirai K, Tisdale MJ. Role of beta3-adrenergic receptors in the action of a tumour lipid mobilizing factor. Br J Cancer 2002; 86:424–428.

173. Bing C, Bao Y, Jenkins J, Sanders P, Manieri M, Cinti S, Tisdale MJ, Trayhurn P. Zinc-alpha2-glycoprotein, a lipid mobilizing factor, is expressed in adipocytes and is up-regulated in mice with cancer cachexia. Proc Natl Acad Sci USA 2004; 101:2500–2505.

174. Bao Y, Yamano Y, Morishima I. A novel lebocin-like gene from eri-silkworm, Samia cynthia ricini, that does not encode the antibacterial peptide lebocin. Comp Biochem Physiol B Biochem Mol Biol 2005; 140:127–131.

175. Gohda T, Makita Y, Shike T, Tanimoto M, Funabiki K, Horikoshi S, Tomino Y. Identification of epistatic interaction involved in obesity using the KK/Ta mouse as a Type 2 diabetes model: is Zn-alpha2 glycoprotein-1 a candidate gene for obesity? Diabetes 2003; 52:2175–2181.

176. Hug C, Lodish HF. Medicine. Visfatin: a new adipokine. Science 2005; 307:366–367.

177. Fruhbeck G, Gomez-Ambrosi J, Muruzabal FJ, Burrell MA. The adipocyte: a model for integration of endocrine and metabolic signaling in energy metabolism regulation. Am J Physiol Endocrinol Metab 2001; 280:E827–847.

178. Trayhurn P, Beattie JH. Physiological role of adipose tissue: white adipose tissue as an endocrine and secretory organ. Proc Nutr Soc 2001; 60:329–339.

179. Dietze D, Koenen M, Rohrig K, Horikoshi H, Hauner H, Eckel J. Impairment of insulin signaling in human skeletal muscle cells by co-culture with human adipocytes. Diabetes 2002; 51:2369–2376.

180. Ehrhart-Bornstein M, Lamounier-Zepter V, Schraven A, Langenbach J, Willenberg HS, Barthel A, Hauner H, McCann SM, Scherbaum WA, Bornstein SR. Human adipocytes secrete mineralocorticoid-releasing factors. Proc Natl Acad Sci USA 2003; 100:14211–14216.

181. Rayner DV, Trayhurn P. Regulation of leptin production: sympathetic nervous system interactions. J Mol Med 2001; 79:8–20.

182. De Ceuninck F, Dassencourt L, Anract P. The inflammatory side of human chondrocytes unveiled by antibody microarrays. Biochem Biophys Res Commun 2004; 323:960–969.

183. Pedersen BK, Steensberg A, Fischer C, Keller C, Keller P, Plomgaard P, Wolsk-Petersen E, Febbraio M. The metabolic role of IL-6 produced during exercise: is IL-6 an exercise factor? Proc Nutr Soc 2004; 63:263–267.

184. Pedersen BK, Steensberg A, Fischer C, Keller C, Ostrowski K, Schjerling P. Exercise and cytokines with particular focus on muscle-derived IL-6. Exerc Immunol Rev 2001; 7:18–31.

185. Spiegelman BM. PPAR-gamma: adipogenic regulator and thiazolidinedione receptor. Diabetes 1998; 47:507–514.

186. Kallen CB, Lazar MA. Antidiabetic thiazolidinediones inhibit leptin (ob) gene expression in 3T3-L1 adipocytes. Proc Natl Acad Sci USA 1996; 93:5793–5796.

187. Greenberg AS. The expanding scope of the metabolic syndrome and implications for the management of cardiovascular risk in type 2 diabetes with particular focus on the emerging role of the thiazolidinediones. J Diabetes Complications 2003; 17:218–228.

188. Calabro P, Samudio I, Safe SH, Willerson JT, Yeh ET. Inhibition of tumor-necrosis-factor-alpha induced endothelial cell activation by a new class of PPAR-gamma agonists. An in vitro study showing receptor-independent effects. J Vasc Res 2005; 42:509–516.

189. Haffner SM, Greenberg AS, Weston WM, Chen H, Williams K, Freed MI. Effect of rosiglitazone treatment on nontraditional markers of cardiovascular disease in patients with type 2 diabetes mellitus. Circulation 2002; 106:679–684.

190. Fryer LG, Parbu-Patel A, Carling D. The Anti-diabetic drugs rosiglitazone and metformin stimulate AMP-activated protein kinase through distinct signaling pathways. J Biol Chem 2002; 277:25226–25232.

191. Tiikkainen M, Hakkinen AM, Korsheninnikova E, Nyman T, Makimattila S, Yki-Jarvinen H. Effects of rosiglitazone and metformin on liver fat content, hepatic insulin resistance, insulin clearance, and gene expression in adipose tissue in patients with type 2 diabetes. Diabetes 2004; 53:2169–2176.

CHAPTER 4

CYCLOOXYGENASE-2 (COX-2) AND THE INFLAMMOGENESIS OF CANCER

RANDALL E. HARRIS

College of Medicine and School of Public Health, Center of Molecular Epidemiology and Environmental Health, The Ohio State University Medical Center, 310 West 10th Avenue, Columbus, Ohio 43210-1240

Abstract: Cohesive scientific evidence from molecular, animal, and human investigations supports the hypothesis that aberrant induction of COX-2 and up-regulation of the prostaglandin cascade play a significant role in carcinogenesis, and reciprocally, blockade of the process has strong potential for cancer prevention and therapy. Supporting evidence

R. E. Harris (ed.), Inflammation in the Pathogenesis of Chronic Diseases, 93–126.
© 2007 *Springer.*

includes the following: [1] expression of constitutive COX-2-catalyzed prostaglandin biosynthesis is induced by most cancer-causing agents including tobacco smoke and its components (polycylic aromatic amines, heterocyclic amines, nitrosamines), essential polyunsaturated fatty acids (unconjugated linoleic acid), mitogens, growth factors, pro-inflammatory cytokines, microbial agents, tumor promoters, and other epigenetic factors, [2] COX-2 expression is a characteristic feature of all premalignant neoplasms, [3] COX-2 expression is a characteristic feature of all malignant neoplasms, and expression intensifies with stage at detection and cancer progression and metastasis, [4] all essential features of carcinogenesis (mutagenesis, mitogenesis, angiogenesis, reduced apoptosis, metastasis, and immunosuppression) are linked to COX-2-driven prostaglandin (PGE-2) biosynthesis, [5] animal studies show that COX-2 up-regulation (in the absence of genetic mutations) is sufficient to stimulate the transformation of normal cells to invasive cancer and metastatic disease, [6] non-selective COX-2 inhibitors, such as aspirin and ibuprofen, reduce the risk of human cancer and precancerous lesions, and [7] selective COX-2 inhibitors, such as celecoxib, reduce the risk of human cancer and precancerous lesions at all anatomic sites thus far investigated. Results confirming that COX-2 blockade is effective for both cancer prevention and therapy have been tempered by observations that some COX-2 inhibitors pose a risk to the cardiovascular system, and more studies are needed in order to determine if certain of these drugs can be taken at dosages that prevent cancer without increasing cardiovascular risk. It is emphasized that the "inflammogenesis model of cancer" is not mutually exclusive and may in fact be synergistic with the accumulation of somatic mutations in tumor suppressor genes and oncogenes or epigenetic factors in the development of cancer

1.   INTRODUCTION

Despite intensive medical and public health efforts, cancer has now surpassed cardiovascular disease as the leading cause of death in people under age 85 in the United States [1]. While some progress has been made, particularly in the treatment of leukemia in children, conventional methods of surgery, chemotherapy, and radiotherapy have not impacted greatly on the general morbidity and mortality due to many forms of cancer in adults.

Cancerous growths result from a complex process known collectively as carcino-genesis. In this chapter, we discuss the hypothesis that aberrant induction of COX-2 and up-regulation of the prostaglandin cascade play a significant role in carcino-genesis, a process designated as the "inflammogenesis of cancer". Because a variety of genetic mutations have been identified through molecular studies of cancerous tissues [2], the process of carcinogenesis is considered by many to result from the accumulation of two or more somatic mutations that impact upon control of the cell cycle or other features of neoplastic development [3]. Nevertheless, many cancers arise without evidence of accumulating somatic mutations, and studies of precancerous and cancerous tissues often fail to disclose either chromosomal aberrations or mutated tumor suppressor genes and oncogenes [4]. Furthermore, mutational events that are identified in cancerous tissues may have occurred late in tumor development as the result of cancer development rather than the cause [5, 6]. The existing evidence is inconsistent with the hypothesis that cancer always arises from a single "mutated" cell and progresses due to accumulation of subsequent mutations that confer a survival advantage to cancer cells. As a consequence, novel models have recently been proposed postulating the presence of mutator genes that heighten the burden of mutations influencing cell division and carcinogenesis [7], and espousing the importance of "epigenetic factors" that deregulate the expression of cancer genes [8, 9].

More than a century ago, Virchow [10, 11, 12] suggested that chronic inflammation leads to cancer development by increasing cellular proliferation. Various models of carcinogenesis have been proposed involving inflammatory stimuli and mediators of wound healing [13, 14, 15]. Discovery of the inducible cyclooxygenase-2 (COX-2) gene has rekindled interest in the causal link between inflammation and cancer [16, 17, 18]. This chapter documents convincing evidence that carcinogenesis often evolves as a progressive series of highly specific cellular and molecular changes in response to induction of constitutive over-expression of COX-2 and the prostaglandin cascade in the "inflammogenesis of cancer".

2. EVOLUTION OF CANCER

Solid cancerous growths (tumors) often develop from cells of the epithelial lining of solid organs, and less often from dividing cells of muscle, bone, and the central nervous system. Hematopoietic cancers (leukemias, lymphomas) arise from lymphocytes, granulocytes, or other dividing cells of the blood. The evolution of cancer is thought to be a long term process spanning many years and often decades. The following paragraphs provide a brief description of some of the cell types that appear during the evolution of cancer [19, 20].

2.1. Dysplasia (Premalignant Lesions)

The evolution of cancer proceeds through a continuum of steps, the first of which is the development of dysplasia wherein normal cells undergo morphological changes of the nucleus and cytoplasm. In dysplasia, the cell nucleus becomes prominent, the cytoplasm appears swollen and vacuolated, and the cells exhibit increased rates of cell division and disordered maturation. Dysplasia invariably precedes the development of cancer, and dysplastic lesions that serve as precursors of cancer can be detected at a number of anatomic sites. Examples of pre-malignant lesions include actinic keratosis of the skin, leukoplakia of the oral cavity, Barrett's esophagus, fibrocystic disease with atypia of the breast, adenomatous polyps of the colon, dysplasia of the prostate and intraepithelial neoplasia of the uterine cervix. Clearly, the early detection and treatment of such lesions is an important component of effective cancer control.

2.2. Carcinoma in situ

When cancers arise, they are at first confined to their original location and have not broken through the basement membranes into surrounding tissues. A confined neoplasm of the epithelial cell layer is thus called "*carcinoma in situ*". Such *in situ* lesions represent a defined step in cancer evolution. They exhibit all of the features of malignancy except invasiveness and metastasis; namely, the cells of *in situ* neoplasms manifest unchecked mitosis and proliferation, maturation failure and resistance to death, and disordered organization of the cell population. And yet, the *in situ* neoplasm is theoretically curable by excision since it has not spread beyond its original location and is in containment by the basement membrane.

2.3.   Invasive Cancer

In contrast to *in situ* neoplasms, invasive cancers have broken through the basement membranes to spread beyond their original location into contiguous tissues. This is a critical step in the evolution of cancer since surgical excision may no longer be effective as a form of cancer therapy. The breach of the basement membranes by cancer cells requires acquisition of certain new functions, e.g., the secretion of enzymes that degrade basement membranes.

2.4.   Metastatic Cancer

Metastatic disease represents the final step in the evolution of cancer. Cancer cells first invade contiguous tissues, and then spread through lymphatic channels and blood vessels to other anatomic sites. Cancer causes death by metastasizing (spreading) to vital organs such as the liver, brain, and spine. It is within these vital organs that the cancer cells overwhelm the normal cellular constituency and produce collapse of their life-sustaining functions. Early detection prior to the development of invasive cancer and metastasis is therefore vitally important to the successful treatment and survival of cancer patients. The entire process of cancer development often goes unheeded and undetected by the human immune system; hence the term "silent killer" has been aptly applied to describe cancer in its various forms.

3.   COX-2 IN MALIGNANT AND PREMALIGNANT NEOPLASMS

Molecular studies reveal that over-expression of COX-2 is a prominent feature of virtually every form of cancer. Furthermore, COX-2 is commonly found in premalignant lesions, carcinoma *in situ*, invasive cancer, and metastatic disease.

Initially, examination of colon and breast tumors revealed high levels of COX-2 expression [21, 22, 23, 24, 25]. Subsequently, molecular biologists from multiple independent laboratories have consistently observed COX-2 over-expression in every type of cancer studied [17, 18]. Remarkably, high levels of COX-2 expression are evident throughout tumorigenesis in every anatomic site that has been examined.

Figure 1. shows the mean frequency of lesions over-expressing COX-2 in the progression of tumorigenesis for selected studies of Barrett's esophagus [26, 27, 28], urinary bladder cancer [29, 30, 31, 32], breast cancer [24, 33, 34, 35, 36, 37, 38], cervical cancer [39, 40, 41, 42, 43, 44, 45], colon cancer [21, 22, 46, 47, 48, 49], lung cancer [24, 50, 51, 52, 53, 54, 55], oral cavity cancer [56, 57, 58, 59], and prostate cancer [60, 61, 62, 63, 64]. High levels of expression are observed in premalignant lesions such as atypia of the mammary gland [38], dysplasia of the uterine cervix [40], adenomatous polyps of the colon [47], leukoplakia of the buccal mucosa [56], and the early stages of cancer, e.g., *carcinoma in situ* [26, 33, 34, 35]. It has been suggested that COX-2 may therefore be a useful biomarker of impending cancer [65].

Overexpression of COX-2 is also a prominent feature in primary cancers of the nasopharynx [66], larynx [67], parotid gland [68], stomach [69, 70], pancreas [71],

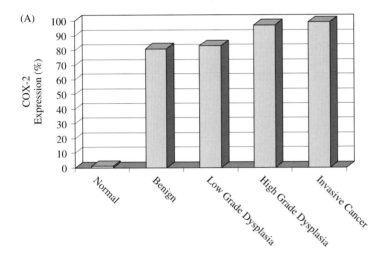

Barrett's Esophagus
Source: (a) Data from references 27,27,28

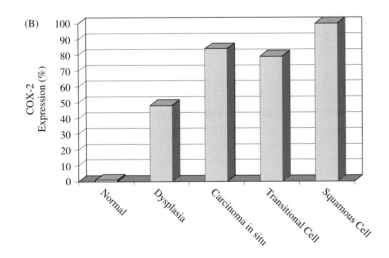

Bladder Cancer
Source: (b) Data from references 29,30,31,32
Figure 1.(Continued)

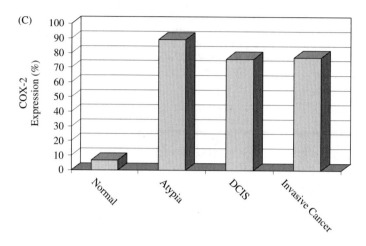

Breast Cancer

Source: (c) Data from references 24,33,34,35,36,37,38

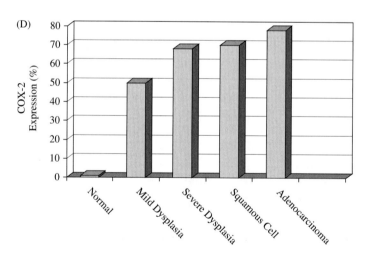

Cervical Cancer

Source: (d) Data from references 39,40,41,42,43,44,45
Figure 1. (Continued)

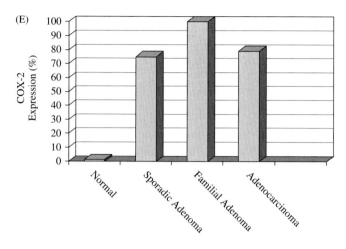

Colon Cancer
Source: (e) Data from references 21,22,46,47,48,49

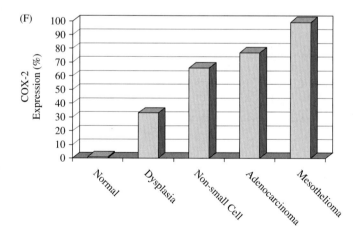

Lung Cancer
Source: (f) Data from references 24,50,51,52,53,54,55
Figure 1.(Continued)

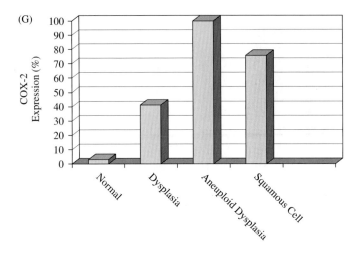

Oral Cavity Cancer
Source: (g) Data from references 56,57,58,59

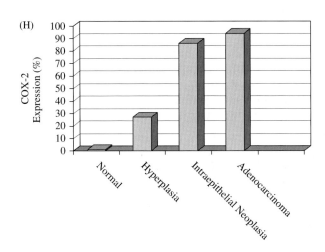

Prostate Cancer
Source: (h) Data from references 60,61,62,63,64
Figure 1. COX-2 expression in the progression of cancer. (A) Barrett's Esophagus. (B) Bladder cancer. (C) Breast cancer. (D) Cervical cancer. (E) Colon cancer. (F) Lung cancer. (G) Oral cavity cancer. (H) Prostate cancer

liver [72], ovary [73], endometrium [74], kidney [75], and skin [76, 77], as well as malignant melanoma [78], multiple myeloma [79], brain tumors [80, 81], retinoblastoma [82], sarcomas [83, 84], leukemias [85], and lymphomas [86, 87], and many studies suggest that expression intensifies with stage at detection, cancer progression and metastasis [28, 34, 40, 43, 44, 49, 52, 53, 59, 66, 69, 70, 74, 79, 81]. Furthermore, several investigators have observed that COX-2 over-expression is sufficient to transform normal cells to malignant neoplasms in animal models of carcinogenesis [88, 90, 91, 92]. These findings support the hypothesis that COX-2 expression is not only an early event in the genesis of cancer, but is required throughout the entire evolutionary process of cancer development and progression.

In contrast to the up-regulation of COX-2 that is associated with the transformation of normal tissue to cancer, COX-2 is usually not detectable in normal tissues, with the exception of the macula densa of the kidney, the brain, the testes, and tracheal epithelium where relatively low levels of constitutive expression are present [93, 94]. It is also noteworthy that mutations of both oncogenes and tumor suppression genes are usually absent in premalignant lesions as well as most cancers [4, 5, 6].

4.   MODEL OF INFLAMMOGENESIS OF CANCER

Various molecular mechanisms may be responsible for the initiation and promotion of carcinogenesis by COX-2. It is indeed remarkable that the induction of constitutive COX-2 expression and prostaglandin (PGE2) biosynthesis are sufficient to stimulate all of the key features of carcinogenesis including *mutagenesis, mitogenesis, angiogenesis, metastasis*, inhibition of *apoptosis* and *immunosupression* with reduced antineoplastic activity of T and B lymphocytes. These mechanisms are thoroughly reviewed and discussed elsewhere, e.g, by Howe et al. [95] and Shiff et al. [96].

As depicted in Figure 2, continuous over-expression of COX-2 can initiate and promote carcinogenesis by [1] increasing production of malondialdehyde and other reactive oxygen species that are carcinogenic *(mutagenesis)*, [2] increasing production of PGE-2 and other prostaglandins that strongly promote cell proliferation e.g., correlative up-regulation of the gene for aromatase (CYP19) and estrogen biosynthesis in stromal cells, or activation of epidermal growth factor receptor (EGFR) that stimulates an intracellular cascade of mitogenic signaling *(mitogenesis)*, [3] stimulation of vascular endothelial growth factor (VEGF) and platelet derived growth factor (PDGF) by PGE-2 resulting in *de novo* formation of blood vessels *(angiogenesis)*, [4] increasing production of matrix metalloproteinases (MMP) via co-expression of COX-2 and the Her-2/Neu gene, thus enhancing invasive potential *(metastasis)*, [5] decreasing bioavailable arachidonic acid pools necessary for conversion of sphingomyelin to ceramide, and stimulation of the Bcl-2 gene and inhibition of the BAX gene thereby reducing cell differentation and apoptosis *(anti-apoptosis)*, and [6] inhibiting proliferation of B and T lymphocytes, particularly natural killer T cells, thus limiting antineoplastic activity *(immunosuppression)*. All of these processes are discussed in some detail below.

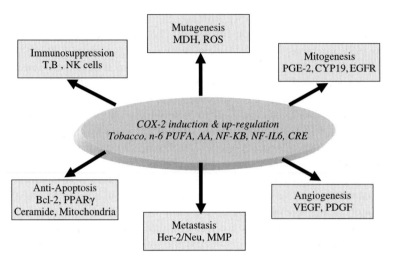

COX-2 in Carcinogenesis

4.1.   Induction of COX-2

A key event in the carcinogenic process is induction of constitutive expression of the COX-2 gene. It is striking that many important risk factors linked to cancer causation have been found capable of inducing COX-2. Important cancer-causing factors that are high on the list of COX-2 inducers are nicotine and its metabolites, nitrosamines, heterocyclic amines, polycyclic aromatic hydro-carbons, and many other inflammatory elements of tobacco smoke [91, 97, 98], certain essential fatty acids of the diet such as unconjugated linoleic acid [99], radiation [100], ultraviolet B [76], free radicals [101], oncogenic proteins [102], growth factors [103, 104], infectious agents such as helicobacter pyloris [105, 106], human papilloma viruses [107], hepatitis viruses [108], and the Epstein Barr virus [109], hypoxia [110], hormones [111], neurotransmitters [112], shear stress [113], and endotoxins [114].

As shown by Karmali and Marsh [115], Rose and Connolly [116], and others, arachidonic acid production, COX-2 expression, and prostaglandin biosynthesis are increased *in vivo* by dietary n-6 polyunsaturated fatty acids (n-6-*PUFAs*) such as unconjugated linoleic acid, and decreased by n-3-*PUFAs* such as linolenic acid. High dietary intake of n-6-*PUFAs* may therefore be an important factor in the induction of constitutive COX-2 expression. This mechanism is compatible with the high rates of cancers of the colon, breast, and prostate (neoplasms that characteristically over-express COX-2) in populations where n-6-*PUFAs*, particularly unconjugated linoleic acid, are abundant in the diet [117].

Molecular studies provide convincing evidence that tobacco smoke is a potent inducer of COX-2 in the lung and upper respiratory tract [91, 118]. It is also noteworthy that tobacco smoke has been found to induce the over-expression of COX-2 in the cells at several other anatomic sites including the oral cavity, esophagus, stomach, colon, breast, urinary bladder, skin, and bone [97, 98, 119, 120, 121, 122, 123].

Castonguay and colleagues [124, 125] demonstrated that the nicotine metabolite, 4-(methylnitrosamino)-1-(3-pyridyl)-1-butanone (NNK), up-regulates COX-2 thereby increasing the production of PGE-2 and promoting the development of pulmonary adenocarcinomas in mice. Induction of COX-2 in this model involves activation of epidermal growth factor receptor (EGFR), tyrosine kinase, and the mitogen-activated protein kinase (MAPK) cascade. Schuller and colleagues [127] found that lung cancer development in the Syrian Golden hamster involves up-regulation of COX-2 by NNK and beta agonists through activation of beta-adrenergic receptors. Dannenberg and colleagues [97] found that the polycyclic aromatic hydrocarbon, benzo[a]pyrene, stimulates up-regulation of COX-2 in association with activation of EGFR and tyrosine kinase activity in human epithelial cells of the oral mucosa. Martey et al. [118] observed that cigarette smoke up-regulates COX-2 in human lung fibroblasts through activation of aryl hydrocarcon hydroxylase receptors.

Induction of constitutive COX-2 expression may also involve many other micro-environmental stimuli such as bacterial lipopolysaccharides (LPS), tumor necrosis factor (TNF), cytokines, growth factors, mitogens, tumor promoters, and byproducts of protein synthesis and degradation. Since the COX-2 gene contains multiple promoter binding sites, nuclear transcription factors such as NFκβ, NF-IL-6, and signal transduction by cyclic AMP response elements (CRE) may also be important mediators of its induction and up-regulation [95, 96]. Notably, *in vitro* studies suggest that mutations at binding sites for these transcription factors in the promoter region of the COX-2 gene effectively inhibit the induction of COX-2 transcription and upregulation [129]. Furthermore, changes in the methylation of C-p-G islands in the promoter region of the COX-2 gene may also play in role in its constitutive expression [130, 131]. Thus, induction of constitutive COX-2 genetic expression may involve synergistic interactions between a number of micro-environmental epigenetic and genetic cofactors.

4.2. Mutagenesis

Accumulated mutagenic damage to DNA is believed to contribute substantially to the etiology of cancer. It is well known that lipid peroxidation in the human system generates reactive electrophilic compounds that have mutagenic potential [131].

Cyclooxygenases (COX) catalyze the two-step oxidation and peroxidation of arachidonic acid to form the intermediate prostaglandin endoperoxides, PGG-2 and PGH-2 [16, 95, 96, 129]. Spontaneous breakdown of PGH-2 yields the mutagen, malondialdehyde (MDA), plus hydroxyheptadecatreionic acid, and specific enzymes of the cytochrome P450 system as well as thromboxane synthetase can also catalyze the breakdown of PGH-2 to MDA [132, 133]. Malondialdehyde reacts with DNA under physiological conditions to form DNA adducts, predominantly pyrimidopurinone adducts of deoxyguanosine [134]. Sharma et al. [135] demonstrated that induction of COX-2 in human non-malignant colon epithelial cells produced increases in PGE-2, MDA, and characteristic DNA adducts that were similar to the levels observed in malignant colon epithelial cells. These findings underscore the potential for carcinogenesis due to oxidative damage and mutagenesis attributable to constitutive over-expression of COX-2.

4.3. Mitogenesis

Induction of constitutive over-expression of COX-2 in a cell predominantly increases the biosynthesis of PGE-2, which is the chief prostaglandin of the inflammatory cascade. This short-lived intercellular hormone is capable of inducing the transcription of specific genes in the nucleus of nearby cells. In particular, PGE-2 has been found to stimulate the transcription of genes that have powerful mitogenic effects.

One such mechanism is PGE-2 activation of EGFR that in turn triggers mitogenic signaling through the MAPK cascade. Pai et al. [136] discovered that PGE-2 rapidly phosphorylates EGFR and triggers the extracellular kinase, ERK-2, thereby activating the mitogenic signaling cascade in normal gastric epithelium and colon cancer. Their studies indicate that PGE-2-induced EGFR transactivation involves signal transduction via transforming growth factor alpha (TGF-alpha) and activated MMP. Other investigators have confirmed that co-expression of COX-2, PGE-2, and EGFR results in mitogenic activation in precancerous and cancerous tissues [103, 104, 137, 138].

Molecular studies from multiple laboratories reveal that adenocarcinoma of the breast is characterized by aberrant over-expression of COX-2 by breast cancer epithelial cells [24, 33–38]. The COX-2 enzyme efficiently catalyzes the conversion of essential dietary fats (principally arachidonic acid and unconjugated linoleic acid) into prostaglandins. Importantly, it has recently been discovered that there is a strong link between prostaglandins and estrogen biosynthesis. This occurs when the chief prostaglandin, PGE-2, activates the promoter II region of the aromatase gene (CYP-19), which is responsible for estrogen biosynthesis catalyzed by aromatase [139]. Furthermore, combined molecular studies of these genes reveal a significant correlation between up-regulation of cyclooxygenase expression and CYP-19 transcription in breast cancer tissues [140, 141]. Notably, this mechanism has been demonstrated in other malignant neoplasms including cancers of the lung [142], colon [143], and prostate [144] and may in fact be a ubiquitous feature in cancer promotion and development. Clearly, the established molecular link between heightened levels of essential polyunsaturated fatty acids, cyclooxygenase, prostaglandins, aromatase, and estrogens, provides a basis for carcinogenesis through unbridled mitogenesis.

Molecular examination of colon cancer reveals accumulation of the cell adhesion molecule, beta-catenin, in the nucleus of malignant cells [92, 145, 146]. Cell adhesion is under the control of the gene for adenomatous polyposis coli (APC) and involves maintenance of the integrity of a molecular cell adhesion complex comprised of beta-catenin, APC protein, T-cell factor (TcF) and actin [147]. Familial adenomatous polyposis (FAP) is caused by a mutation of the APC gene that causes dissociation of these cell adhesion complexes and the migration of beta-catenin to the cell nucleus where it activates one of the peroxisome proliferator-activated receptors (PPAR gamma) on the nuclear membrane. Castellone et al. [148] conducted a series of experiments demonstrating that inhibition of PGE-2 biosynthesis by NSAIDs effectively reduces the accumulation of beta-catenin and the progression of colon cancer. Based on their results, over-expression of COX-2 with increased PGE-2 biosynthesis and binding to its receptor in turn activates a cytoplasmic G-protein receptor that binds axin thereby reducing phosphorylation of beta-catenin. This chain of molecular events leads to dissociation of the adhesion complex, accumulation of unphosphorylated beta-catenin in the cell nucleus, activation of the nuclear receptor, PPAR-gamma, and stimulation of cell proliferation through transcription of cell cyclin genes. Recent molecular studies suggest that this mechanism is not limited to the colon; that is, induction of cyclooxygenase and increased prostaglandins (PGE-2) can result in cellular beta-catenin accumulation, nuclear PPAR-gamma activation, and subsequent cell proliferation and carcinogenesis in a variety of tissues [149].

4.4. Angiogenesis

Vascular Epidermal Growth Factor (VEGF) is a potent stimulant of *de novo* blood vessel formation (angiogenesis) in a variety of tissues. Once believed present only in the endothelial lining of blood vessels, VEGF has now been discovered in virtually all types of cancers [150]. Gallo *et al.* [151] and subsequently several other investigators [17, 65, 93, 117, 150] have linked the expression of COX-2 to increased levels of VEGF and angiogenesis in the promotion of tumor growth and development. Results suggest that COX-2-derived prostaglandins such as PGE-2 up-regulate the synthesis of VEGF and delimit its effects by increasing vascular permeability. Furthermore, VEGF (and other growth factors) may further amplify COX-2 expression in a positive feedback loop. Notably, inhibition of this vicious cycle by COX-2 inhibiting agents such as celecoxib has been found to limit angiogenesis and halt the progression and metastatic spread of tumors in animals [17, 150, 151, 152, 153].

4.5. Metastasis

The HER-2/neu oncogene is a member of the epidermal growth factor receptor (EGFR) family. It is an important mediator of cancer cell growth and metastasis. Koki *et al.* [17] and Subbaramaiah *et al.* [154] demonstrated that COX-2 and HER-2/neu are co-expressed in breast cancer. Co-expression of COX-2 and Her-2/neu involves the mitogen-activated protein kinase (MAPK/AP-1) signaling cascade. When the HER-2/neu receptor protein is activated, multiple other factors are activated that promote tumor development and metastatic spread of cancer cells including VEGF (angiogenesis) and matrix metalloproteinases (degradation of cell membranes) [17]. Over-expression of HER-2/neu is now widely used by clinicians as a biomarker of poor prognosis and metastasis for patients with invasive breast cancer [155].

Induction and up-regulation of COX-2 in cancer tissue is tightly correlated with increased activity of matrix metalloproteinases (MMP) [156, 157, 158, 159]. These enzymes degrade cell membranes and basement membrane and are thus associated with tumor invasiveness, metastasis, and poor survival. Reciprocally, NSAIDs that inhibit COX-2 have been demonstrated to reduce MMP levels thereby decreasing the metastasis of colon cancer in animals [160, 161, 162].

4.6.   Suppression of Apoptosis

Apoptosis or controlled cell death is an important regulatory mechanism for the maintenance of homeostasis in cell populations. Dysfunctional apoptosis results in immortalization of cells, a key feature of cancer cells. Inflammation, COX-2 over-expression, and increased PGE-2 are clearly anti-apoptotic, whereas, anti-inflammatory compounds that inhibit COX-2 are pro-apoptotic [95, 163, 164, 165, 166, 167, 168, 169].

Apoptosis is regulated by an intrinsic pathway that originates inside the cell and an extrinsic pathway that originates outside the cell. Notably, both pathways are inhibited by COX-2 over-expression. The intrinsic pathway involves mitochondrial release of cytochrome c and activation of caspase 9 and other enzymes that destroy the cell. Intrinsic apoptosis is triggered when the expression of two nuclear genes, Bcl-2 and BAX, favors BAX. Notably, COX-2 over-expression and prostaglandin biosynthesis promotes Bcl-2 and inhibits BAX, thereby blocking intrinsic apoptosis [95, 163, 164, 165, 166].

The extrinsic pathway involves activation of death receptors on the cell membrane by tumor necrosis factors, alpha and beta, and other epigenetic factors. This results in activation of caspase 8 and other enzymes that destroy the cell. Over-expression of COX-2 attenuates activation of this mechanism thereby blocking extrinsic apoptosis [95, 167, 168, 169, 170].

Compounds that inhibit COX-2 and PGE-2 appear to enhance both intrinsic and extrinsic apoptosis [163], and as a consequence, COX-2 inhibitors used in combination with radiation show beneficial synergism in the elimination of cancer cells in inoperable solid tumors [100, 165]. Nonsteroidal anti-inflammatory drugs also increase apoptosis by increasing bioavailable arachidonic acid pools necessary for conversion of sphingomyelin to ceramide since ceramide accumulation in the cell triggers apoptosis [92, 171, 172].

4.7.   Immunosuppression

Immunosuppression is a characteristic feature of cancer patients that correlates with disease promotion and progression. It is an interesting paradox that COX-2 overexpression and prostaglandin biosynthesis empowers cancer cell proliferation, immortalization, and metastasis on the one hand, while suppressing the function of important cells of the immune system on the other, thereby creating an immuno-suppressed host with little ability to mount an immune defense against a developing tumor. Indeed, the induction of T cell anergy is an early event in the course of tumor progression [173].

Prostaglandins, particularly PGE-2, are important modulators of immunosuppression. Pockaj *et al.* [174] found that increased levels of PGE-2 suppress the immunocompetence of helper T-cells and dendritic cells in newly diagnosed breast cancer patients. Specifically, elevated levels of PGE-2 were associated with reduced secretion of anti-tumor factors by T-cells (interferon-gamma, tumor necrosis factor-alpha, and interleukins IL-2 and IL-12) and loss of immunocompetence in dendritic cells (reduced secretion of stimulatory molecules, loss of antigen-sensitizing function, reduced phagocytic activity, and lack of maturation potential). Defective T-cell and dendritic cell function due to COX-2 driven PGE-2 biosynthesis is therefore an important mechanism by which tumors evade immunosurveillance.

5.   COX-2 BLOCKADE IN CANCER PREVENTION AND THERAPY

The molecular evidence suggests that aberrant induction and upregulation of COX-2 and the prostaglandin cascade play a significant role in carcinogenesis. But if inflammogenesis of cancer is to be upheld as a viable model, then the reciprocal relationship must also be true, *vis a vis.*, blockade of COX-2 should have significant inhibitory impact against carcinogenesis at multiple anatomic sites. Below, we consider the evidence from animal and human investigations.

5.1.   Animal Studies

In the past quarter century, scores of independent investigations employing animal models of carcinogenesis have generated compelling evidence that NSAIDs have significant and consistent effects against cancer development at several anatomic sites. Early investigations in the 1980's by Pollard et al. [175, 176] and Reddy et al. [177, 178] showed that administration of indomethacin and piroxicam significantly inhibited colon carcinogenesis. Karmali *et al.* [179] discovered similar effects of NSAIDs against breast cancer, and also elucidated differential effects of essential dietary fatty acids in prostaglandin (PG) biosynthesis and tumor promotion. Her studies showed that dietary supplementation with the n-6 fatty acid, linoleic acid, promoted tumor growth and development via enhanced arachidonic acid metabolism and elevated levels of PG activity, whereas the n-3 essential fatty acid, linolenic acid, had the opposite effect. Subsequent investigations have confirmed these early findings not only for colon and breast cancer, but also for lung cancer [180], prostate cancer [181], and a variety of other tumors that have been investigated in animal models [182]. In these studies of chemically induced tumors, supplemental administration of general NSAIDs such as aspirin, ibuprofen, piroxicam, sulindac, and others, in the diet or drinking water consistently reduced the growth and development of malignant neoplasms by 25 to 75%. It is important to note that recent preclinical studies have demonstrated even stronger antineoplastic effects of selective COX-2 inhibitors such as celecoxib, rofecoxib, valdecoxib, and nimesulide against colon cancer [89, 183] and breast cancer [90, 184], as well as other malignancies. Animal models of carcinogenesis therefore provide compelling evidence that NSAIDs inhibit tumor growth and development. Preclinical investigations provide consistent evidence that both selective and non-selective NSAIDs effectively inhibit chemically induced carcinogenesis of epithelial tumors.

5.2.   Human Studies of Non-Selective COX-2 Inhibitors

Recently, we comprehensively reviewed the published scientific literature on nonsteroidal anti-inflammatory drugs (NSAIDs) and cancer and evaluated results based upon epidemiologic criteria of judgment: consistency of results, strength of association, dose response, molecular specificity, and biological plausibility [185]. At the time of publication, sufficient data from 91 epidemiologic studies were available to examine the association of relative risk and NSAID intake for ten human malignancies.

In Figure 3, results have been updated to summarize the findings of 104 publications on NSAIDs and cancer [186–290]. Results show decreases in cancer risk ranging from 25 -75% with intake of NSAIDs (primarily aspirin or ibuprofen). Significant risk reductions were observed for each of the four major types of cancer: colon, breast, lung, and prostate cancer. Daily intake of NSAIDs (325 mg aspirin or 200 mg ibuprofen) produced risk reductions of 63% for colon cancer, 39% for breast cancer, 36% for lung cancer, and 39% for prostate cancer. Significant risk reductions were also observed for esophageal cancer (73%), stomach cancer (62%), and ovarian cancer (47%). NSAID effects became apparent after five or more years

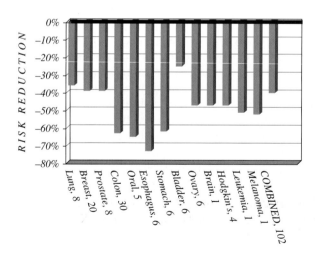

Relative cancer risk: Over the counter NSAIDs
Source: Data from Harris et al., Oncology Reports, 2005 [185]

of use and were stronger with longer duration. Observed protective effects were also consistently stronger for gastrointestinal malignancies (esophagus, stomach, and colon). Though the estimates for pancreatic cancer, urinary bladder cancer, and renal cancer showed heterogeneity among studies, the combined results for each of these malignancies also suggested a downward trend in the risk. Initial epidemiologic studies of malignant melanoma, Hodgkin's disease, and adult leukemia also found that NSAIDs were protective.

Our review of the epidemiologic literature therefore provides compelling evidence that regular intake of NSAIDs that non-selectively block cyclooxygenase-2 (COX-2) protects against the development of many types of cancer. When results are combined according to the relative incidence of these malignancies, it is estimated that regular NSAID intake is associated with a 36% reduction in overall cancer risk. This estimate is in close agreement with the findings of Gonzalez-Perez, et al. [291] who reported a 33% reduction in overall cancer risk with NSAID use.

5.3. Human Studies of Selective COX-2 Inhibitors

Epidemiologic studies of sporadic adenomatous polyps have consistently observed that intake of aspirin, ibuprofen, or other NSAIDs reduces the risk of polyp development [294, 295, 296, 297, 298, 299]. Subsequently, clinical studies confirmed that regular and continuing intake of an NSAID (aspirin, ibuprofen, piroxicam, sulindac) suppresses the formation of adenomatous polyps [300] and causes regression of existing polyps in patients with Familial Adenomatous Polyposis [301, 302, 303]. These studies which are thoroughly reviewed elsewhere [206, 304, 305] provide convincing evidence that sustained intake of compounds with COX-2 blocking activity not only inhibit the development of colon cancer *per se*, but also interrupt the evolution of preneoplastic lesions of the colonic mucosa.

Based upon results of the early studies, a number of clinical trials have been initiated to examine the effects of selective COX-2 inhibitors such as celecoxib (Celebrex) and rofecoxib (Vioxx) in preventing the development of precancerous lesions at various anatomic sites. Trial results reflect antineoplastic effects of these compounds: e.g., daily doses of selective COX-2 inhibitors effectively reduced the development of precancerous polyps of the colon [306, 307, 308], leukoplakia in the oral cavity [309], and dysplasia in Barett's esophagus [310]. But these encouraging results are tempered by concerns about cardiovascular risk associated with taking compounds that inhibit COX-2 [185, 311]. Before recommendations can be made, more studies are needed to determine if certain COX-2 inhibiting drugs can be taken at dosages that prevent cancer without increasing the risk of heart conditions.

Based on the epidemiologic evidence that nonselective NSAIDs reduce human cancer risk, we recently initiated case control studies of selective COX-2 inhibitors to assess their effects on the relative risk of breast cancer, prostate cancer, colon cancer, and lung cancer. In brief, we observed a significant risk reduction for each type of malignancy associated with daily use of a COX-2 inhibitor (celecoxib or rofecoxib) during the relatively short window of exposure between 1999–2005.

Regular intake of a COX-2 inhibitor produced a 79% risk reduction in breast cancer [312], and a 70% composite risk reduction across all four malignancies. Detailed results of these studies are given in chapter 9 of this book.

6. SUMMARY AND CONCLUSIONS

Cohesive scientific evidence from molecular, animal, and human investigations supports the hypothesis that aberrant induction of COX-2 and up-regulation of the prostaglandin cascade play a significant role in carcinogenesis, and reciprocally, blockade of the process has strong potential for cancer prevention and therapy. A summary of the evidence supporting the "inflammogenesis of cancer" is given below.

1. Expression of constitutive COX-2-catalyzed prostaglandin biosynthesis is induced by a plethora of cancer-causing agents including tobacco smoke and its components (e.g., polycylic aromatic amines, heterocyclic amines, nitrosamines), essential polyunsaturated fatty acids (e.g., unconjugated linoleic acid), mitogens, growth factors, pro-inflammatory cytokines, microbial agents, tumor promoters, and other epigenetic factors.
2. COX-2 expression is a characteristic feature of all premalignant neoplasms.
3. COX-2 expression is a characteristic feature of all malignant neoplasms, and expression tends to intensify with stage at detection and cancer progression and metastasis.
4. All essential features of carcinogenesis (mutagenesis, mitogenesis, angiogenesis, reduced apoptosis, metastasis, and immunosuppression) are linked to COX-2-driven prostaglandin (PGE-2) biosynthesis.
5. Animal studies show that COX-2 upregulation (in the absence of genetic mutations) is sufficient to stimulate the transformation of normal cells to invasive cancer and metastatic disease.
6. Non-selective COX-2 inhibitors, such as aspirin and ibuprofen, used on a regular basis reduce the risk of human cancer and precancerous lesions at all anatomic sites thus far investigated.
7. Selective COX-2 inhibitors, such as celecoxib, used on a regular basis reduce the risk of human cancer and precancerous lesions at all anatomic sites thus far investigated.

Results confirming that COX-2 blockade is effective for both cancer prevention and therapy have been tempered by recent observations that some COX-2 inhibitors may pose a risk to the cardiovascular system due to the imbalance created in prostaglandin biosynthesis. More studies are needed in order to determine if certain COX-2 inhibiting drugs can be taken at dosages that prevent cancer without increasing the risk of cardiovascular conditions. It should be emphasized that the "inflammogenesis model of cancer" is not mutually exclusive. Indeed, mutagenesis may in fact be an early consequence of the inflammatory process, and accumulation of cancer-causing mutations may be synergistic with inflammatory mediators in the evolution of cancer.

REFERENCES

1. Ahmedin J, Siegel R, Ward E, Murray T, Xu J, Smigal C, Thun MJ. Cancer Statistics, 2006. *CA Cancer J Clin* 56: 106–130, 2006.
2. Fearon ER, Vogelstein B. A genetic model for colorectal tumorigenesis. *Cell* 61 (5): 759–767, 1990.
3. Knudson AG. Two genetic hits (more or less) to cancer. *Nat Rev Cancer* 1 (2): 157–162, 2001.
4. Soto AM, Sonnenschein C. The somatic mutation theory of cancer: growing problems with the paradigm? *Biosessays* 26 (10): 1097–1107, 2004.
5. Lijinsy W. A view of the relation between carcinogenesis and mutagenesis. *Environ Mol Mutagen* 14 (16): 78–84, 1989.
6. Prehn RT. Cancers beget mutations versus mutations beget cancers. *Cancer Research* 54: 5296–5300, 1994.
7. Loeb LA, Loeb KR, Anderson JP. Multiple mutations and cancer. *Proc Natl Acad Sci USA* 100: 776–781, 2003.
8. Verma M, Maruvada P, Srivastara S. Epigenetics and cancer. *Crit Rev Clin Lab Sci* 41: 5–6, 2004.
9. Momparler RL. Cancer epigenetics. *Oncogene* 22(42): 6479–6483, 2003.
10. Virchow R. Reizung and Reizbarkeit. *Arch Pathol Anat Klin Med* 14: 1–63, 1858.
11. Virchow R. Aetiologie der neoplastischen Geschwulst/Pathogenie der neoplastischen Geschwulste. In: Die Krankhaften Geschwulste. Berlin: Verlag von August Hirschwald, pp. 57–101, 1863.
12. Balkwill F, Mantovani A. Inflammationand cancer: back to Virchow? *Lancet* 357: 539–545, 2001.
13. Schrieber H, Rowley DA. Inflammation and cancer. In: JI Gallin, R Snyderman, eds. Inflammation: Basic Principles and Clinical Correlates, third ed. Philadelphia: Lippincott Williams & Wilkins, pp. 1117–1129, 1999.
14. Coussens LM, Werb Z. Inflammation and cancer. *Nature* 420: 860–867, 2002.
15. Philip M, Rowley DA, Schreiber H. Inflammation as a tumor promoter in cancer induction. *Seminars in Cancer Biology* 14: 433–439, 2004.
16. Herschman HR. Historical Aspects of COX-2. In: RE Harris, ed. COX-2 Blockade in Cancer Prevention and Therapy. Human Press, Totowa, NJ, 2002.
17. Koki AT, Leahy KM, Harmon JM, Masferrer JL. Cyclooxygenase-2 and cancer. In: RE Harris, ed. COX-2 Blockade in Cancer Prevention and Therapy. Human Press, Totowa, NJ, 2002.
18. Harris RE. Cyclooxygenase-2 blockade in cancer prevention and therapy: widening the scope of impact. In: RE Harris, ed. COX-2 Blockade in Cancer Prevention and Therapy. Human Press, Totowa, NJ, 2002.
19. Robbins SL, Cotran RS. Pathologic Basis of Disease. 2nd edn, WB Saunders Company, Philadelphia, PA, 1979.
20. Kumar V, Fausto N, Abbas AK. Robbins and Cotran Pathologic Basis of Disease. 7th edn, WB Saunders Company, Philadelphia, PA, 2004.
21. Eberhart CE, Coffey RJ, Radhika A, Giardiello FM, Ferrenbach S, DuBois RN. Up-regulation of cyclooxygenase-2 gene expression in human colorectal adenomas and adenocarcinomas. *Gastroenterology* 107: 1183–1188, 1994.
22. Sano H, Kawahito Y, Wilder RR, Hashiramoto A, Mukai S, Asai K, Kimura S, Kato H, Kondo M, Hla T. Expression of cyclooxygenase-1 and -2 in colorectal cancer. *Cancer Res* 55: 3785–3789, 1995.
23. Dubois RN, Smalley WE. Cyclooxygenase, NSAIDs, and colorectal cancer. *J Gastroenterology* 31: 898–906, 1996.
24. Parrett ML, Harris RE, Joarder FS, Ross MS, Clausen KP, Robertson FM. Cyclooxygenase-2 gene expression in human breast cancer. *International Journal of Oncology* 10: 503–507, 1997.
25. Hwang D, Scollard D, Byrne J, Levine E. Expression of cyclooxygenase-1 and cyclooxygenase-2 in human breast cancer. *J Natl Cancer Inst* 90 (6): 455–460, 1998.
26. Morris CD, Armstrong GR, Bigley G, Green H, Attwood SE. Cyclooxygenase-2 expression in the Barrett's metaplasia-dysplasia-adnocarcinoma sequence. *Am J Gastroenterol* 96 (4): 991–996, 2001.

27. Lagorce C, Paraf F, Vidaud D, Couvelard A, Wendum D, Martin A, Flejou JF. Cyclooxygenase-2 is expressed frequently and early in Barrett's eosophagus and associated adenocarcinoma. *Histopathology* 42 (5): 457–465, 2003.

28. Buskens CJ, Van Rees BP, Sivula A, Reitsma JB, Haglund C, Bosma PJ, Offerhaus GJ, Van Lanschot JJ, Ristimaki A. Prognostic significance of elevated cyyclooxygenase-2 expression in patients with adenocarcinoma of the esophagus. *Z Gastroenterol* 41 (7): 678–681, 2003.

29. Shirahama T, Sakakura C. Overexpression of cyclooxygenase-2 in squamous cell carcinoma of the urinary bladder. *Clin Cancer Res* (3): 558–561, 2001.

30. Shirahama T. Cyclooxygenase-2 expression is up-regulated in transitional cell carcinoma and its preneoplastic lesions in the human urinary bladder. *Clin Cancer Res* 6 (6): 2424–2430, 2000.

31. Mohammed SI, Knapp DW, Bostwick DG, Foster RS, Khan KN, Masferrer JL, Woerner BM, Snyder PW, Koki AT. Expression of cyclooxygenase-2 (COX-2) in human invasive transitional cell carcinoma (TCC) of the urinary bladder. *Cancer Res* 59 (22): 5647–5650, 1999.

32. Oku S, Higashi M, Imazono Y, Sueyoshi K, Enokida H, Kubo H, Yonezawa S, Shirahama T. Overexpression of cyclooxygenase-2 in high-grade human transitional cell carcinoma of the upper urinary tract. *BJU Int* 91 (1): 109–114, 2003.

33. Barnes N, Haywood P, Flint P, Knox WF, Bundred NJ. Survivin expression in *in situ* and invasive breast cancer relates to COX-2 expression and DCIS recurrence. *Br J Cancer* 94 (2): 253–258, 2006.

34. Perrone G, Santini D, Vincenzi B, Zagami M, La Cesa A, Bianchi A, Altomare V, Primavera A, Battista ZC, Vetrani A, Tonini G, Rabitti C. Cox-2 expression in DCIS: correlation with VEGF, HER-2/neu, prognostic molecular markers and clinico-pathological features. *Histopathology* 46 (5): 561–568, 2005.

35. Boland GP, Butt IS, Prasad R, Knox WF, Bundred NJ. COX-2 expression is associated with an aggressive phenotype in ductal carcinoma in situ. *Br J Cancer* 90 (2): 423–429, 2004.

36. Nakopoulou L, Mylona E, Papadaki I, Kapranou A, Giannopoulou I, Markaki S, Keramopoulous A. Overexpression of cyclooxygenase-2 is associated with a favorable prognostic phenotype in breast carcinoma. *Pathobiology* 72 (5): 241–249, 2005.

37. Mehrotra S, Morimiya A, Agarwal B, Konger R, Badve S. Microsomal prostaglandin E2 synthase-1 in breast cancer: a potential target for therapy. *J Pathol* 208 (3): 356–363, 2006.

38. Hartmann LC, Lingle W, Frost MH, Shaun D, Maloney RA, Vierkant V, Pankratz S, Tisty T, Degnim AC, Visscher DW. COX-2 expression in atypia: correlation with breast cancer risk. Abstract No. 2353, *American Association for Cancer Research*, 97th Annual Meeting, 2006.

39. Kim JY, Lim SJ, Park K, Lee CM, Kim J. Cyclooxygenase-2 and c-erbB-2 expression in uterine cervical neoplasm assessed using tissue microarrays. *Gynecol Oncol* 97 (2): 337–341, 2005.

40. Farley J, Uyehara C, Hashiro G, Belnap C, Birrer M, Salminen E. Cyclooxygenase-2 expression predicts recurrence of cervical dysplasia following loop electrosurgical excision procedure. *Gynecol Oncol* 92 (2): 596–602, 2004.

41. Sales KJ, Katz AA, Davis M, Hinz S, Soeters RP, Hofmeyr MD, Millar RP, Jabbour HN. Cyclooxygenase-2 expression and prostaglandin E(2) synthesis are up-regulated in carcinomas of the cervix. *J Clin Endocrinol Metab* 86 (5): 2243–2249, 2001.

42. Lee JS, Choi YD, Lee JH, Nam JH, Choi C, Lee MC, Parck CS, Juhng SW, Kim HS, Min KW. Expression of cyclooxygenase-2 in adenocarcinomas of the uterine cervix and its relation to angiogenesis and tumor growth. *Gynecol Oncol* 95 (3): 523–529, 2004.

43. Chen HH, Su WC, Chou CY, Gui HR, Ho SY, Que J, Lee WY. Increased expression of nitric oxide synthase and cylooxygenase-2 is associated with poor survival in cervical cancer treated with radiotherapy. *Int J Radiat Oncol Biol Phys* 63 (4): 1093–1100, 2005.

44. Manchana T, Triratanachat S, Sirisabya N, Vasuratna A, Termrungruanglert W, Tresukosol D. Prevalence and prognostic significance of COX-2 expression in stage IB cervical cancer. *Gynecol Oncol* 100 (3): 556–560, 2006.

45. Kulkarni S, Rader JS, Zhang F, Liapis H, Koki AT, Masferrer JL, Subbaramaiah K, Dannenberg AJ. Cyclooxygenase-2 is overexpressed in human cervical cancer. *Clin Cancer Res* 7 (2): 429–434, 2001.

46. Soslow RA, Dannenberg AJ, Rush D, Woerner BM, Khan KN, Masferrer JL, Koki AT. COX-2 is expressed in human pulmonary, colonic, and mammary tumors. *Cancer* 89 (12): 2637–2645, 2000.

47. Khan KN, Masferrer JL, Woerner BM, Soslow R, Koki AT. Enhanced cyclooxygenase-2 expression in sporadic and familial adenomatous polyposis of the human colon. *Scand J Gastroenterol* 36 (8): 865–869, 2001.

48. Nasir A, Kaiser HE, Boulware D, Hakam A, Zhao H, Yeatman T, Barthel J, Coppola D. Cyclooxygenase-2 expression in right and left-sided colon cancer. *Clin Colorectal Cancer* 3 (4): 243–247, 2004.

49. Soumaoro LT, Uetake H, Takagi Y, Iida S, Higuchi T, Yasuno M, Enomoto M, Sugihara K. Co-expression of VEGF-C and COX-2 in human colorectal cancer and its association with lymph node metastasis. *Dis Colon Rectum* 49 (3): 393–398, 2006.

50. Hida T, Yatabe Y, Achiwa H, Muramatsu H, Kozaki K, Nakamura S, Ogawa M, Mitsudomi T, Sugiura T, Takahashi T. Increased expression of cyclooxygenase-2 occurs frequently in human lung cancers, specifically in adenocarcinomas. *Cancer Res* 58 (17): 3761–3764, 1998.

51. Wolff H, Saukkonen K, Anttila S, Karjalainen A, Vainio H, Ristimaki A. Expression of cyclooxygenase-2 in human lung carcinoma. *Cancer Res* 58 (22): 4997–5001, 1998.

52. Khuri FR, Wu H, Lee JJ, Kemp BL, Lotan R, Lippman SM, Feng L, Hong WK, Xu XC. Cyclooxygenase-2 overexpression is a marker of poor prognosis in stage I non-small cell lung cancer. *Clin Cancer Res* 7 (4): 861–867, 2001.

53. Achiwa H, Yatabe Y, Hida T, Kuroishi T, Kozaki K, Nakamura S, Ogawa M, Sugiura T, Mitsudomi T, Takahasi T. Prognostic significance of elevated cyclooxygenase-2 expression in primary, resected lung adenocarcinomas. *Clin Cancer Res* 5 (5): 1001–1005, 1999.

54. Marrogi AJ, Travis WD, Welsh JA, Khan MA, Rahim H, Tazelaar H, Pairolero P, Trastek V, Jett J, Caporaso NE, Liotta LA, Harris CC. Nitric oxide synthase, cyclooxygenase-2, and vascular endothelial growth factor in the angiogenesis of non-small cell lung carcinoma. *Clin Cancer Res* 6 (12): 4739–4744, 2000.

55. Marrogi A, Pass HI, Khan M, Metheny-Barlow LJ, Harris CC, Gerwin BI. Human mesothelioma samples overexpress both cyclooxygenase-2 (COX-2) and inducible nitric oxide synthase (NOS2): *in vitro* antiproliferative effects of a COX-2 inhibitor. *Cancer Res* 60 (14): 3696–3700, 2000.

56. Sudbo J, Ristimaki A, Sondresen JE, Kildal W, Goysen M, Koppang HS, Reith A, Risberg B, Nesland JM, Bryne M. Cyclooxygenease-2 (COX-2) expression in high-risk premalignant oral lesions. *Oral Oncol* 39 (5): 497–505, 2003.

57. Pannone G, Bufo P, Caiaffa MF, Serpco R, Lanza A, Lo Muzio L, Rubini C, Staibano S, Petruzzi M, De Benedictis M, Tursi A, De Rosa G, Macchia L. Cyclooxygenase-2 expression in oral squamous cell carcinoma. *Int J Immunopathol Pharmacol* 17 (3): 273–282, 2004.

58. Tang DW, Lin SC, Chang KW, Chi CW, Chang CS, Liu TY. Elevated expression of COX-2 in oral squamous cell carcinoma. *J Oral Pathol Med* 32 (9): 522–529, 2003.

59. Chang BW, Kim DH, Kowalski DP, Burleson JA, Son YH, Wilson LD, Haffty BG. Prognostic significance of cyclooxygenase-2 in oropharyngeal squamous cell carcinoma. *Clin Cancer Res* 10 (5): 1678–1684, 2004.

60. Gupta S. Srivastava M, Ahmad N, Bostwick DG, Mukhtar H. Overexpression of cyclooxygenase-2 in human prostate adenocarcinoma. *Prostate* 42: 73–78, 2000.

61. Yoshimura R, Sano H, Masuda C, Kawamura M, Tsubouchi Y, Charui J. Expression of cyclooxygenease-2 in prostate carcinoma. *Cancer* 89: 589–596, 2000.

62. Wang W, Bergh A, Damber JE. Cyclooxygenase-2 expression correlates with local chronic inflammation and tumor neovascularization in human prostate cancer. *Clin Cancer Res* 11 (9): 3250–3256, 2005.

63. Edwards J, Mukherjee R, Munro AF, Wells AC, Almushatat A, Bartlett JM. HER2 and COX2 expression in human prostate cancer. *Eur J Cancer* 40 (1): 50–55, 2004.

64. Kirschenbaum A, Liu X, Yao S, Levine AC. The role of cyclooxygenase-2 in prostate cancer. *Urology* 58 (2 Suppl 1): 127–131, 2001.

65. Masferrer JL, Leahy KM, Koki AT, Aweifel BS, Settle SL, Woerner BM, Edwards DA, Flickinger AG, Moore RJ, Seibert K. Antiangiogenic and antitumor activities of cyclooxygenase-2 inhibitors. *Cancer Res* 60 (5): 1306–1311, 2000.
66. Peng JP, Chang HC, Hwang CF, Hung WC. Overexpression of cyclooxygenase-2 in nasopharyngeal carcinoma and association with lymph node metastasis. *Oral Oncol* 41 (9): 903–908, 2005.
67. Lu H, Gong S. Expression of cyclooxygenase-2 and p53 and their correlation in carcinoma of larynx. *Lin Chuang Er Bi Yan Hou Ke Za Zhi* 18 (7): 421–423, 2004.
68. Sakamoto T, Kondo K, Yamasoba T, Sugasawa M, Kaga K. Elevated expression of cyclooxygenase-2 in adenocarcinomas of the parotid gland: insights into malignant transformation of pleomorphic adenoma. *Ann Otol Rhinol Laryngol* 113 (11): 930–935, 2004.
69. Liu J, Yu HG, Yu JP, Wang XL, Zhou XD, Luo HS. Overexpression of cylooxygenase-2 in gastric cancer correlated with the high abundance of vascular endothelial growth factor-C and lymphatic metastasis. *Med Oncol* 22 (4): 389–397, 2005.
70. Mrena J, Wiksten JP, Thiel A, Kokkola A, Pohjola L, Lundin J, Nordling S, Ristimaki A, Haglund C. Cyclooxygenase-2 is an independent prognostic factor in gastric cancer and its expression is regulated by the messenger RNA stability factor HuR. *Clin Cancer Res* 11 (20): 7362–7368, 2005.
71. Tucker ON, Dannenberg AJ, Yang EK, Zhang F, Teng L, Daly JM, Soslow RA, Masferrer JL, Woerner BM, Koki AT, Fahey TJ. 3rd. Cyclooxygenase-2 expression is up-regulated in human pancreatic cancer. *Cancer Res* 59 (5): 987–990, 1999.
72. Shiota G, Ikubo M, Noumi T, Goguchi N, Oyama K, Takano Y. Cyclooxygenase-2 expression in hepatocellular carcinoma. *Hepatogastroenterology* 46 (25): 407–412, 1999.
73. Ferrandina G, Zannoni GF, Ranelletti FO, Legge F, Gessi M, Salutari V, Gallotta V, Lauriola L, Scambia G. Cyclooxygenase-2 expression in borderline ovarian tumors. *Gynecol Oncol* 95 (1): 46–51, 2004.
74. Ferrandina G, Legge F, Ranelletti FO, Zannoni GF, Maggiano N, Evangelisti A, Mancuso S, Scambia G, Lauriola L. Cyclooxygenase-2 expression in endometrial carcinoma: correlation with clinicopathologic parameters and clinical outcome. *Cancer* 95 (4): 801–807, 2002.
75. Ristimaki A, Nieminen O, Saukkonen K, Hotakainen K, Nordling S, Haglund C. Expression of cyclooxygenase-2 in human transitional cell carcinoma of the urinary bladder. *Am J Pathol* 158 (3): 849–853, 2001.
76. Buckman SY, Gresham A, Hale P, Hruza G, Anast J, Masferrer J. COX-2 expression is induced by UVB exposure in human skin: implications for the development of skin cancer. *Carcinogenesis* 19 (5): 723–729, 1998.
77. Muller-Decker K. Cyclooxygenases in the skin. *J Dtsch Dermatol* Ges 2 (8): 668–675, 2004.
78. Kuzbicki L, Sarneck A, Chwirot BS. Expression of cyclooxygenase-2 in benign nevi and during human cutaneous melanoma progression. *Melanoma Res* 16 (1): 29–36, 2006.
79. Ladetto M, Vallet S, Trojan A, Dell' Aquila M, Monitillo L, Rosato R, Santo L, Drandi D, Bertola A, Falco P, Cavallo F, Ricca I, De Marco F, et al. Cyclooxygenase-2 (COX-2) is frequently expressed in multiple myeloma and is an independent predictor of poor outcome. *Blood* 105 (12): 4784–4791, 2005.
80. Sminia P, Stoter TR, van der Valk P, Elkhuizen PH, Tadema TM, Kuipers GK, Vandertop WP, Lafleur MV, Slotman BJ. Expression of cyclooxygenase-2 and epidermal growth factor receptor in primary and recurrent gliobastoma multiforme. *J Cancer Res Clinc Oncol* 131 (10): 653–661, 2005.
81. Buccoliero AM, Caldarella A, Arganini L, Mennonna P, Gallina P, Taddei A, Taddei GL. Cyclooxygenase-2 in oligodendroglioma: possible prognostic significance. *Neuropathology* 24 (3): 201–207, 2004.
82. Karin MM, Hayashi Y, Inoie M, Imai Y, Ito H, Yamamoto M. COX-2 expression in retinoblastoma. *Am J Opthamol* 129 (3): 398–401, 2000.
83. Dickens DS, Kozielski R, Khan J, Forus A, Cripe TP. Cyclooxygenase-2 expression in pediatric sarcoma. *Pediatr Dev Pathol* 5 (4): 356–364, 2002.

84. Lassus P, Ristimaki A, Huuhtanen R, Tukiainen E, Asko-Seljavaara S, Andersson LC, Miettinen M, Blomqvist C, Haglund C, Bohling T. Cyclooxygenase-2 expression in human soft-tissue sarcomas is related to epithelial differentiation. *Anticancer Res* 25 (4): 2669–2674, 2005.

85. Secchiro P, Barbarotto E, Gonelli A, Tiribelli M, Zerbinati C, Celeghini C, Agostinelli C, Pileri SA, Zauli G. Potential pathogenetic implication of cylcooxygenase-2 overexpression in B chronic lymphoid leukemia cells. *Am J Pathol* 167 (6): 1599–1607, 2005.

86. Hazar B, Ergin M, Sevrek E, Erdogan S, Tuncer I, Hakverdi S. Cyclooxygenase-2 (COX-2) expression in lymphoma. *Leuk Lymphoma* 45 (7): 1395–1399, 2004.

87. Li HL, Sun BZ, Ma FC. Expression of COX-2, iNOS, p. 53, and Ki-67 in gastric mucosa-associated lymphoid tissue lymphoma. *World J Gastroenterol* 10 (13): 1862–1866, 2004.

88. Liu CH, Chang SH, Narko K, Trifan OC, Wu MT, Smith E, Haudenschild C, Lane TF, Hla T. Overexpression of cyclooxygnease-2 is sufficient to induce tumorigenesis in transgenic mice. *J Biol Chem* 276 (21): 18563–18569, 2001.

89. Reddy BS, Rao CV. Role of synthetic and naturally occurring cyclooxygenase inhibitors in colon cancer prvention. In: RE Harris, ed. COX-2 Blockade in Cancer Prevention and Therapy. Human Press, Totowa, NJ, pp. 71–83, 2002.

90. Abou-Issa HM, Alshafie GA, Harris RE. Chemoprevention of breast cancer by nonsteroidal anti-inflammatory drugs and selective COX-2 blockade in animals. In: RE Harris, ed. COX-2 Blockade in Cancer Prevention and Therapy. Human Press, Totowa, NJ, pp. 85–98, 2002.

91. Schuller HM. The role of cyclooxygenase-2 in the prevention and therapy of lung cancer. In: RE Harris, ed. COX-2 Blockade in Cancer Prevention and Therapy. Human Press, Totowa, NJ, pp. 99–116, 2002.

92. Whelan J, McEntee MF. Nonsteroidal anti-inflammatory drugs, prostaglandins, and *Apc*-driven intestinal tumorigenesis. In: RE Harris, ed. COX-2 Blockade in Cancer Prevention and Therapy. Human Press, Totowa, NJ, pp. 117–145, 2002.

93. DuBois RN, Abramson SB, Rofford L, Gupta RA, Simon LS, Van De Putte LB, Lypsky PE. Cyclooxygenase in biology and disease. *FASEB J* 12: 1063–1073, 1998.

94. Wu KK. Cyclooxygenase-2 induction: molecular mechanisms and pathophysiologic roles. *J Lab Clin Med* 128: 242–245, 1996.

95. Shiff SJ, Rigas B. The role of cyclooxygenase inhibition in the antineoplastic effects of nonsteroidal anti-inflammatory drugs (NSAIDs). *J Exp Med* 190: 445–450, 1999.

96. Howe LR, Subbaramaiah K, Brown AMC, Dannenberg AJ. Cyclooxygenase-2: a target for the prevention and treatment of breast cancer. *Endocrine-Related Cancer* 8: 97–114, 2001.

97. Kelley DJ, Mestre JR, Subbaramaiah K, Sacks PG, Schantz SP, Tanabe T, Inoue H, Ramonetti JT, Dannenberg AJ. Benzo[a]pyrene up-regulates cyclooxygenase-2 gene expression in oral epithelial cells. *Carcinogenesis* 18 (4): 795–799, 1997.

98. Song S, Lippman SM, Zouj Y, Ye X, Ajani JA, Xu XC. Induction of cyclooxygenase-2 by benzo[a]pyrene diol epoxide through inhibiton of retinoic acid receptor-beta 2 expression. *Oncogene* 24 (56): 8268–8276, 2005.

99. Karmali RA. Dietary fatty acids, COX-2 blockade, and carcinogenesis. In: RE Harris, ed. COX-2 Blockade in Cancer Prevention and Therapy. Human Press, Totowa, NJ, pp. 3–12, 2002.

100. Burd R, Choy H, Dicker A. Potential for inhibitors of cyclooxygenase-2 to enhance tumor radioresponse. In: RE Harris, ed. COX-2 Blockade in Cancer Prevention and Therapy. Human Press, Totowa, NJ, pp. 301–311, 2002.

101. Jaimes EA, Tian RX, Pearse D, Raij L. Up-regulation of glomerular COX-2 by angiotensin II: role of reactive oxygen species. *Kidney Int* (5): 2143–2153, 2005.

102. Chang YW, Putzer K, Ren L, Kaboord B, Chance TW, Qoronfleh MW, Jakobi R. Differential regulation of cyclooxygenase 2 expression by small GTPases Ras, Rac1, and RhoA. *J Cell Biochem* 96(2): 314–329, 2005.

103. Coffey RJ, Hawkey CJ, Damstrup L, Graves-Deal R, Daniel VC, Dempsey PJ, Chinery R, Kirkland SC, DuBois RN, Jetton TL, Morrow JD. Epidermal growth factor receptor activation induces nuclear targeting of cylooxygenase-2, basolateral realease of prostaglandins, and mitogenesis in polarizing colon cancer cells. *Proc Natl Acad Sci USA* 94 (2): 657–662, 1997.

104. Moraitis D, Du B, De Lorenzo MS, Boyle JO, Weksler BB, Cohen EG, Carew JF, Altorki NK, Kopelovich L, Subbaramaiah K, Dannenberg AJ. Levels of cyclooxygenase-2 are increased in the oral mucosa of smokers: evidence for the role of epidermal growth factor receptor and its ligands. *Cancer Res* 65 (2): 664–670, 2005.

105. Chang YJ, Wu MS, Lin JT, Chen CC. Helicobacter pylori-induced invasion and angiogenesis of gastric cells is mediated by cyclooxygenase-2 induction through TLR2/TLR9 and promoter regulation. *J Immunol* 175 (12): 8242–8252, 2005.

106. Konturek PC, Hartwich A, Zuchowicz M, Labza H, Pierzchalski P. Helicobacter pylori, gastrin and cyclooxygenase in gastric cancer. *J Physiol Pharmacol* 51 (4, Pt 1): 737–749, 2000.

107. Singh A, Sharma H, Salhan S, Gupta SD, Bhatla N, Jain SK, Singh N. Evaluation of expression of apoptosis-related proteins and their correlation with HPV, telomerase activity, and apoptotic index in cervical cancer. *Pathobiology* 71 (6): 314–322, 2004.

108. Cheng AS, Chan HL, Leung WK, To KF, Go MY, Chan JY, Liew CT, Sung JJ. Expression of HBx and COX-2 in chronic hepatitis B, cirrhosis and hepatocellular carcinoma: implication of HBx in upregulation of COX-2. *Mod Pathol* 17 (10): 1169–1179, 2004.

109. Kaul R, Verma SC, Murakami M, Lan K, Choudhuri T, Robertson ES. Epstein-Barr virus protein can upregulate cyclo-oxygenase-2 expression through association with the suppressor of metastasis Nm23-H1. *J Virol* 80 (3): 1321–1331, 2006.

110. Ji YS, XI Q, Schmedtje JF Jr. Hypoxia induced high-mobility group protein I(Y) and transcription of the cyclooxygenase-2 gene in human vascular endothelium. *Circ Res* 83 (3): 295–304, 1998.

111. Diaz-Cruz ES, Brueggemeier RW. Interrelationships between cyclooxygenases and aromatase: unraveling the relevance of cyclooxygenase inhibitors in breast cancer. *Anticancer Agents Med Chem* 6(3): 221–232, 2006.

112. Muller N, Riedel M, Schwarz MJ. Psychotropic effects of COX-2 inhibitors–a possible new approach for the treatment of psychiatric disorders. *Pharmacopsychiatry* 37(6): 266–269, 2004.

113. Inoue H, Taba Y, Miwa Y, Yokota C, Miyagi M, Sasaguri T. Transcriptional and posttranscriptional regulation of cyclooxygenase-2 expression by fluid shear stress in vascular endothelial cells. *Arterioscler Thromb Vasc Biol* 22(9): 1415–1420, 2002.

114. Bezugla Y, Kolada A, Kamionka S, Bernard B, Scheibe R, Dieter P. COX-1 and COX-2 contribute differentially to the LPS-induced release of PGE2 and TxA2 in liver macrophages. *Prostaglandins Other Lipid Mediat* 79 (1–2): 93–100, 2006.

115. Karmali RA, Marsh J. Antitumor activity in rat mammary adenocarcinoma: effects of cyclooxygenase inhibitors and immunization against prostaglandin E2. *Prostaglandins Leukotrienes and Medicine* 23: 11–14, 1986.

116. Rose DP, Connolly JM. Omega-3 fatty acids as cancer chemopreventive agents. *Pharmacology and Therapeutics* 83: 217–244, 1999.

117. Harris RE, Robertson FM, Farrar WB, Brueggemeier RW. Genetic induction and upregulation of cyclooxygenase (COX) and aromatase (CYP-19): an extension of the dietary fat hypothesis of breast cancer. *Medical Hypotheses* 52 (4): 292–293, 1999.

118. Martey CA, Baglole CJ, Gasiewicz TA, Sime PJ, Phipps RP. The aryl hydrocarbon receptor is a regulator of cigarette smoke induction of the cyclooxygenase and prostaglandin pathways in human lung fibrobasts. *Am J Physiol Lung Cell Mol Physiol* 289 (3): 391–399, 2005.

119. Shin VY, Liu ES, Ye YN, Koo MW, Chu KM, Cho CH. A mechanistic study of cigarette smoke and cyclooxygenase-2 on proliferation of gastric cancer cells. *Toxicol Appl Pharmacol* 195(1): 103–112, 2004.

120. Liu ES, Shin VY, Ye YN, Luo JC, Wu WK, Cho CH. Cyclooxygenase-2 in cancer cells and macrophages induces colon cancer cell growth by cigarette smoke extract. *Eur J Pharmacol* 518(1): 47–55, 2005.

121. Cakir Y, Plummer HK 3rd, Tithof PK, Schuller HM. Beta-adrenergic and arachidonic acid-mediated growth regulation of human breast cancer cell lines. *Int J Oncol* J 1: 153–157, 2002.

122. Badawi AF, Habib SL, Mohammed MA, Abadi AA, Michael MS. Influence of cigarette smoking on prostaglandin synthesis and cyclooxygenase-2 gene expression in human urinary bladder cancer. *Cancer Invest* 20 (5–6): 651–656, 2002.

123. Izzotti A, Cartiglia C, Longobardi M, Balansky RM, D'Agostini F, Lubet RA, De Flora S. Alterations of gene expression in skin and lung of mice exposed to light and cigarette smoke. *FASEB J* 18 (13):1559–1561, 2004.

124. Rioux N, Castonaguay A. Prevention of NNK-induced lung tumorigenesis in A? J mice by acetylsalicylic acid and NS-398. *Cancer Res* 58: 5354–5360, 1998.

125. Castonguay A, Rioux N, Duperron C, Jalbert G. Inhibition of lung tumorigenesis by NSAIDs: a working hypothesis. *Exp Lung Res* 24: 605–615, 1998.

126. Tsai KS, Yang RS, Liu SH. Benzo[a]pyrene regulates osteoblast proliferation through an estrogen receptor-related cyclooxygenase-2 pathway. *Chem Res Toxicol* (5): 679–684, 2004.

127. Schuller HM, Plummer HK III, Bochsler PN, Dudrick P, Bell JL, Harris RE. Co-expression of beta-adrenergic receptors and cyclooxygenase-2 in pulmonary adenocarcinomas. *Int J Oncol* 19: 445–449, 2001.

128. Jang B-C, Hla T. Regulation of expression and potential carcinogenic role of cylcooxygenase-2. In: RE Harris, ed. COX-2 Blockade in Cancer Prevention and Therapy. Human Press, Totowa, NJ, pp. 3–12, 2002.

129. Ogino S, Brahmandam M, Kawasaki T, Kirkner GJ, Loda M, Fuchs CS. Combined Analysis of COX-2 and p53 Expressions Reveals Synergistic Inverse Correlations with Microsatellite Instability and CpG Island Methylator Phenotype in Colorectal Cancer. *Neoplasia* 8 (6): 458–464, 2006.

130. Chow LW, Zhu L, Loo WT, Lui EL. Aberrant methylation of cyclooxygenase-2 in breast cancer patients. *Biomed Pharmacother* 59 (2): S264–267, 2005.

131. Marnett LJ. Lipid peroxidation-DNA damage by malondialdehyde. *Mutat Res* 424: 83–95, 1999.

132. Hendrickse CW, Kelly RW, Radley S, Donovan IA, Beighley MRB, Neoptolemos JP. Lipid peroxidation and prostaglandins in colorectal cancer. *Br J Surg* 81: 1219–1223, 1994.

133. Plastara JP, Guengerich FP, Nebert DW, Marnett LJ. Xenobiotic-metabolizing cytochromes P450 convert prostaglandin endoperoxide to hydroxyheptadecatienoic acid and the mutagen, malondialdehyde. *J Biol Chem* 275: 11784–11790, 2000.

134. Marnett LJ, Basu AK, O'hara SM, Weller PE, Rahman AFMM, Oliver JP. Reaction of malon-dialdehyde with guanine nucleosides: formation of adducts containing oxadraza-bicyclononene residues in the base-pairing region. *J Am Chem Soc* 108: 1348–1350, 1986.

135. Sharma RA, Gescher A, Plastaras JP, Ceuratti C, Singh R, Gallacher-Horley B, Offord E, Marnett LJ, Steward WP, Plummer SM. Cyclooxygenase-2, malondialdehyde and pyrimidop-urinone adducts of deoxyguanosine in human colon cells. *Carcinogensis* 22 (9): 1557–1560, 2001.

136. Pai R, Soreghan B, Szabo IL, Pavelka M, Baatar D, Tarnawski AS. Prostaglandin E2 transacti-vates EGF receptor: a novel mechanism for promoting colon cancer growth and gastrointestinal hypertrophy. *Nat Med* 8 (3): 289–293, 2002.

137. Mestre JR, Subbaramaiah K, Sacks PG, Schantz SP, Tanabe T, Inoue H, Dannenberg AJ. Retinoids suppress epidermal growth factor-induced transcription of cyclooxygenase-2 in human oral squamous carcinoma cells. *Cancer Res* 57 (14): 2890–2895, 1997.

138. Kinoshita T, Takahashi Y, Sakashita T, Inoue H, Tanabe T, Yoshimoto T. Growth stimulation and induction of epidermal growth factor receptor by overexpression of cyclooxygenases 1 and 2 in human colon carcinoma cells. *Biochim Biophys Acta* 1438 (1): 120–130, 1999.

139. Zhao Y, Agarwal VR, Mendelson CR, Simpson ER. Estrogen biosynthesis proximal to a breast tumor is stimulated by PGE2 via cyclic AMP, leading to activation of promoter II of the CYP19 (aromatase) gene. *Endocrinology* 137 (12): 5739–5742, 1996.

140. Brueggemeier RW, Quinn AL, Parrett ML, Joarder FS, Harris RE, Robertson FM. Correlation of aromatase and cyclooxygenase gene expression in human breast cancer specimens. *Cancer Lett* 140 (1–2): 27–35, 1999.

141. Richards JA, Brueggemeier. Interactions of cyclooxygenase and aromatase pathways in normal and malignant breast cells. In: RE Harris, ed. COX-2 Blockade in Cancer Prevention and Therapy. Human Press, Totowa, NJ, 2002.

142. Weinberg OK, Marquez-Garban DC, Fishbein MC, Goodglick L, Garban HJ, Dubinett SM, Pietras RJ. Aromatase inhibitors in human lung cancer therapy. *Cancer Res* 65 (24): 11287–11291, 2005.

143. Fiorelli G, Picariello L, Martineti V, Tonelli F, Brandi ML. Estrogen synthesis in human colon cancer epithelial cells. *J Steroid Biochem Mol Biol* 71 (5–6): 223–230, 1999.
144. Ellem SJ, Risbridger GP. Aromatase and prostate cancer. *Minerva Endocrinol* 31 (1): 1–12, 2006.
145. Polakis P. The oncogenic activation of beta-catenin. *Curr Opin Genet Dev* 9 (1): 15–21, 1999.
146. Henderson BR. Nuclear-cytoplasmic shuttling of APC regulates beta-catenin subcellular localization and turnover. *Nat Cell Biol* 2 (9): 653–660, 2000.
147. Clevers H. Colon cancer-understanding how NSAIDs work. *NEJM* 354 (7): 761–763, 2006.
148. Castellone MD, Teramoto H, Williams BO, Druey KM, Gutkind JS. Prostaglandin E2 promotes colon cancer cell growth through a GS-axin-beta-catenin signaling axis. *Science* 310: 1504–1510, 2005.
149. He T-C. Association of COX-2 and PPARs in carcinogenesis and chemoprevention. In: RE Harris, ed. COX-2 Blockade in Cancer Prevention and Therapy. Human Press, Totowa, NJ, 2002.
150. Folkman J. Angiogenesis. *Annu Rev Med* 57: 1–18, 2006.
151. Gallo O, Franchi A, Magnelli L, Sardi I, Vannacci A, Boddi V, Chiarugi V, Masini E. Cyclooxygenase-2 pathway correlates with VEGF expression in head and neck cancer. Implications for tumor angiogenesis and metastasis. *Neoplasia* 3: 53–61, 2001.
152. Masferrer JL, Koki A, Seibert K, Zweifel BS, Settle SL, Woerner BM. Antiangiogenic and antitumor acivities of cyclooxygenase-2 inhibitors. *Cancer Res* 60: 1306–1311, 2000.
153. Gupta RA, DuBois RN. Cyclooxygenase-2, prostaglandins, and colorectal carcinogenesis. In: RE Harris, ed. COX-2 Blockade in Cancer Prevention and Therapy. Human Press, Totowa, NJ, 2002.
154. Subbaramaiah K, Norton L, Gerald W, Dannenberg AJ. Cyclooxygenase-2 is overexpressed in HER-2/neu-positive breast cancer-evidence for involvement of AP-1 and PEA3. *J Biol Chem* 277: 18649–18657, 2002.
155. Benoit V, Relic BG, Leval Xd X, Chariot A, Merville MP, Bours V. Regulation of HER-2 oncogene expression by cyclooxygenase-2 and prostaglandin E2. *Oncogene* 23 (8): 1631–1635, 2004.
156. Tsuji M, Kuwano S, DuBois RN. Cyclooxygenase-2 expression in human colon cancer cells increases metastatic potential. *Proc Natl Acad Sci USA* 94: 3336–3340, 1997.
157. Sivula A, Talvensaari-Mattila A, Lundin J, Joensuu H, Haglund C, Ristimaki A, Turpeenniemi-Hujanen T. Association of cyclooxygenase-2 and matrix metalloproteinase-2 expression in human breast cancer. *Breast Cancer Res Treat* 89 (3): 215–220, 2005.
158. Byun JH, Lee MA, Roh SY, Shim BY, Hong SH, Ko YH, Ko SJ, Woo IS, Kang JH, Hong YS, Lee KS, Lee AW, Park GS, Lee KY. Association between cyclooxygenase-2 and matrix metalloproteinase-2 expression in non-small cell lung cancer. *Jpn J Clin Oncol* 36 (5): 263–268, 2006.
159. Sun WH, Sun YL, Fang RN, Shao Y, Xu HC, Xue QP, Ding GX, Cheng YL. Expression of cyclooxygenase-2 and matrix metalloproteinase-9 in gastric carcinoma and its correlation with angiogenesis. *Jpn J Clin Oncol* 35 (120): 707–713, 2005.
160. Larkins TL, Nowell M, Singh S, Sanford GL. Inhibition of cyclooxygenase-2 decreases breast cancer cell motility, invasion and matrix metalloproteinase expression. *BMC Cancer* 6 (1): 181, 2006.
161. Kinugasa Y, Hatori M, Ito H, Jurihara Y, Ito D, Nagumo M. Inhibition of cyclooxygenase-2 suppresses invasiveness of oral squamous cell carcinoma cell lines via down-regulation of matrix metalloproteinase-2 and CD44. *Clin Exp Metastasis* 21 (8): 737–745, 2004.
162. Pan MR, Chuang LY, Hung WC. Nonsteroidal anti-inflammatory drugs inhibit matrix metalloproteinase-2 expression via repression of transcription in lung cancer cells. *FEBS Lett* 508 (3): 365–368, 2001.
163. Rigas B, Shiff SJ. Nonsteroidal anti-inflammatory drugs and the induction of apoptosis in colon cells: evidence for PHS-dependent and PHS-independent mechanisms. *Apoptosis* 4 (5): 373–381, 1999.
164. Battu S, Rigaud M, Beneytout JL. Resistance to apoptosis and cyclooxygenease-2 expression in a human adenocarcinoma cell line HT29 CL19A. *Anticancer Res* 18 (5A): 3579–3583, 1998.

165. Petersen C, Petersen S, Milas L, Lang FF, Tofilon PJ. Enhancement of intrinsic tumor cell radiosensitivity induced by a selective cyclooxygenase-2 inhibitor. *Clin Cancer Res* 6 (6): 2513–2520, 2000.

166. Johnsen JI, Lindskog M, Ponthan F, Pettersen I, Elfman L, Orrego A, Sveinbjornsson B, Kogner P. Cyclooxygenase-2 is expressed in neuroblastoma, and nonsteroidal anti-inflammatory drugs induce apoptosis and inhibit tumor growth *in vivo*. *Cancer Res* 64 (20): 7210–7215, 2004.

167. Tsujii M, Dubois RN. Alterations in cellular adhesion and apoptosis in epithelial cells overexpressing prostaglandin endoperoxide synthase 2. *Cell* 83: 493–501, 1995.

168. Tang X, Sun YJ, Half E, Kuo MT, Sinicrope F. Cyclooxygenase-2 overexpression inhibits death receptor 5 expression and confers resistance to tumor necrosis factor-related apoptosis-inducing ligand-induced apoptosis in human colon cancer cells. *Cancer Res* 62 (17): 4903–4908, 2002.

169. Totzke G, Schulze-Osthoff K, Janicke RU. Cyclooxygenase-2 (COX-2) inhibitors sensitize tumor cells specifically to death receptor-induced apoptosis independently of COX-2 inhibition. *Oncogene* 22 (39): 8021–8030, 2003.

170. Yamanaka Y, Shiraki K, Inoue T, Miyashita K, Fuke H, Yamaguchi Y, Yamamoto N, Ito K, Sugimoto K, Nakano T. Cox-2 inhibitors sensitize human hepatocellular carcinoma cells to TRAIL-induced apoptosis. *Int J Mol Med* 18 (1): 41–47, 2006.

171. Subbaramaiah K, Chung WJ, Dannenberg AJ. Ceramide regulates the transcription of cyclooxygenase-2: evidence for involvement of extracellular signal regulated kinase/c-jun N-terminal kinase and p38 mitogen-activated protein kinase pathways. *J Biol Chem* 273: 32943–32949, 1998.

172. Martin S, Phillips DC, Szekely-Szucs K, Elghazi L, Desmots F, Houghton JA. Cyclooxygense-2 inhibition sensitizes human colon carcinoma cells to Trail-induced apoptosis through clustering of DR5 and concentrating death-inducing signaling complex components into ceramide-enriched caveolae. *Cancer Res* 65 (24): 11447–11458, 2005.

173. Staveley-O'Carroll K, Sotomayor E, Montgomery J. Induction of antigen-specific T cell anergy: an early event in the course of tumor progression. *Proc Natl Acad Sci USA* 95: 1178–1183, 1998.

174. Pockaj BA, Basu GD, Pathangey LB, Gray RJ, Hernandez JL, Gendler SJ, Mukherjee P. Reduced T-cell and dendritic cell function is related to cyclooxygenase-2 overexpression and prostaglandin E2 secretion in patients with breast cancer. *Ann Surg Oncol* 11: 328–339, 2004.

175. Pollard M, Luckert PH. Prolonged antitumor effect of indomethacin on autochthonous intestinal tumors in rats. *J Natl Cancer Inst* 70: 1103–5, 1983.

176. Pollard M, Luckert PH. Prevention and treatment of primary intestinal tumors in rats by piroxicam. *Cancer Res* 49: 6471–3, 1989.

177. Reddy BS, Maruyama H, Kelloff G. Dose related inhibition of colon carcinogenisis by dietary piroxicam, a nonsteroidal antiinflammatory drug, during different stages of rat colon tumor development. *Cancer Res* 47: 5340–6, 1987.

178. Reddy BS, Tokumo K, Kulkarni N, Aligia C, Kelloff G. Inhibition of colon carcinogenesis by prostaglandin synthesis inhibitors and related compounds. *Carcinogenesis* 13: 1019–23, 1992.

179. Karmali RA, Marsh J, Fuchs C. Effect of omega-3 fatty acids on growth of a rat mammary tumor. *J Natl Cancer Inst* 73: 457–461, 1984.

180. Duperron C, Castonguay A. Chemopreventive efficacies of aspirin and sulindac against lung tumorigenesis in A/J mice. *Carcinogenesis* 18: 1001–1006, 1997.

181. Rose DP, Connolly JM. Effects of fatty acids and eicosanoid synthesis inhibitors on the growth of two human prostate cancer cell lines. *Prostate* 18: 243–254, 1991.

182. Kelloff GJ, Steele VE, Sigman CC. Chemoprevention of cancer by NSAIDs and selective COX-2 blockade. In: RE Harris, ed. COX-2 Blockade in Cancer Prevention and Therapy. Humana Press, Totowa, NJ, pp. 279–300, 2002.

183. Kawamori T, Rao CV, Siebert K, Reddy BS. Chemopreventive activity of celecoxib, a specific cyclooxygenase 2 inhibitor, against colon carcinogenesis. *Cancer Res* 58: 409–412, 1998.

184. Harris RE, Alshafie GA, Abou-Issa H, Seibert K. Chemoprevention of breast cancer in rats by celecoxib, a specific cyclooygenase-2 (COX-2) inhibitor. *Cancer Res* 60: 2101–2103, 2000.

185. Harris RE, Beebe-Donk J, Doss H, Burr-Doss D. Aspirin, ibuprofen, and other non-steroidal anti-inflammatory drugs in cancer prevention: a critical review of non-selective COX-2 blockade (Review). Oncology Reports 13: 559–583, 2005.

186. Paganini-Hill A, Chao A, Ross RK, Henderson BE. Aspirin use and chronic diseases: a cohort study of the elderly. *Br Med J* 299: 1247–1250, 1989.

187. Thun MJ, Namboodiri MM, Heath CW Jr. Aspirin use and reduced risk of fatal colon cancer. *N Engl J Med* 325: 1593, 1991.

188. Gridley G, McLaughlin JK, Ekbom A. Incidence of cancer among patients with rheumatoid arthritis. *J Natl Cancer Inst* 85: 307–311, 1993.

189. Pinczowski D, Ekbom A, Baron J, Yuen J, Adami H-O. Risk factors for colorectal cancer in patients with ulcerative colitis: a case-control; study. *Gastroentology* 107: 117–120, 1994.

190. Schreinemachers DM, Everson RB. Aspirin use and lung, colon, and breast cancer incidence in a prospective study. *Epidemiology* 5: 138–146, 1994.

191. Giovannucci E, Rimm EB, Stampfer MJ, Colditz GA, Asherio A, Willett WC. Aspirin use and the risk for colorectal cancer and adenoma in male health professionals. *Ann Intern Med* 121: 241–246, 1994.

192. Giovannucci E, Egan KM, Hunter DJ, Stampfer MJ, Colditz GA, Willett WC, Speizer FE. Aspirin and the risk of colorectal cancer in women. *N Engl J Med* 333: 609–614, 1995.

193. Kauppi M, Pukkala E, Isomaki H. Low incidence of colorectal cancer in patients with rheumatoid arthritis. *Clin Exp Rheumatol* 14: 551–553, 1996.

194. Smalley W, Ray WA, Daugherty J, Griffin MR. Use of nonsteroidal anti-inflammatory drugs and incidence of colorectal cancer. *Arch Intern Med* 159: 161–166, 1999.

195. Collet JP, Sharpe C, Belzile E, Boivin J-F, Hanley J, Abenhaim L. Colorectal cancer prevention by nonsteroidal anti-inflammatory drugs: effects of dosage and timing. *Br J Cancer* 81: 62–68, 1999.

196. Langman MJ, Cheng KK, Gilman EA, Lancashire RJ. Effect of anti-inflammatory drugs on overall risk of common cancer: case-control study in a general practice research database. *Br Med J* 320: 1642–1646, 2000.

197. Garcia Rodriguez LA, Huerta-Alvarez C. Reduced risk of colorectal cancer among long-term users of aspirin and non-aspirin nonsteroidal anti-inflammatory drugs. *Epidemiology* 12: 88–93, 2001.

198. Peleg I, Maibach H, Brown SH, Wilcox CM. Aspirin and nonsteroidal anti-inflammatory drug use and the risk of subsequent colorectal cancer. *Arch Intern Med* 154: 394–399, 1994.

199. Muscat J, Stellman SD, Wynder EL. Nonsteroidal anti-inflammatory drugs and colorectal cancer. *Cancer* 74: 1847–1854, 1994.

200. Reeves MJ, Newcomb PA, Trentham-Diez A, Storer BE, Remington P. Nonsteroidal anti-inflammatory drug use and protection against colorectal cancer in women. *Cancer Epidemiol Biomarkers Prev* 5: 955–960, 1996.

201. LaVecchia C, Negri E, Franceschi S, Conti E, Montella M, Giacosa A, et al. Aspirin and colorectal cancer. Br J Cancer 76: 675–677, 1997.

202. Rosenberg L, Louik C, Shapiro S. Nonsteoridal anti-inflammatory drug use and reduced risk of large bowel carcinoma. *Cancer* 82: 3236–33, 1998.

203. Friedman GD, Coates AO, Potter JD, Slattery ML. Drugs and colon cancer. *Pharmacoepidemol Drug Safety* 7: 99–106, 1998.

204. Coogan PF, Rosenberg L, Louik C, Zauber AG, Stolley PD, Strom BL, et al. NSAIDs and risk of colorectal cancer according to presence or absence of family history of the disease. *Cancer Causes Control* 11: 249–255, 2000.

205. Rahme E, Barkum AN, Goubouti Y, Bardou M. The cyclooxygenase2 selective inhibitors rofecoxib and celecoxib prevent colorectal neoplasia occurrence and recurrence. *Gastroenterology* 125 (2): 404–412, 2003.

206. Thun MJ, Henley SJ. Epidemiology of nonsteroidal anti-inflammatory drugs in colorectal cancer. In: RE Harris, ed. COX-2 Blockade in Cancer Prevention and Therapy. Humana Press, Totowa, NJ, pp. 35–55, 2002.

207. Slattery ML, Samowitz W, Hoffman M, Ma KN, Levin TR, Neuhausen S. Aspirin, NSAIDs, and colorectal cancer: possible involvement in an insulin-related pathway. *Cancer Epidemiol Biomarkers Prev* 13 (4): 538–545, 2004.

208. Thun MJ, Namboodiri MM, Calle EE, Flanders WD, Heath CW. Aspirin use and risk of fatal cancer. *Cancer Res* 53: 1322–1327, 1993.

209. Egan KM, Stampfer MJ, Giovannucci E, Rosner BA, Colditz GA. Prospective study of regular aspirin use and the risk of breast cancer. *J Natl Cancer Inst* 88: 988–993, 1996.

210. Harris RE, Kasbari S, Farrar WB. Prospective study of nonsteroidal anti-inflammatory drugs and breast cancer. *Oncology Reports* 6: 71–73, 1999.

211. Johnson TJ, Anderson KI, Lazovich D, Folsom AR. Association of aspirin and other nonsteroidal anti-inflammatory drug use with incidence of postmenopausal breast cancer. *Proc Amer Assoc Cancer Res* 42: Abstract 4098, 763, 2001.

212. Harris RE, Chlebowski RT, Jackson RD, Frid DJ, Ascensco JL, Anderson G, Loar A, Rodabough RJ, White E, McTiernan A. Breast cancer and nonsteroidal anti-inflammatory drugs: prospective results from the Women's Health Initiative. *Cancer Research* 63: 6096–6101, 2003.

213. Harris RE, Namboodiri KK, Farrar WB. Epidemiologic study of non-steroidal anti-inflammatory drugs and breast cancer. *Oncology Reports* 2: 591–592, 1995.

214. Rosenberg L. Nonsteroidal anti-inflammatory drugs and cancer. *Prev Med* 24: 107–109, 1995.

215. Harris RE, Namboodiri KK, Farrar WB. Nonsteroidal anti-inflammatory drugs and breast cancer. *Epidemiology* 7: 203–205, 1996.

216. Neuget AI, Rosenbert DJ,Ahsan H, Jacobson JS, Wahid N, Hagan M, Rahman MI, Khan ZR, Chen L, Pablos-Mendez A, Shea S. Association between coronary heart disease and cancers of the breast, prostate, and colon. *Cancer Epidemiol Biomarker Prev* 7: 869–873, 1998.

217. Coogan PF, Rao Sr, Rosenberg L, Palmer JR, Strom BL, Zauber AG, Stolley PD, Shapiro S. The relationship of nonsteroidal anti-inflammatory drug use to the risk of breast cancer. *Prev Med* 29 (2): 72–76, 1999.

218. Sharpe CR, Collet JP, McNutt M, Belzille E, Boivin JF, Hanley JA. Nested case control study of the effects of nonsteroidal anti-inflammatory drugs on breast cancer risk and stage. *Br J Can* 83: 112–120, 2000.

219. Cotterchio M, Kreiger N, Steingart A, Buchan G. Nonsteroidal anti-inflammatory drug (NSAID) use and breast cancer. *SER Abstract, Amer J Epidemiol* 151: S72, 2000.

220. Langman MJ, Chen KK, Gilman EA, Lancashire RJ. Effect of anti-inflammatory drugs on the overall risk of common cancer: case control study in general practice research database. *Br Med J* 320: 1642–1646, 2000.

221. Meier CR, Schmitz S, Jeck H. Association between acetaminophen or nonsteroidal anti-inflammatory drugs and risk of developing ovarian, breast, or colon cancer. *Pharmacotherapy* 22 (3): 303–309, 2002.

222. Moorman PG, Grubber JM, Millikan RC, Newman B. Association between nonsteroidal anti-inflammatory drugs (NSAIDs) and invasive breast cancer and carcinoma *in situ* of the breast. *Cancer Causes and Control* 14: 915–922, 2003.

223. Terry MB, Gammon MD, Zang FF, Tawfik H, Teitelbaum SL, Britton JA, Subbaramaiah K, Dannenberg AJ, Neuget AI. Association of frequency and duration of aspirin use and hormone receptor status with breast cancer risk. *JAMA* 291 (20): 2433–2440, 2004.

224. Zhang Y, Coogan PF, Palmer JR, Strom BL, Rosenberg L. Use of nonsteroidal anti-inflammatory drugs and risk of breast cancer: the Case-Control Surveillance Study revisited. *Am J Epidemiol* 162 (2): 165–170, 2005.

225. Peto R, Gray R, Collins R, Wheatley K, Hennekens C, Jamrozik K, Warlow C, Hafner B, Thompson E, Norton S. Randomised trial of prophylactic daily aspirin in British male doctors. *Br Med J (Clin Res Ed)* 296 (6618): 313–316, 1988.

226. Harris RE, Beebe-Donk J, Schuller HM. Chemoprevention of lung cancer by nonsteroidal anti-inflammatory drugs among cigarette smokers. *Oncology Reports* 9: 693–695, 2002.

227. Akhmedkhanov A, Toniolo P, Zeleniuch-Jacquotte A, Koenig KL, Shore RE. Aspirin and lung cancer in women. *Br J Cancer* 87 (11): 1337–1338, 2002.

228. Moysich KB, Menezes RJ, Ronsani A, Swede H, Reid ME, Cummings KM, Falkner KL, Loween GM, Bepler G. Regular aspirin use and lung cancer risk. *BMC Cancer* 2(1): 31, 2002.

229. Holick CN, Michaud DS, Leitzmann MF, Willett WC, Giovannucci E. Aspirin use and lung cancer in men. *Br J Cancer* 89 (9): 1705–1708, 2003.

230. Muscat JE, Chen SQ, Richie JP Jr, Altorki NK, Citron M, Olson S, Neugut AI, Stellman SD. Risk of lung carcinoma among users of nonsteroidal anti-inflammatory drugs. *Cancer* 97 (7): 1732–1736, 2003.

231. Roberts RO, Jacobson DJ, Girman CJ, Rhodes T, Lieber MM, Jacobsen SJ. A population based study of daily nonsteroidal anti-inflammatory drug use and prostate cancer. *Mayo Clin Proc* 77 (3): 219–225, 2002.

232. Leitzman MF, Stampfer MJ, Ma J, Chan JM, Colditz GA, Willett WC, Giovannucci E. Aspirin use in relation to risk of prostate cancer. *Cancer Epidemiol Biomarkers Prev* (101): 1108–1111, 2002.

233. Habel LA, Zhao W, Stanford JL. Daily aspirin use and prostate cancer risk in a large, multiracial cohort in the US. *Cancer Causes Control* 13 (5): 427–434, 2002.

234. Nelson JE, Harris RE. Inverse association of prostate cancer and nonsteroidal anti-inflammatory drugs (NSAIDs): results of a case control study. *Oncology Reports* 7: 169–170, 2000.

235. Norrish AE, Jackson RT, McRae CU. Nonsteroidal anti-inflammatory drugs and prostate cancer progression. *International Journal of Cancer* 77: 511–515, 1998.

236. Irani J, Ravery V, Pariente JL, Chartier-Kastler E, Lechevallier E, Soulie M, Chautar D, Coloby P, Fontaine E, Bladou F, Desgradnchampls F, Lahillot O. Effect of nonsteroidal anti-inflammatory agents and finasteride on prostate cancer risk. *J Urol* 168 (5): 1985–1988, 2002.

237. Perron L, Bairati I, Moore L, Meyer F. Dosage, duration and timing of nonsteroidal anti-inflammatory drug use and risk of prostate cancer. *Int J Cancer* 106 (3): 409–415, 2003.

238. Garcia Rodriguez LA, Gonzalez-Perez A. Inverse association between nonsteroidal anti-inflammatory drugs and prostate cancer. *Cancer Epidemiol Biomarkers Prev* 13 (4): 649–653, 2004.

239. Funkhouser EM, Sharp GB. Aspirin and reduced risk of esophageal carcinoma. *Cancer* 76 (7): 1116–1119, 1995.

240. Farrow DC, Vaughan TL, Hansten PD, Stanford JL, Risch HA, Gammon MD, Chow WH, Dubrow R, Ahsan H, Mayne ST, Schoenberg JB, West AB, Rotterdam H, Fraumeni JF Jr, Blot WJ. Use of aspirin and other nonsteroidal anti-inflammatory drugs and risk of esohpageal and gastric cancer. *Cancer Epidemiol Biomarkers Prev* 7 (2): 97–102, 1998.

241. Garidou A, Tzonou A, Lipworth L, Signorello LB, Kalapothaki V, Trichopoulos D. Lifestyle factors and medical condition in relation to esophageal cancer by histologic type in a low risk population. *Int J Cancer* 68 (3): 295–299, 1996.

242. Cheng KK, Sharp L, McKinney PA, Logan RF, Chilvers CE, Cook-Mosaffari P, Ahmed A, Day NE. A case control study of oesophageal adenocarcinoma in women: a preventable disease. *Br J Cancer* 83 (1): 127–132, 2000.

243. Gammon MD, Terry MB, Arber N, Chow WH, Risch HA, Vaughan TL, Schoenberg JB, Mayne ST, Stanford JL, Dubrow R, Rotterdam H, West AB, Fraumeni JF Jr, Weinstein IB, Hibshoosh H. Nonsteroidal anti-inflammatory drug use associated with reduced incidence of adenocarcinomas of the esophagus and gastric cardia that overexpress cyclin D1: a population-based study. *Cancer Epidemiology, Biomarkers & Prevention* 13: 34–39, 2004.

244. Farrow DC, Vaughan TL, Hansten PD, Stanford JL, Risch HA, Gammon MD, Chow WH, Dubrow R, Ahsan H, Mayne ST, Schoenberg JM, West AB, Rotterdam H, Fraumeni JF Jr, Blot WJ. Use of aspirin and other nonsteroidal anti-inflammatory drugs and risk of esophageal and gastric cancer. *Cancer Epidemiol Biomarkers Prev* 7 (2): 97–102, 1998.

245. Coogan PF, Rosenberg L, Palmer JR, Strom BL, Zauber AG, Stolley PD, Shapiro S. Nonsteroidal anti-inflammatory drugs and risk of digestive cancers at sites other than the large bowel. *Cancer Epidemiol Biomarkers Prev* 9 (1): 119–123, 2000.

246. Zaridze D, Borisova E, Maximovitch D, Chkhikvadze V. Aspirin protects against gastric cancer: results of a case-control study from Moscow, Russia. *Int J Cancer* 82 (4): 473–476, 1998.

247. Akre K, Ekstrom AM, Signorello LB, Hansson LE, Nyren O. Aspirin and risk for gastric cancer: a population-based case-control study in Sweden. *Br J Cancer* 84 (7): 965–968, 2001.

248. Anderson KE, Johnson TW, Lazovich D, Folsom AR. Association of aspirin and other nonsteroidal anti-inflammatory drug use with incidence of pancreatic cancer in a cohort of postmenopausal women. *Proc Amer Assoc Cancer Res, 92d Ann Meeting, Abstract 4095*, 42: 763, 2001.

249. Menezes RJ, Huber KR, Mahoney MC, Moysich KB. Regular use of aspirin and pancreatic cancer risk. *BMC Public Health* 2(1): 18, 2002.

250. Schernhammer ES, Kang JH, Chan AT, Michaud DS, Skinner HG, Giovannucci E, Colditz GA, Fuchs CS. A prospective study of aspirin use and the risk of pancreatic cancer in women. *J Natl Cancer Inst* 96: 22–28, 2004.

251. Jacobs EJ, Connell CJ, Rodriguez C, Patel AV, Calle EE, Thun MJ. Aspirin use and pancreatic cancer mortality in a large United States cohort. *J Natl Cancer Inst* 96 (7): 524–528, 2004.

252. Fairfield KM, Hunter DJ, Fuchs CS, Colditz GA, Hankinson SE. Aspirin, other NSAIDs, and ovarian cancer risk (United States). *Cancer Causes Control* 13 (6): 535–542, 2002.

253. Tzonou A, Polychronopoulou A, Hsieh CC, Rebelakos A, Karakatsani A, Trichopoulos D. Hair dyes, analgesics, tranquilizers and perineal talc application as risk factors for ovarian cancer. *Int J Cancer* 44 (3): 408–410, 1993.

254. Cramer DW, Harlow BL, Titus-Ernstoff L, Bohlke K, Welch WR, Greer ER. Over-the-counter analgesics and risk of ovarian cancer. *Lancet* 351 (9096): 104–1097, 1998.

255. Tavani A, Gallus S, La Vecchia C, Conti E, Montella M, Franceschi S. Aspirin and ovarian cancer, and Italian case-control study. *Ann Oncol* 11 (9): 1171–1173, 2000.

256. Rosenberg L, Palmer JR, Rao RS, Coogan PF, Strom BL, Zauber AG, Shapiro S. A case-control study of analgesic use and ovarian cancer. *Cancer Epidemiol Biomarkers Prev* (9): 933–937, 2000.

257. Moysich KB, Mettlin C, Piver MS, Natarajan N, Menezes RJ, Swede H. Regular use of analgesic drugs and ovarian cancer risk. *Cancer Epidemiol Biomarkers Prev* 10(8): 903–906, 2001.

258. Akhmedkhanov A, Toniolo P, Zeleniuch-Jacquotte A, Kato I, Koening KL, Shore RE. Aspirin and epithelial ovarian cancer. *Prev Med* 33 (6): 682–687, 2001.

259. Lacey JV, Sherman ME, Hartge P, Schatzkin A, Schairer C. Medication use and risk of ovarian carcinoma: a prospective study. *Int J Cancer* 108: 281–286, 2004.

260. Castelao JE, Yuan J-M, Gago-Dominguez, Yu MC, Ross RK. Nonsteroidal anti-inflammatory drugs and bladder cancer prevention. *British J Cancer* 82(7): 1364–1369, 2000.

261. McCredie M, Ford J, Taylor JS, Stewart JH. Analgesics and cancer of the renal pelvis in New South Wales. *Cancer* 49 (12): 2617–2725, 1982.

262. McCredie M, Stewart JH, Fort JM. Analgesics and tobacco as risk factors for cancers of the ureter and renal pelvis. *J Urol* 130 (1): 28–30, 1983.

263. McLaughlin KJ, Blot WJ, Mehl ES, Fraumeni JF Jr. Relation of analgesic use to renal cancer: population-based findings. *Natl Cancer Inst Monogr* 69: 217–222, 1985.

264. Ross RK, Paganini-Hill A, Landolph J, Gerkins V, Henderson BE. Analgesics, cigarette smoking, and other risk factors for cancers of the renal pelvis and ureter. *Cancer Res* 49 (4): 1045–1048, 1989.

265. Chow WH, McLaughlin KJ, Linet MS, Niwa S, Madel JS. Use of analgesics and risk of renal cell cancer. *Int J Cancer* 59 (4): 467–470, 1994.

266. Derby LE, Jick H. Acetaminophen and bladder cancer. *Epidemiology* 7 (4): 358–362, 1996.

267. Jensen OM, Knudsen JB, Tomasson H, Sorensen BL. The Copenhagen case-control study of renal pelvis and ureter cancer: role of analgesics. *Int J Cancer* 44 (6): 965–968, 1989.

268. Rosenberg L, Rao RS, Palmer JR, Strom BL, Zauber A, Warshauer ME, Stolley PD, Shapiro S. Transitional cell cancer of the urinary tract and renal cell cancer: relation to acetaminophen use (United States). *Cancer Causes Control* 9 (1): 83–88, 1998.

269. Gago-Dominguez M, Yuan JM, Castelao JE, Ross RK, Yu MC. Regular use of analgesics is a risk factor for renal cell carcinoma. *Br J Cancer* 81 (3): 542–548, 1999.

270. Linet MS, Chow WH, McLaughlin JK, Wacholder S, Yu MC, Schoenberg JB, Lynch C, Fraumeni JF Jr. Analgesics and cancers of the renal pelvis and ureter. *Int J Cancer* 62 (1): 15–18, 1995.

271. McCredie M, Pommer W, McLaughlin JK, Stewart JH, Lindblad P, Mandel JS, Mellemgaard A, Schlehofer B, Niwa S. International renal cell cancer study. II. Analgesics. *Int J Cancer* 60 (3): 345–349, 1995.

272. Pommer W, Bronder E, Klimpel A, Helmert U, Greiser E, Molzahn M. Urothelial cancer at different tumor sites: role of smoking and habitual intake of analgesics and laxatives. Results of the Berlin Urothelial Cancer Study. *Nephrol Dial Transplant* 14 (12): 2892–2997, 1999.

273. Harris RE, Beebe-Donk J, Namboodiri KK. Inverse association of nonsteroidal anti-inflammatory drugs and malignant melanoma among women. *Oncology Reports* 8: 655–657, 2001.

274. Prior P, Symmons DPM, Hawkins CF, Scott DL, Brown R. Cancer morbidity in rheumatoid arthritis. *Ann Rheum Dis* 43: 128–131, 1984.

275. Gridley G, McLaughlin JK, Ekbom A, Klareskog L, Adami HO, Hacker DG, Hoover R, Fraumeni JF Jr. Incidence of cancer among patients with rheumatoid arthritis. *J Natl Cancer Inst* 85 (4): 258–259, 1993.

276. Cerhan JR, Wallace RB, Folsom AR, Potter JD, Sellers TA, Zheng W, Langley CT. Medical history risk factors for non-Hodgkins's lymphoma in older women. *J Natl Cancer Inst* 89 (11): 816–817, 1997.

277. Mellemkjaer L, Linet MS, Gridley G, Frisch M, Moller H, Olsen JH. Rheumatoid arthritis and risk of cancer. *Ugeskr Laeger* 160 (21): 3069–3073, 1998.

278. Thomas E, Brewster DH, Black RJ, Macfarlane GJ. Risk of malignancy among patients with rheumatic conditions. *Int J Cancer* 88 (3): 497–502, 2000.

279. Tavani A, La Vecchia C, Franceschi S, Serraino D, Carbone A. Medical history and risk of Hodgkin's and non-Hodgkin's lymphomas. *Eur J Cancer Prev* 9 (1): 59–64, 2000.

280. Baecklund E, Ekbom A, Sparen P, Fetelius N, Kareskog L. Disease activity and risk of lymphoma in patients with rheumatoid arthritis: nested case-control study. *BMJ* 317: 180–181, 1998.

281. Tennis P, Andrews E, Bombardier C, Wang Y, Strand L, West R, Tilson R, Doi P. Record linkage to conduct an epidemiologic study on the association of rheumatoid arthritis and lymphoma in the Province of Saskatchewan, Canada. *J Clin Epidemiol* 46 (7): 685–695, 1993.

282. Bendix G, Bjell A, Holmberg E. Cancer morbidity in rheumatoid arthritis patients treated with Proresid or parenteral gold. *Scand J Rheumatol* 24 (2): 79–84, 1995.

283. Jones M, Symmons D, Finn J, Wolfe F. Does exposure to immunosuppressive therapy increase the 10 year malignancy and mortality risks in rheumatoid arthritis? A matched cohort study. *Br J Rheumatol* 35 (8): 738–745, 1996.

284. Bernstein L, Ross RK. Prior medication use and health history as risk factors for non-Hodgkin's lymphoma: preliminary results from a case-control study in Los Angeles County. *Cancer Res* 52 (19): 5510–5515, 1992.

285. Cerhan JR, Anderson KE, Janney CA, Vachon CM, Witzig TE, HabermannTM. Association of aspirin and other nonsteroidal anti-inflammatory drug use with incidence of non-Hodgkin's lymphoma, *Int J Ca*ncer 106: 784–788, 2003.

286. Kato I, Koenig KL, Shore RE, Baptiste MS, Lillquist PP, Grizzera G, Burke JS, Watanabe H. Use of anti-inflammatory and non-narcotic analgesic drugs and risk of non-Hodgkin's lymphoma (NHL) (United States). *Cancer Causes and Control* 13: 965–974, 2002.

287. Holly EA, Lele C, Bracci PM, McGrath MS. Case-control study of non-Hodgkin's lymphoma among women and heterosexual men in the San Francisco Bay Area, California. *Am J Epidemiol* 150 (4): 375–389, 1999.

288. Chang ET, Zheng T, Weir EG, Borowitz M, Mann RB, Spiegelman D, Mueller NE. Aspirin and the risk of Hodgkin's lymphoma in a population-based case-control study. *J Natl Cancer Inst* 96 (4): 305–315, 2004.

289. Kasum CM, Blair CK, Folsom AR, Ross JA. Nonsteroidal anti-inflammatory drug use and risk of adult leukemia. *Cancer Epidemiol Biomarkers Prev* 12 (6): 534–537, 2003.

290. Zheng W, Linet MS, Shu XO, Pan RP, Gao YT, Fraumeni JF Jr. Prior medical conditions and the risk of adult leukemia in Shanghai People's Republic of China. *Cancer Causes Control* 4 (4): 361–368, 1993.

291. Gonzalez-Perez A, Garcia Rodriguez LA, Lopez-Ridaura R. Effects of non-steroidal anti-inflammatory drugs on cancer sites other than the colon and rectum: a meta-analysis. *BMC Cancer* 3: 28, 2003.

292. Waddell WR, Loughry RW. Sulindac for polyposis of the colon. *J Surg Oncol* 24: 83–7, 1983.

293. Giardiello FM. NSAID-induced polyp regression in Familial Adenomatous Polyposis patients. *Gastroenterology Clinics of North America* 25: 349–61, 1996

294. Suh O, Mettlin C, Petrelli N. Aspirin use, cancer, and polyps of the large bowel. *Cancer* 72: 1171–1177, 1993.

295. Peleg I, Maibach H, Brown SH, Wilcox CM. Aspirin and nonsteroidal anti-inflammatory drug use and the risk of subsequent colorectal cancer. *Arch Intern Med* 154: 394–399, 1994.

296. Greenberg ER, Baron JA, Freeman DH Jr, Mandel JS, Haile R. Reduced risk of large bowel adenomas among aspirin users. The Polyp Prevention Study Group. *J Natl Cancer Inst* 85: 912–916, 1993.

297. Logan RF, Litte J, Hawtin PG, Hardcastle JD. Effect of aspirin and nonsteroidal anti-inflammatory drugs on colorectal adenomas: case-control study of subjects participating in the Nottingham faecal occult blood screening program. *BMJ* 307: 285–289, 1993.

298. Martinez M, McPherson RS, Levin B, Annegers JF. Aspirin and other nonsteroidal anti-inflammatory drugs and risk of colorectal adenomatous polyps among endoscoped individuals. *Cancer Epidemiol Biomarkers Prev* 4: 703–707, 1995.

299. Sandler RS, Galanko JC, Murray SC, Helm JF, Woosley JT. Aspirin and nonsteroidal anti-inflammatory agents and risk for colorectal adenomas. *Gastroenterology* 114: 441–448, 1998.

300. Breuer-Katschinski B, Nemes K, Rump B, Leiendecker B, Marr A, Breuer N, et al. Long-term use of nonsteroidal anti-inflammatory drugs and the risk of colorectal adenomas. The Colorectal Adenoma Study Group. *Digestion* 61: 129–134, 2000.

301. Labayle D, Fischer D, Vielh P, Drouhin F, Pariente A, Bories C, Duhamel O, Troussett M, Attali P. Sulindac causes regression of rectal polyps in familial adenomatous polyposis. *Gastroenterology* 101: 635–639, 1991.

302. Giardiello FM, Hamilton SR, Krush AJ, Piantadosi S, Hylind LM, Celano P, Booker SV, Robinson CR, Offerhaus JA. Treatment of colonic and rectal adenomas with sulindac in familial adenomatous polyposis. *N Engl J Med* 328: 1313–6, 1993.

303. Nugent KP, Farmer KC, Spigelman AD, Williams CB, Phillips RK. Randomized controlled trial of the effect of sulindac on duodenal and rectal polyposis and cell proliferation in patients with familial adenomatous polyposis. *Br J Surg* 80: 1618–9, 1993.

304. Thun MJ, Henley SJ, Patrono C. Nonsteroidal anti-inflammatory drugs as anticancer agents: mechanistic, pharmacologic, and clinical issues. *J Natl Cancer Inst* 94 (Feb 20): 252–266, 2002.

305. Anderson WF, Umar A, Viner JL, Hawk ET. Potential role of NSAIDs in COX-2 blockade in cancer therapy. In: RE Harris, ed. COX-2 Blockade in Cancer Prevention and Therapy. Humana Press, Totowa, NJ, pp. 313–340, 2002.

306. Steinbach G, Lynch PM, Phillips RK, Wallace MB, Hawk E, Gordon G, al et. The effect of celecoxib, a cyclooxygenase-2 inhibitor, in familial adenomatous polyposis. *New Engl J Med* 342: 1946–52. 2000.

307. Bertagnolli MM, Eagle CJ, Hawk ET. Celecoxib recduces spradic colrectal adenomas: results from the Adenoma Prevention with Celecoxib (APC) trial. *American Association for Cancer Research*, 97th Annual Meeting, Abstract CP-3, page 186, 2006.

308. Arber N, Racz I, Spicak J, Zavoral M, Lechuga MJ, Gerletti P, Eagle CJ, Levin B. Chemoprevention of colorectal adenomas with celecoxib in an international randomized, placebo-controlled, double-blind trial. *American Association for Cancer Research*, 97th Annual Meeting, Abstract CP-4, page 186, 2006.

309. Mulshine JL, Atkinson JC, Greer RO, Papadimitrakopoulou VA, Van Waes C, Rudy S, Martin JW, Steinberg SM, Liewehr DJ, Avis I, Linnoila RI, Hewitt S, Lippman SM, Frye R, Cavanaugh PF Jr. Randomized, double-blind, placebo-controlled phase IIb trial of the cyclooxygenase inhibitor ketorolac as an oral rinse in orpharyngeal leukoplakia. *Clin Cancer Res* 10 (5): 1565–1671, 2004.

310. Kaur BS, Khamnehei N, Iravani M, Namburu SS, Lin O, Triadofilopoulos G. Rofecoxib inhibits cyclooxygenase-2 expression and activity and reduces cell proliferation in Barrett's esophagus. *Gastroenterology* 123 (1): 60–67, 2002.
311. Mukherjee D, Nissen SE, Topol EJ. Risk of cardiovascular events associated with selective COX-2 inhibitors. *JAMA* 286 (8): 954–959, 2001.
312. Harris RE, Beebe-Donk J, Alshafie GA. Reduction in the risk of human breast cancer by selective cyclooygenase-2 (COX-2) inhibitors. *BMC Cancer* 6: 27, 2006.

CHAPTER 5

ROLE OF COX-2 IN INFLAMMATORY AND DEGENERATIVE BRAIN DISEASES

LUISA MINGHETTI

Department of Cell Biology and Neurosciences, Istituto Superiore di Sanità, Rome, Italy

Abstract: In the last decade, the potential role of cyclooxygenase-2 (COX-2) and prostaglandins (PGs) in brain diseases has been extensively studied. COX-2 over-expression has been associated with neurotoxiticy in acute conditions, such as hypoxia/ischemia and seizures, as well as in inflammatory chronic diseases, including Creutzfeldt-Jakob disease (CJD) and Alzheimer's disease (AD). However, the role played by COX-2 in neurodegenerative diseases is still controversial and further clinical and experimental studies are warranted. In addition, the emerging role of COX-2 in behavioural and cognitive functions strongly indicates that studies aimed at improving our knowledge of the physiological role of COX-2 in the central nervous system are crucial to fully understand the pros and cons of its manipulation in disabling neurological diseases

1.   INTRODUCTION

Since its discovery in the early 1990s, COX-2 has emerged as a major factor in inflammatory reactions in peripheral tissues (Hinz and Brune, 2002). By extension, COX-2 expression in brain has been associated with pro-inflammatory activities, which are thought to be instrumental in the neurodegenerative processes occurring in acute and chronic diseases. However, there are some major issues that have to be considered when approaching the complexity of COX-2 in brain diseases.

R. E. Harris (ed.), Inflammation in the Pathogenesis of Chronic Diseases, 127–141.
© 2007 *Springer.*

First, in the central nervous system, COX-2 is expressed under physiological conditions and contributes to fundamental behavioral and cognitive functions. Second, inflammation is more tightly regulated in the brain than in peripheral tissues. In many cases, brain inflammation is a local process that is triggered and sustained by resident cells in the absence of overt leukocyte infiltration from the blood stream. Among the resident cellular elements, microglial cells, the macrophages of brain parenchyma, are of primary importance in regulating inflammation. In normal conditions, microglia exhibit a down-regulated or quiescent phenotype, but they react to subtle microenvironment alterations by changing morphology and acquiring an array of functions typical of activated macrophages such as phagocytosis and secretion of inflammatory mediators (Minghetti and Levi, 1998; Streit, 2002). In addition to microglia, reactive astrocytes contribute to the inflammatory process by limiting the area of lesions and releasing local mediators.

Like inflammation in peripheral organs and tissues, "neuroinflammation" is a two-edged sword, being a self-defensive reaction aimed at eliminating injurious stimuli and restoring tissue integrity, but contributing to tissue damage when exceeding critical thresholds. Inflammation is a complex process that requires a tight regulation. Excess as well as deficiency of response will result in pathological conditions such as chronic inflammation or uncontrolled infection, respectively. Regardless of the nature of primary pathogenetic events, inflammation per se is one of the main therapeutic targets and often the best choice to treat diseases. This explains why anti-inflammatory drugs account for the largest number of prescriptions in developed countries.

Over the last few decades, there has been increasing interest in research on neurodegenerative diseases (Forman et al., 2004). Although the primary causes of neurodegenerative diseases are varied, neuroinflammation and microglial activation are common features in most of these diseases and the use of anti-inflammatory strategies to prevent neurodegeneration has been intensively investigated and recommended as a promising approach.

From this perspective, COX-1 and COX-2 have received intensive attention and COX inhibition is currently believed to be neuroprotective in different settings of neurotoxicity and neurodegeneration. COX-2 inhibitors have been found neuroprotective in several models of ischemia, as well as in in vitro and in vivo models of amyotrophic lateral sclerosis, Parkinson's disease, and Alzheimer's disease (Minghetti, 2004). However, in several of these models, the mechanisms of neuroprotection mediated by COX-2 inhibitors are not fully elucidated or not clearly related to the abrogation of COX-2 activity. Furthermore, in spite of the classical pro-inflammatory activities attributed to COX-2, in vitro and in vivo evidence supports anti-inflammatory and protective functions. During systemic infection, suppression of COX activity by non selective or COX-2-selective inhibitors enhances the transcriptional activation of pro-inflammatory genes in vascular-associated cells of the brain and in microglial cells (Blais et al., 2002; Blais et al., 2005). This paradoxical pro-inflammatory effect of COX-2 inhibition is explained by the crucial role of COX-2-derived PGE_2 in increasing the levels of glucocorticoids during systemic inflammation. Glucocorticoids are potent anti-inflammatory molecules, which mediate the physiological feed-back regulation of innate immunity by the hypothalamic-pituitary-adrenal axis (Simard and Rivest, 2006; Sternberg, 2006). Brain PGE_2 may also exert local anti-inflammatory activities by limiting microglia activation thus contributing to restore tissue homeostasis (Levi et al., 1998; Zhang and Rivest, 2001).

While an excessive inflammatory reaction clearly contributes to brain damage, increasing evidence suggests that a controlled inflammatory response is instrumental for the resolution of pathological events in order to preserve or restore proper neuronal function. The same concept, if applied to COX-2 activity, could help explain the apparent conflicting results reported in the literature on the role of COX-2 in brain physiology and pathology.

This chapter will review some of the recent data in this area, focusing on the emerging role of COX-2 in normal brain functions as well as in some major human neurological diseases, such as Creutzfeldt-Jakob disease and Alzheimer's disease. Other important brain diseases will be discussed in other chapters of this book.

2. COX ISOFORMS IN THE BRAIN

The CNS represents an interesting exception to the general rule that describes COX-1 as the only COX isoform constitutively expressed. Indeed, in mammalian brain, both COX-1 and COX-2 are expressed in specific neuronal populations under normal physiological conditions (Yamagata et al., 1993; Breder et al., 1995; O'Neill and Ford-Hutchinson, 1993; Yasojima et al., 1999). In rat brain, COX-2 mRNA and immunoreactivity are found in dentate gyrus granule cells, pyramidal cell neurons in the hippocampus, the piriform cortex, superficial cell layers of neocortex, the amygdala, and at low levels in the striatum, thalamus and hypothalamus. In other regions, such as midbrain, pons and medulla, COX-1 immunoreactivity prevails (Yamagata et al., 1993; Breder et al., 1995). Similar patterns have been described for COX-1 and COX-2 mRNAs in human brain (O'Neill and Ford-Hutchinson, 1993; Yasojima et al., 1999).

In addition, a third variant named COX-3 has been identified from canine and human cerebral cortex cDNAs (Chandrasekharan eta al., 2002). COX-3 is a product of the COX-1 gene retaining intron 1 in its mRNA. The expression of COX-3 appears tissue-specific, with the highest expression in the brain followed by the heart. Within the brain, the highest levels are in the cerebral cortex, where the expression of COX-3 accounts for $\sim 5\%$ of COX-1. As its counterpart COX-1, COX-3 is not induced by acute inflammatory stimulation (Shaftel et al., 2003). COX-3 exhibits glycosylation-dependent enzymatic activity and is especially sensitive to the inhibitory activity of paracetamol (acetaminophen). Thus, it has been proposed that COX-3 could represent the brain specific COX isoform hypothesized a few decades ago to explain the potent analgesic and antipyretic actions of paracetamol, in spite of its poor inhibitory activity on purified preparations of COX-1 and COX-2 at therapeutic concentrations (Botting, 2000). At present, this hypothesis is not supported by solid experimental evidence and the functional role of COX-3 in human brain remains uncertain (Kis et al, 2005; Quin et al., 2005).

The relative contribution of COX-1 and COX-2 activity to brain pathology and physiology is another open question that deserves some attention. It has been pointed out that COX-1 activity in brain diseases has been overlooked. This claim is supported, among other findings, by the observations that COX-1 plays a role in inflammation and that preferential COX-1 inhibitors are beneficial in Alzheimer's disease and in some models of this disease (Schwab and Schluesener, 2003). On the other side, mandatory evidence suggests that COX-2 plays a special role in normal neuronal function and in neurotoxiticy (Graham and Hickey, 2003). Recent in vivo studies using isoform-selective inhibitors have shown that both isoforms contribute to the brain levels of PGs triggered by excitotoxic events, although COX-2 is the prominent isoform (Candelario-Jalil et al., 2003; Pepicelli et al. 2005). Although the debate will be solved only by further studies, increasing evidence indicates that the popular paradigm by which COX-1 serves physiological functions and COX-2 is responsible for "pathological" PGs, is an over generalized and misleading concept (Parente and Perretti 2003).

3.   COX-2 IN BRAIN FUNCTIONS

In normal brain, neuronal COX-2 expression is exclusively localized to excitatory glutamatergic neurons and is dependent on normal synaptic activity (Kaufmann et al., 1996). Thus, rather than constitutive, the physiological expression of COX-2 in neurons should most properly be regarded as dynamically regulated and sustained by normal synaptic activity.

The dependence of COX-2 expression on natural excitatory synaptic activity is consistent with the presence of COX-2 immunoreactivity in distal dendrites and dendritic spines, which are involved in synaptic signaling, and with the heterogeneous distribution within a specific neuronal population, which is similar to that described for other immediate early genes activated by excitatory stimulation (Kaufmann et al., 1997a).

Neuronal COX-2 expression appears to be developmentally regulated. In rat brain, neuronal COX-2 mRNA and protein are detectable after the first postnatal week, reach a peak of expression during the third and the fourth week, and decrease to adult levels by 2 months. COX-2 immunoreactivity is first detected in the cell body, and by the third postnatal week it begins to appear in dendrites. At adulthood, COX-2 is localized to the most distal dendrites and spines. The comparison of COX-2 expression with markers of dendritic maturation in rat neocortex suggests that the post-synaptic localization of COX-2 is related to the final activity-dependent processes during dendritic development (Kaufmann et al., 1996). In the neocortex, COX-2 positive neurons show a typical laminar distribution that is heavily disrupted in subjects affected by Rett' syndrome, a neurodevelopmental disorder characterized by a defective development of cortical neurons and abnormalities of dendritric branching (Kaufmann et al., 1997b). In rats subjected to selective destruction of basal forebrain cholinergic neurons during the fist post-natal week, the hippocampal levels of COX-2 mRNA are decreased at adulthood, whereas the COX-1 mRNA levels are unaffected. From a behavioral point of view, these animals show impairment in social memory, suggesting that the early loss of hippocampal cholinergic input may impact on the expression of COX-2 in hippocampal neurons and on the functional role of PGs in synaptic activity (Ricceri et al., 2004).

Several studies have investigated the effect of COX inhibition on behavioral and cognitive functions. Systemic administration or hippocampal infusion of COX-2 selective inhibitors shortly after training in the Morris water maze, a hippocampal dependent learning task, have been shown to impair spatial memory in rats (Teather et al., 2002; Sharifzadeh et al., 2005). In addition, pre-training infusion of the COX-2 selective inhibitor celecoxib in the hippocampus of adult rats impaired acquisition of the Morris water maze, suggesting that in rats COX-2 activity in the hippocampus is necessary for both memory and learning of a spatial task (Rall et al., 2003). Similarly, intracerebral injection of COX inhibitors in chicks attenuated memory of a passive avoidance response (Holscher, 1995). In a recent study, Sharifzadeh et al., (2006) have shown that the impairment of spatial memory retention by hippocampal infusion of celecoxib is transient, with maximal effect at 72h after infusion and with a concomitant reduction of COX-2 immunoreactive neurons.

Peripheral administration of the COX-2 selective inhibitor, parecoxib, decreased the firing rate and burst firing activity of dopamine neurons in the ventral tegmental area, involved in the control of motivational processes and control of emotions, such as reward and reinforcement (Schwieler et al., 2006). This action was attributed to a decrease in brain concentration of kynurenic acid, an endogenous glutamate receptor antagonist with a preferential action on the glycine site of the NMDA glutamate receptor. The opposite effect on both kynurenic acid level and dopamine neuron firing rate was observed after administration of the non selective COX inhibitor indomethacin.

In line with experiments indicating the involvement of COX-2 in spatial learning and memory, systemic administration of ibuprofen, a non-selective COX inhibitor, caused deficits in spatial learning in the water maze and in the induction of long-term potentiation (LTP), a major model of synaptic plasticity. Ibuprofen did not affect non-hippocampal tasks or baseline synaptic transmission, but it abolished the increase in PGE_2 and brain derived growth factor (BDNF) levels following LTP and spatial learning (Shaw et al., 2003).

Several lines of evidence converge on attributing to PGE_2 a prominent role in the COX-2 dependent brain functions. PGE_2 is preferentially formed by the enzymatic activity of COX-2 rather than COX-1, as suggested by observations of COX-1 and COX-2 knock out mice (Bosetti et al., 2004). The functional coupling of COX-2 and PGE synthase (PGES), the enzyme converting the inter-mediated product PGH_2 into PGE_2, is further supported by their intracellular colocalization (Vazquez-Tello et al., 2004) and their co-induction in endothelial and perivascular macrophages upon systemic inflammatory stimulation (Ek et al.,

2001; Blais et al., 2005). PGES exists in three distinct forms, a cytosolic PGES and two microsomal forms (mPGES-1 and mPGES-2). Of these forms, mPGES-1 is functionally coupled with COX-2 and is essential for PGE_2 synthesis during inflammation.

Bazan and co-workers have shown that exogenous application of PGE_2, but not PGD_2 or $PGF_{2\alpha}$, reversed the suppression of LTP induced by COX-2-inhibition in hippocampal dentate granule neurons in vitro (Chen et al., 2002). More recently, they have demonstrated the post-synaptic localization of both COX-2 and mPGES-1 and the presence of pre-synaptic PGE_2 receptor EP2 in dendritic spines in the hippocampus and provided evidence for a role of PGE_2 as a retrograde messenger (Sang et al., 2005).

Other mechanisms by which PGE_2 could indirectly contribute to synaptic plasticity include modulation of adrenergic, noradrenegic and glutamatergic neuro-transmission and regulation of membrane excitability (Bazan, 2003 and references therein). Moreover, COX-2-derived PGs are involved in the coupling of synaptic plasticity with cerebral blood flow, as suggested by attenuation of the increase in neocortical blood flow in response to vibrissal stimulation by the COX-2 selective inhibitor NS 398 (Niwa et al., 2000).

4.   COX-2 IN CHRONIC DEGENERATIVE DISEASES

4.1.   Alzheimer's Disease

Alzheimer's disease (AD) is the most common cause of dementia in the elderly and one of the best characterized chronic neurodegenerative disorders. The main neuropathological feature of the disease is the formation of extracellular amyloid plaques and intracellular neurofibrillary tangles. The involvement of inflammatory mechanisms in the loss of neurons in AD is supported by several lines of evidence, including the finding of activated microglia around amyloid plaques and increased levels of inflammatory mediators including cytokines, chemokines and elements of complement system in AD brains as well as in animal models of the human disease (McGeer and McGeer, 2001).

The use of anti-inflammatory drugs to treat AD was proposed in the early 1990s (McGeer and Rogers, 1992). Since then, a multitude of studies have been undertaken to test this theory. Retrospective epidemiological studies have reported an association between long-term NSAID use and reduced risk of AD, although not every investigation has found the same protective effect (in t' Veld et al., 2001; Aisen, 2002).

The beneficial effect of NSAIDs led the way to the hypothesis that COX activity, and in particular that of the inducible isoform COX-2, is involved in the cascade of events leading to neurodegeneration in AD. Several studies have analyzed COX-1 and COX-2 expression in animal models and post mortem AD brain tissues and have provided a substantial but still controversial body of evidence.

The levels of COX-1 mRNA and protein were found not significantly altered in AD brains (Yasojima et al., 1999; Yermakova et al., 1999). COX-1 immuno-reactivity is mainly localized to microglial cells associated with Aβ-deposits, regardless of their ramified or activated morphology (Yermakova et al., 1999). By contrast, COX-2 mRNA levels in AD brains were reported as either decreased or increased (Yasojima et al., 1999; Chang et al., 1996), possibly because of the short half-life of COX-2 transcripts or individual variability of inflammatory-related processes (Lukiw and Bazan, 1997). Similarly, analyses of post-mortem specimens have produced apparently conflicting results. Several studies reported increased neuronal COX-2 immunoreactivity compared to control brain tissues (Yasojima et al., 1999; Pasinetti and Aisen, 1998). In other studies, in which COX-2 expression was related to specific hallmarks of the disease, such as clinical dementia rating and Braak stage of disease, the number of COX-2 positive neurons decreased with the severity of dementia. In end stage AD, COX-2 positive neurons were significantly fewer than in non-demented controls (Yermakova et al., 2001, Hoozemans et al., 2002). In more recent studies (Hoozemans et al., 2004; 2005), the number of neurons expressing COX-2 negatively correlated with the Braak score for Aβ-deposits and the highest levels of neuronal COX-2 was observed in the first stages of AD pathology, prior to maximal glial activation.

Neuronal COX-2 expression has been reported to correlate with cell cycle regulators involved in controlling the G_0/G_1 phase, such as cyclin D1 and E and the retinoblastoma protein (Hoozemans et al., 2004; 2005). Cell cycle control disruption has been proposed as a primary mechanism by which post-mitotic neurons undergo apoptotic death in AD (Nagy et al., 1998; Webber et al., 2005) and some evidence indicates that COX-2 might regulate cell cycle progression (Hoozemans et al., 2004 and references therein). It is therefore possible that COX-2 is involved in early steps leading to neurodegeneration, but the functional link between COX-2 and cell cycle alteration remains elusive.

The dependence of COX-2 expression on disease stage may explain the contro-versial findings reported in the literature, recently reviewed by Firuzi and Praticò, (2006). Moreover, analyses of post mortem tissues may be affected by several biases due to the occurrence of terminal systemic infections, variable post mortem delay times, and manipulation of dissected tissues. Ex vivo cerebrospinal fluid (CSF) studies may avoid some of these confounding factors.

In an early study, Montine et al. (1999) reported elevated CSF PGE_2 levels in patients with probable AD. More recently, we performed a longitudinal study, in which control subjects and AD patients were examined for at least three annual visits, to evaluate the CSF levels of PGE_2 in relation to cognitive decline and survival (Combrinck et al., 2006). We found that CSF PGE_2 declines with the increasing dementia severity. PGE_2 levels were higher in patients with mild memory impairment, but lower in those with more advanced AD, in line with the disease stage-dependent expression of COX-2 shown in AD brains (Yermakova et al., 1999; Hoozemans et al., 2002, 2004). Interestingly, patients with higher initial CSF PGE_2 levels survived longer. The result was not affected by cognitive score, sex or age at the time of CSF sampling (Combrinck et al., 2006). These observations weigh against the idea that PGE_2 and/or COX activity are neurotoxic, and suggest that CSF PGE_2 may reflect the survival of COX-positive neurons. Notably, in normal brain, COX-2 is expressed by neuronal populations that are known to be particularly vulnerable to degeneration in AD. Alternatively, PGE_2 levels could reflect early inflammatory processes that may impede the later progression of AD.

Although in vitro and in vivo AD experimental models have shown increased vulnerability to excitotoxiticy of COX-2 over-expressing neurons and neuroprotection by COX-2 inhibition, the causal role of COX-2 in human pathology is far from being established. Taking into account the positive and negative effects of inhibition of COX-2 activity and the emerging role of COX-2 derived PGs in brain function, it is difficult to predict the final outcome of long-term therapeutic COX-2 inhibition. At present, clinical trials of selective COX-2 inhibitors have not been as convincing as expected (Aisen et al., 2003; Reines et al., 2004), but these failures may be related to drug selection and dose, duration of treatment and state of disease of selected patients. The recent withdrawal from the market of the COX-2 selective inhibitor, rofecoxib, due to increased risk of adverse cardiovascular events is a further indication that the pros and cons of selective COX-2 inhibition in neurodegenerative diseases have not yet been fully investigated.

4.2.   Creutzfeldt-Jakob Disease

Creutzfeldt-Jakob disease (CJD) is the best known human form of transmissible spongiform encephalopathies or prion diseases, a heterogeneous group of infectious, sporadic and genetic disorders characterized by rapidly progressive dementia and more than 90% mortality within one year from the onset (Will et al., 1998). As with AD, the neuropathological hallmarks of the disease are the presence of amyloid plaques generated by deposition of the pathological form of the prion protein (proteinase-resistant prion protein PrP^{res} or PrP^{sc}) and extensive microglial activation, both of which suggest that a local non-immune mediated chronic inflammatory response plays a role in development (Perry et al., 2002). Although the interest in prion diseases intensified after the variant CJD was recognized in the UK in 1996 as a novel human transmissible spongiform encephalopathy (TSE) caused by the same agent as bovine spongiform encephalopathy (Will et al., 1996), this group of human diseases are not as well characterized as AD. Nevertheless, the roles of inflammation and microglial activation have been thoroughly investigated (Perry et al., 2002).

We explored the involvement of COX activity in prion diseases by measuring PGE_2 levels in the CSF in a group of subjects affected by sporadic or genetic CJD (Minghetti et al., 2000). The levels of PGE_2 were significantly higher in CJD patients than in a control group of age-matched subjects undergoing subdural anesthesia or affected by non-inflammatory neurological diseases. The levels of PGE_2 measured in the CSF of CJD patients were over 5 fold higher than those reported in AD patients (Combrinck et al., 2006). In contrast to what has been observed in AD patients, higher PGE_2 levels were associated with shorter survival in CJD patients. PGE_2 levels were not dependent on the time of CSF sampling during the course of the disease, suggesting that PGE_2 may be an index of disease severity rather than progression (Minghetti et al., 2000).

We later confirmed the elevated CSF levels of PGE_2 in a group of 18 cases of variant CJD (Minghetti et al., 2002). This disease is mainly confined to young people showing early psychiatric symptoms and sensory disturbances. Later, the disease evolves in a clinic picture more typical of CJD including involuntary movements, severe dementia and, eventually, akinetic mutism. The levels of PGE_2 in variant CJD patients were comparable to those measured in the other two forms, sporadic and genetic CJD. They were also similar to those measured in an age-matched group of subjects affected by psychiatric disorders with a known inflammatory component.

The increased CSF PGE_2 levels found in sporadic, genetic, and variant CJD were consistent with the increased levels of PGE_2 in brain homogenates from mice infected by the mouse-adapted ME7 strain of the ovine prion agent or scrapie, a well characterized prion disease model (Betmouni et al., 1996). These mice develop the disease with a well defined time course and pathology and typical clinical signs are observed by 20–23 weeks post injection (p.i.). Intense COX-2-immunoreactivity was associated with microglial-like cells in brains of ME7 injected mice. COX-2-positive cells were particularly dense in areas of typical spongiform degeneration and their number increased with disease progression. In control brains from mice injected with normal brain homogenate, sporadic COX-2-immunoreactivity was found associated with cells characterised by a small cell body and fine processes typical of parenchymal resting microglia (Walsh et al., 2000).

Since microglial activation occurs with considerable variation in CJD and in animal models of the disease (Baker et al., 1999; Puoti et al., 2005), we verified that expression of COX-2 is elevated using a second model in which C3H mice were infected with brain homogenates obtained from subjects who died by genetic or sporadic CJD. In this model, several COX-2-positive microglial cells were detected in areas of intense spongiform degeneration. The intensity of COX-2 immunoreactivity was variable among infected animals, but was significantly increased compared to control mice (Minghetti et al., 2005).

The similar findings obtained in the two mouse models, which are characterized by different mouse strains (C3H and C57BL/6J), type of prion agent used (CJD and mouse-adapted scrapie), and time of incubation necessary to develop the disease (> 90 and 22–24 weeks), suggest that the selective up-regulation of COX-2 in microglial cells is a consistent feature of prion disease and not characteristic of a specific prion agent or mouse strain. Nevertheless, in a human study of sporadic CJD, COX-1 and COX-2 were both increased in the cortex of patients who died with disease(Deininger et al., 2003). COX-1 immunoreactivity was present in macrophages/microglial cells whereas COX-2 was predominantly in neurons. Messenger RNAs and proteins of both isoforms were higher in tissue from the temporal lobe of one CJD patient when compared to one neuropathologically unaltered control case. At present, it remains to be established whether COX over-expression is a cause or a consequence of neuronal death in CJD or whether CSF levels of PGE_2 represent an index of disease severity.

Experimental evidence suggests that PGE_2 synthesis and COX-2 expression in microglial cells are promoted by microglial clearance of apoptotic, but not necrotic, neurons (De Simone et al., 2004). In CJD, abundance of apoptotic neurons correlated well with microglial activation (Gray et al., 1999), supporting the hypothesis that the increased levels of PGE_2 in the CSF of CJD patients and the high expression of COX-2 in microglial cells in experimental prion diseases may be associated with the clearance of apoptotic neurons.

At opposed to AD, there is very little information available on anti-inflammatory treatment of prion diseases. In neuroblastoma cells, COX-1 inhibitors were beneficial against PrP peptide toxicity (Bate et al., 2002). In a rat model of CJD, oral administration of indomethacin, begun soon after infection, had a moderate effect on the onset of clinical signs, but not on survival time. In the same model, dapsone, an antibiotic used to treat leprosy and skin infections, significantly delayed clinical signs and extended disease duration (Manuelidis et al., 1998). Dapsone did not ameliorate the course of disease nor the postmortem histopathology in scrapie infected mice (Guenther et al., 2001).

5.   CONCLUSIONS

In spite of intensive research over the past years, evidence of a direct role of COX-2 in neurodegenerative events is still controversial and further experimental and clinical studies are required before anti-inflammatory therapies aimed to inhibit COX-2 are recommended for preventing or limiting neurodegeneration.

Numerous features contribute to the complexity of the role of COX-2 in brain physiology and pathology. Specific neuronal populations express COX-2 under physiological condition and such expression is central to important tasks such as synaptic plasticity, and cognitive and behavioral functions. Several cell types, including resident cells (neurons, glia, and endothelial cells) and infiltrating blood cells, can express COX-2 following pathological events. Expression or over-expression of COX-2 in each of these cells may have different functional conse-quences and the final outcome is likely to depend on the prevailing product of COX-2 activity, including PGs with different functions and free radicals, as well as on the specific PG receptors expressed by target cells. COX-2 induction and/or over-expression in particular cell types, is likely to be dependent on specific signals (glutamate, cytokines, amyloid deposits, damaged neurons) which may be related to disease or to a stage of disease, thus explaining some of the discordance in the reported results. The comparison of similar but distinct chronic degenerative diseases such as AD and CJD exemplifies the complexity of the problem and illustrates how over generalization of the role of COX activity can be misleading. Increased levels of PGE_2 in the CSF of subjects affected by these two diseases are likely to reflect distinct phenomena with opposite predictive values for subject survival (Figure 1).

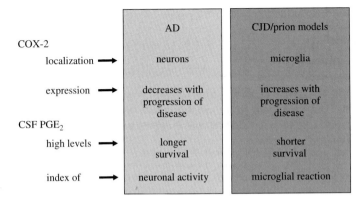

	AD	CJD/prion models
COX-2		
localization ➡	neurons	microglia
expression ➡	decreases with progression of disease	increases with progression of disease
CSF PGE₂		
high levels ➡	longer survival	shorter survival
index of ➡	neuronal activity	microglial reaction

Figure 1. COX-2 expression and PGE$_2$ CSF levels in chronic inflammatory diseases: comparison between Alzheimer's disease and Creutzfeldt-Jakob disease

A final consideration concerns the beneficial effects of COX inhibitors in several experimental models and epidemiological studies. These beneficial effects, which are exerted by several but not all COX inhibitors, provide indirect proof of the causative role of COX-2 in neurodegeneration. COX-independent mechanisms including free radical scavenging activity, peroxisome proliferator-activated receptor-γ activation, anti-amyloidogenic activity by some non selective NSAIDs, as well as actions interfering with systemic inflammatory processes, which in turn can influence central inflammation, cannot be excluded.

REFERENCES

Aisen P.S., Schafer K.A., Grundman M., Pfeiffer E., Sano M., Davis K.L., Farlow M.R., Jin S., Thomas R.G., Thal L.J. Alzheimer's Disease Cooperative Study. Effects of rofecoxib or naproxen vs placebo on Alzheimer disease progression: a randomized controlled trial. JAMA 2003; 289:2819–2826.

Aisen P.S. The potential of anti-inflammatory drugs for the treatment of Alzheimer's disease. The Lancet Neurology 2002; 1:279–284.

Baker C.A., Lu Z.Y., Zaitsev I., Manuelidis L. Microglial activation varies in different models of Creutzfeldt-Jakob disease. J Virol 1999; 73:5089–5097.

Bate C., Rutherford S., Gravenor M., Reid S., Williams A. Cyclo-oxygenase inhibitors protect against prion-induced neurotoxicity in vitro. Neuroreport 2002; 13:1933–1938.

Bazan N.G. Synaptic lipid signaling: significance of polyunsaturated fatty acids and platelet-activating factor. J Lipid Res 2003; 44:2221–2233.

Betmouni S., Perry V.H., Gordon J.L. Evidence for an early inflammatory response in the central nervous system of mice with scrapie. Neuroscience 1996; 74:1–5.

Blais V., Zhang J., Rivest S. In altering the release of glucocorticoids, ketorolac exacerbates the effects of systemic immune stimuli on expression of proinflammatory genes in the brain. Endocrinology. 2002; 143:4820–4827.

Blais V., Turrin N.P., Rivest S. Cyclooxygenase 2 (COX-2) inhibition increases the inflammatory response in the brain during systemic immune stimuli. J Neurochem 2005; 95:1563–1574.

Bosetti F., Langenbach R., Weerasinghe G.R. Prostaglandin E2 and microsomal prostaglandin E synthase-2 expression are decreased in the cyclooxygenase-2-deficient mouse brain despite compensatory induction of cyclooxygenase-1 and Ca^{2+}-dependent phospholipase A2. J Neurochem 2004; 91:1389–1397.

Botting R.M. Mechanism of action of acetaminophen: is there a cyclooxygenase 3? Clin Infect Dis 2000; 31:S202–S210.

Breder C.D., Dewitt D., Kraig R.P. Characterization of inducible cyclooxygenase in rat brain. J Comp Neurol 1995; 355:296–315.

Candelario-Jalil E., Gonzalez-Falcon A., Garcia-Cabrera M., Alvarez D., Al-Dalain S., Martinez G., Leon O.S., Springer J.E. Assessment of the relative contribution of COX-1 and COX-2 isoforms to ischemia-induced oxidative damage and neurodegeneration following transient global cerebral ischemia. J Neurochem 2003; 86:545–555.

Chandrasekharan N.V., Dai H., Roos K.L., Evanson N.K., Tomsik J., Elton T.S., Simmons D.L. COX-3, a cycloxygenase-1 variant inhibited by acetaminophen and other analgesic/antipyretic drugs: cloning, structure and expression. Proc. Natl Acad Sci USA 2002; 99:13926–13931.

Chang J.W., Coleman P.D., O'Banion M.K. Prostaglandin G/H synthase-2 (cyclooxygenase-2) mRNA expression is decreased in Alzheimer's disease. Neurobiol Aging 1996; 17:801–808.

Chen C., Magee J.C., Bazan N.G. Cyclooxygenase-2 regulates prostaglandin E_2 signaling in hippocampal long-term synaptic activity. J Neurophysiol 2002; 87:2851–2857.

Combrinck M., Williams J., De Berardinis M.A., Warden D., Puopolo M., Smith A.D., Minghetti L. Levels of CSF prostaglandin E2, cognitive decline, and survival in Alzheimer's disease. J Neurol Neurosurg Psychiatry. 2006; 77:85–88.

De Simone R., Ajmone-Cat M.A., Minghetti L. Atypical antiinflammatory activation of microglia induced by apoptotic neurons: possible role of phosphatidylserine-phosphatidylserine receptor interaction. Mol Neurobiol 2004; 29:197–212.

Deininger M.H., Bekure-Nemariam K., Trautmann K., Morgalla M., Meyermann R., Schluesener H.J. Cyclooxygenase-1 and -2 in brains of patients who died with sporadic Creutzfeldt-Jakob disease. J Mol Neurosci 2003; 20:25–30.

Ek M., Engblom D., Saha S., Blomqvist A., Jakobsson P., Ericsson-Dahlstrand A. Inflammatory response: pathway across the blood-brain barrier. Nature 2001; 410:430–431.

Firuzi O., Pratico D. Coxibs and Alzheimer's disease: should they stay or should they go? Ann Neurol 2006; 59:219–228.

Forman M.S., Trojanowski J.Q., Lee V.M. Neurodegenerative diseases: a decade of discoveries paves the way for therapeutic breakthroughs. Nat Med 2004; 10:1055–1063.

Graham S.H., Hickey R.W. Cyclooxygenases in central nervous system diseases: a special role for cyclooxygenase 2 in neuronal cell death. Arch Neurol 2003; 60:628–630.

Gray F., Chretien F., Adle-Biassette H., Dorandeu A., Ereau T., Delisle M.B., Kopp N., Ironside J.W., Vital C. Neuronal apoptosis in Creutzfeldt-Jakob disease. J Neuropathol Exp Neurol 1999; 58:321–328.

Guenther K., Deacon R.M., Perry V.H., Rawlins J.N. Early behavioural changes in scrapie-affected mice and the influence of dapsone. Eur J Neurosci 2001; 14:401–409.

Hinz B., Brune K. Cyclooxygenase-2 – 10 years later. J Pharm Exp Ther 2002; 300:367–75.

Holscher C. Inhibitors of cyclooxygenase produce amnesia for passive avoidance task in the chick. Eur J Neurosci 1995; 7:1360–1365.

Hoozemans J.J., Bruckner M.K., Rozemuller A.J., Veerhuis R., Eikelenboom P., Arendt T. Cyclin D1 and cyclin E are co-localized with cyclo-oxygenase 2 (COX-2) in pyramidal neurons in Alzheimer disease temporal cortex. J Neuropathol Exp Neurol 2002; 61:678–688.

Hoozemans J.J., Veerhuis R., Rozemuller A.J., Arendt T., Eikelenboom P. Neuronal COX-2 expression and phosphorylation of pRb precede p38 MAPK activation and neurofibrillary changes in AD temporal cortex. Neurobiol Dis 2004; 15:492–499.

Hoozemans J.J., van Haastert E.S., Veerhuis R., Arendt T., Scheper W., Eikelenboom P., Rozemuller A.J. Maximal COX-2 and ppRb expression in neurons occurs during early Braak stages prior to the maximal activation of astrocytes and microglia in Alzheimer's disease. J Neuroinflammation. 2005; 2:27.

in t' Veld B.A., Ruitenberg A., Hofman A., Launer L.J., van Duijn C.M., Stijnen T., Breteler M.M., Stricker B.H. Nonsteroidal antiinflammatory drugs and the risk of Alzheimer's disease. N Engl J Med 2001; 345:1515–1521.

Kaufmann W.E., Andreasson K.I., Isakson P.C., Worley P.F. Cyclooxygenases and the central nervous system. Prostaglandins 1997; 54:601–624.

Kaufmann W.E., Worley P.F., Pegg J., Bremer M., Isakson P. COX-2, a synaptically induced enzyme, is expressed by excitatory neurons at postsynaptic sites in rat cerebral cortex. Proc Natl Acad Sci U S A 1996; 93:2317–2321.

Kaufmann W.E., Worley P.F., Taylor C.V., Bremer M., Isakson P.C. Cyclooxygenase-2 expression during rat neocortical development and in Rett syndrome. Brain Dev 1997; 19:25–34.

Kis B., Snipes J.A., Busija D.W. Acetaminophen and the cyclooxygenase-3 puzzle: sorting out facts, fictions, and uncertainties. J Pharmacol Exp Ther 2005; 315:1–7.

Levi G., Minghetti L., Aloisi F. Regulation of prostanoid synthesis in microglial cells and effects of prostaglandin E2 on microglial functions. Biochimie. 199; 80:899–904.

Lukiw W.J., Bazan N.G. Cyclooxygenase 2 RNA message abundance, stability, and hypervariability in sporadic Alzheimer neocortex. J Neurosci Res 1997; 50:937–945.

Manuelidis L., Fritch W., Zaitsev I. Dapsone to delay symptoms in Creutzfeldt-Jakob disease. Lancet 1998; 352:456.

McGeer P.L., McGeer E.G. Inflammation, autotoxicity and Alzheimer disease. Neurobiol Aging. 2001; 22:799–809.

McGeer P.L., Rogers J. Anti-inflammatory agents as a therapeutic approach to Alzheimer's disease. Neurology. 1992; 42:447–449.

Minghetti L., Cardone F., Greco A., Puopolo M., Levi G., Green A.J., Knight R., Pocchiari M. Increased CSF levels of prostaglandin E_2 in variant Creutzfeldt-Jakob disease. Neurology 2002; 58:127–129.

Minghetti L., Greco A., Cardone F., Puopolo M., Ladogana A., Almonti S., Cunningham C., Perry V.H., Pocchiari M., Levi G. Increased brain synthesis of prostaglandin E_2 and F_2-isoprostane in human and experimental transmissible spongiform encephalopathies. J Neuropathol Exp Neurol 2000; 59:866–871.

Minghetti L., Levi G. Microglia as effector cells in brain damage and repair: focus on prostanoids and nitric oxide. Prog Neurobiol 1998; 54:99–125.

Minghetti L., Sbriccoli M., Geloso M.C., Ingrosso L., Di Bari M.A., Greco A., Cardone F., Pocchiari M. Cyclooxygenases and prostaglandin E2 in animal and human prion diseases. Proceedings VII European Meeting on glial cell functions. 2005 May 17–21, Amsterdam. Medimond International Proceeding Publishers, 2005.

Minghetti L. Cyclooxygenase-2 (COX-2) in inflammatory and degenerative brain diseases. J Neuropathol Exp Neurol 2004; 63:901–910.

Montine T.J., Sidell K.R., Crews B.C., Markesbery W.R., Marnett L.J., Roberts L.J. 2nd, Morrow J.D. Elevated CSF prostaglandin E2 levels in patients with probable AD. Neurology 1999; 53:1495–1498.

Nagy Z., Esiri M.M., Smith A.D. The cell division cycle and the pathophysiology of Alzheimer's disease. Neuroscience 1998; 87:731–739.

Niwa K., Araki E., Morham S.G., Ross M.E., Iadecola C. Cyclooxygenase-2 contributes to functional hyperemia in whisker-barrel cortex. J Neurosci 2000; 20:763–770.

O'Neill G.P., Ford-Hutchinson A.W. Expression of mRNA for cyclooxygenase-1 and cyclooxygenase-2 in human tissues. FEBS Lett. 1993; 330:156–160.

Parente L., Perretti M. Advances in the pathophysiology of constitutive and inducible cyclooxygenases: two enzymes in the spotlight. Biochem Pharmacol 2003; 65:153–159.

Pasinetti G.M., Aisen P.S. Cyclooxygenase-2 expression is increased in frontal cortex of Alzheimer's disease brain. Neuroscience 1998; 87:319–324.

Pepicelli O., Fedele E., Berardi M., Raiteri M., Levi G., Greco A., Ajmone-Cat M.A., Minghetti L. Cyclo oxygenase-1 and -2 differently contribute to prostaglandin E_2 synthesis and lipid peroxidation after in vivo activation of N-methyl-D-aspartate receptors in rat hippocampus. J Neurochem 2005; 93:1561–1567.

Perry V.H., Cunningham C., Boche D. Atypical inflammation in the central nervous system in prion disease. Curr Opin Neurol 2002; 15:349–354.

Puoti G., Giaccone G., Mangieri M., Limido L., Fociani P., Zerbi P., Suardi S., Rossi G., Iussich S., Capobianco R., Di Fede G., Marcon G., Cotrufo R., Filippini G., Bugiani O., Tagliavini F. Sporadic Creutzfeldt-Jakob disease: the extent of microglia activation is dependent on the biochemical type of PrPSc. J Neuropathol Exp Neurol 2005; 64:902–909.

Qin N., Zhang S.P., Reitz T.L., Mei J.M., Flores C.M. Cloning, expression, and functional characterization of human cyclooxygenase-1 splicing variants: evidence for intron 1 retention. J Pharmacol Exp Ther. 2005; 315:1298–305.

Rall J.M., Mach S.A., Dash P.K. Intrahippocampal infusion of a cyclooxygenase-2 inhibitor attenuates memory acquisition in rats. Brain Res 2003; 968:273–276.

Reines S.A., Block G.A., Morris J.C., Liu G., Nessly M.L., Lines C.R., Norman B.A., Baranak C.C. Rofecoxib Protocol 091 Study Group. Rofecoxib: no effect on Alzheimer's disease in a 1-year, randomized, blinded, controlled study. Neurology. 2004; 62:66–71.

Ricceri L., Minghetti L., Moles A., Popoli P., Confaloni A., De Simone R., Piscopo P., Scattoni M.L., di Luca M., Calamandrei G. Cognitive and neurological deficits induced by early and prolonged basal forebrain cholinergic hypofunction in rats. Exp Neurol. 2004; 189:162–172.

Sang N., Zhang J., Marcheselli V., Bazan N.G., Chen C. Postsynaptically synthesized prostaglandin E2 (PGE2) modulates hippocampal synaptic transmission via a presynaptic PGE2 EP2 receptor. J Neurosci. 2005; 25:9858–9870.

Sharifzadeh M., Naghdi N., Khosrovani S., Ostad S.N., Sharifzadeh K., Roghani A. Post-training intrahippocampal infusion of the COX-2 inhibitor celecoxib impaired spatial memory retention in rats. Eur J Pharmacol. 2005; 511:159–166.

Sharifzadeh M., Tavasoli M., Soodi M., Mohammadi-Eraghi S., Ghahremani M.H., Roghani A. A time course analysis of cyclooxygenase-2 suggests a role in spatial memory retrieval in rats. Neurosci Res. 2006; 54:171–179.

Schwab J.M., Schluesener H.J. Cyclooxygenases and central nervous system inflammation: conceptual neglect of cyclooxygenase 1. Arch Neurol 2003; 60:630–632.

Schwieler L., Erhardt S., Nilsson L., Linderholm K., Engberg G. Effects of COX-1 and COX-2 inhibitors on the firing of rat midbrain dopaminergic neurons–possible involvement of endogenous kynurenic acid. Synapse. 2006; 59:290–298.

Shaftel S.S., Olschowka J.A., Hurley S.D., Moore A.H., O'Banion M.K. COX-3: a splice variant of cyclooxygenase-1 in mouse neural tissue and cells. Brain Res Mol Brain Res 2003; 119:213–215.

Shaw K.N., Commins S., O'Mara S.M. Deficits in spatial learning and synaptic plasticity induced by the rapid and competitive broad-spectrum cyclooxygenase inhibitor ibuprofen are reversed by increasing endogenous brain-derived neurotrophic factor. Eur J Neurosci 2003; 17:2438–46.

Simard A.R., Rivest S. Neuroprotective properties of the innate immune system and bone marrow stem cells in Alzheimer's disease. Mol Psychiatry 2006; 11:327–335.

Sternberg E.M. Neural regulation of innate immunity: a coordinated nonspecific host response to pathogens. Nat Rev Immunol. 2006; 6:318–328.

Streit W.J. Microglia as neuroprotective, immunocompetent cells of the CNS. Glia. 2002; 40:133–139.

Teather L.A., Packard M.G., Bazan N.G. Post-training cyclooxygenase-2 (COX-2) inhibition impairs memory consolidation. Learn Mem 2002; 9:41–47.

Vazquez-Tello A., Fan L., Hou X., Joyal J.S., Mancini J.A., Quiniou C., Clyman R.I., Gobeil F. Jr, Varma D.R., Chemtob S. Intracellular-specific colocalization of prostaglandin E2 synthases and cyclooxygenases in the brain. Am J Physiol Regul Integr Comp Physiol. 2004; 287:R1155–R1163.

Walsh D.T., Perry V.H., Minghetti L. Cyclooxygenase-2 is highly expressed in microglial-like cells in a murine model of prion disease. Glia 2000; 29:392–396.

Webber K.M., Raina A.K., Marlatt M.W., Zhu X., Prat M.I., Morelli L., Casadesus G., Perry G., Smith M.A. The cell cycle in Alzheimer disease: a unique target for neuropharmacology. Mech Ageing Dev. 2005; 126:1019–1025.

Will R.G., Alperovitch A., Poser S., Pocchiari M., Hofman A., Mitrova E., de Silva R., D'Alessandro M., Delasnerie-Laupretre N., Zerr I., van Duijn C. Descriptive epidemiology of Creutzfeldt-Jakob disease in six European countries, 1993–1995. EU Collaborative Study Group for CJD. Ann Neurol. 1998; 43:763–767.

Will R.G., Ironside J.W., Zeidler M., Cousens S.N., Estibeiro K., Alperovitch A., Poser S., Pocchiari M., Hofman A., Smith P.G. A new variant of Creutzfeldt-Jakob disease in the UK. Lancet 1996; 347:921–925

Yamagata K., Andreasson K.I., Kaufmann W.E., Barnes C.A., Worley P.F. Expression of a mitogen-inducible cyclooxygenase in brain neurons: regulation by synaptic activity and glucocorticoids. Neuron 1993; 11:371–386.

Yasojima K., Schwab C., McGeer E.G., McGeer P.L. Distribution of cyclooxygenase-1 and cyclooxygenase-2 mRNAs and proteins in human brain and peripheral organs. Brain Res 1999; 830:226–236.

Yermakova A.V., O'Banion M.K. Downregulation of neuronal cyclooxygenase-2 expression in end stage Alzheimer's disease. Neurobiol Aging 2001; 22:823–836.

Yermakova A.V., Rollins J., Callahan L.M., Rogers J., O'Banion M.K. Cyclooxygenase-1 in human Alzheimer's, and control brain: quantitative analysis of expression by microglia and CA3 hippocampal neurons. J Neuropathol Exp Neurol 1999; 58:1135–1146.

Zhang J., Rivest S. Anti-inflammatory effects of prostaglandin E2 in the central nervous system in response to brain injury and circulating lipopolysaccharide. J Neurochem 2001; 76:855–64.

SECTION III

**INFLAMMATION AND CARDIOVASCULAR
DISEASE: THE COXIB CONTROVERSY**

CHAPTER 6

CARDIOVASCULAR EFFECTS OF THE SELECTIVE CYCLOOXYGENASE-2 INHIBITORS

WILLIAM B. WHITE*

Professor of Medicine and Chief, Division of Hypertension and Clinical Pharmacology, Pat and Jim Calhoun Cardiology Center, University of Connecticut School of Medicine, 263 Farmington Avenue, Farmington, Connecticut 06030-3940

Abstract: The data that have accumulated in recent years underscore the importance of carefully weighing the risks and benefits of traditional NSAIDs and COX-2 selective inhibitors before making therapeutic decisions for the management of chronic arthritis. In clinical practice, the majority of patients with moderate to severe arthritis who might benefit from NSAID or COX-2 therapy are likely to be elderly and, therefore, at higher risk for gastrointestinal and cardiovascular adverse events than younger persons.

*E-mail: wwhite@nso1.uchc.edu

R. E. Harris (ed.), Inflammation in the Pathogenesis of Chronic Diseases, 145–158.
© 2007 *Springer.*

Thus, these patients are more likely to be taking low-dose aspirin and using over-the-counter NSAIDs for pain.

Selecting a combination of therapies that provides relief from arthritis-related symptoms, minimizes cardiovascular risk, and preserves the gastrointestinal mucosa is complex. Factors to consider include the interference of certain NSAIDs, such as ibuprofen or naproxen, with the antiplatelet effects of aspirin; direct effects of non-selective NSAIDs and of COX-2 selective inhibitors on fluid retention and blood pressure; emerging data about cardiovascular risks associated with these drugs; differences between these agents with regard to associated gastrointestinal adverse event rates; and the feasibility of co-administration of anti-inflammatory therapies with gastro-protective agents

1.   INTRODUCTION

Cyclooxyenase-2 (COX-2) selective inhibitors were developed to create a new class of nonsteroidal anti-inflammatory drugs (NSAIDs) with properties similar to those of nonselective NSAIDs but without their potential COX-1-mediated gastrointestinal toxicity. [1, 2] Studies of COX-2 selective inhibitors have shown that they are in fact associated with a significantly lower risk of upper and lower gastrointestinal complications than traditional NSAIDs, except in patients who are taking concomitant aspirin.

Recent evidence also suggests that at least some of the COX-2 selective inhibitors, and perhaps some traditional NSAIDs as well, are associated with an increased risk of adverse cardiovascular (CV) events at certain doses. For example, reports of a higher incidence of myocardial infarction (MI) among patients with arthritis taking the COX-2 selective inhibitor rofecoxib than those taking the NSAID naproxen [2, 4] have heightened concerns since 2001 about COX-2 inhibitor safety. Additionally, elevated CV event rates were reported in patients with spontaneous adenomatous polyps who were taking celecoxib [5] and in patients who received parecoxib and valdecoxib immediately after coronary artery bypass graft surgery. [6]

This chapter summarizes findings concerning the effects of both nonselective and selective NSAIDs – first to highlight some differences on the GI tract and subsequently on the CV system that must be taken into account in order to fully understand the complexities of the data that have accumulated during the past several years.

2.   EFFECTS OF COX-2 SELECTIVE INHIBITORS
ON THE GASTROINTESTINAL TRACT

The gastrointestinal adverse effects of aspirin and traditional NSAIDs are well defined and include development of gastric or duodenal ulcers, hospitalizations due to gastrointestinal bleeding complications, perforated ulcers or gastric obstruction, and gastrointestinal-related deaths. [7] Gastric and duodenal ulcers and complications arising from them occur frequently in regular users of aspirin and traditional NSAIDs. According to one estimate, more than 100,000 hospitalizations and 16,500 deaths occur annually in the United States because of NSAID-related ulcer complications. [8] Fortunately, the risk of serious NSAID gastropathy has declined substantially in the past decade. Among the reasons are use of lower nonselective-NSAID doses, concomitant use of proton-pump inhibitors, and the introduction of COX-2 selective inhibitors, which are fundamentally COX-1-sparing drugs. [9]

The gastrointestinal toxicity of traditional NSAIDs is due in part to nonselective inhibition of both COX-1 and COX-2 isoenzymes involved in prostaglandin synthesis. [10] By selectively suppressing prostaglandin production by the COX-2 enzyme, COX-2 selective agents provide anti-inflammatory and analgesic benefits while conceptually sparing the gastroprotective activity of COX-1. [10] Data from large-scale clinical trials have confirmed that COX-2 inhibitors are associated with substantial reductions in gastrointestinal risk in the majority of patients who do not use aspirin.

3.   GASTROINTESTINAL RISK WITH COX-2 SELECTIVE INHIBITORS IS REDUCED

Clinical studies suggest that COX-2 inhibitors are associated with a reduction in risk of gastrointestinal adverse events equivalent to that achieved by adding proton pump inhibitor therapy to traditional NSAID therapy. Also, endoscopic evidence indicates that COX-2 selective inhibitors are associated with a lower incidence of gastroduodenal ulcers than conventional NSAIDs. In a study conducted by Laine and colleagues, 742 patients with osteoarthritis were randomly assigned to receive rofecoxib (25 mg or 50 mg/day), ibuprofen, or placebo. [11] Patients were allowed to take acetaminophen, non-NSAID pain medications, or an antacid during the trial. Patients in the rofecoxib and placebo groups had lower rates of endoscopic ulcers than patients in the ibuprofen group at 12 weeks; patients in both rofecoxib groups also had lower rates of endoscopic ulcers at 24 weeks ($P < .001$ for comparisons with ibuprofen). The rofecoxib and placebo groups did not differ for any GI outcome, whereas efficacy or relief of arthritis-related symptoms was similar in the rofecoxib and ibuprofen groups. Similarly, Simon and coworkers showed that patients with rheumatoid arthritis who took celecoxib (100 mg, 200 mg, or 400 mg twice daily) had significantly fewer clinically important ulcers (3 mm or greater with obvious depth) than those who took naproxen 500 mg twice daily over a 12-week period. Further, regardless of the dose of the COX-2 selective inhibitor, these findings were not significantly different from those observed for placebo. [12]

The Vioxx Gastrointestinal Outcomes Research (VIGOR) [2] study was the first large-scale trial to provide evidence that COX-2 selective inhibitors minimize the risk of upper gastrointestinal adverse effects in older ($\geq$ aged 50) patients with rheumatoid arthritis. [2] Over 9 months of follow-up, rofecoxib and naproxen showed equivalent efficacy; however, the incidence of confirmed upper gastrointestinal adverse events per 100 patient-years in the rofecoxib group was less than half that observed in the naproxen group. Of interest, a *post hoc* analysis of the trial indicated that about 40% of the serious events occurred in the lower gastrointestinal tract; these events were also reduced by more than half in patients who received rofecoxib. [13] It is noteworthy that there is no evidence that proton pump inhibitors decrease the incidence of lower GI tract complications.

The Celecoxib Arthritis Safety Study (CLASS) provided additional evidence that COX-2 inhibitors reduce risk of gastrointestinal events in adults with osteoarthritis or rheumatoid arthritis. [1] Patients enrolled in CLASS were randomly assigned to receive celecoxib, ibuprofen, or diclofenac and were also permitted to take low-dose aspirin if indicated for cardiovascular prophylaxis. During the 6-month treatment period, the annualized incidence of upper gastrointestinal complications alone and in combination with symptomatic ulcers was nearly twice as high among patients who received conventional NSAIDs as among those who received celecoxib. Preliminary data suggest that, in addition to minimizing ulcers and their complications, celecoxib is better tolerated than traditional NSAIDs. [12]

Similar or even greater reductions in gastrointestinal risk than those noted in CLASS have been observed with the newer COX-2s etoricoxib, lumiracoxib, and valdecoxib. [15, 18]

In comparative trials, no differences in efficacy have been observed between COX-2 selective agents and NSAID comparators. Thus, COX-2s should not be viewed as replacements for traditional NSAIDs based on efficacy for inflammatory symptoms; instead, after a careful risk/benefit analysis, clinicians should consider using COX-2 inhibitors in appropriately selected patients at high risk for gastrointestinal adverse effects or in patients who require anti-inflammatory therapy for arthritis but who may not tolerate the gastrointestinal effects of ns-NSAIDs.

4.   COX-2 INHIBITORS IN PATIENTS WITH HYPERTENSION

Arthritis and hypertension represent common co-morbid conditions in older patients that often result in the co-administration of non-steroidal anti-inflammatory drugs (NSAIDs) or COX-2 selective inhibitors with antihypertensive agents. Meta-analyses of the NSAIDs from the early 1990s showed that many agents within the class (eg, ibuprofen, indomethacin, and naproxen) could increase mean arterial pressure by as much as 5 to 6 mm Hg in hypertensive patients. [19, 20] Increases in blood pressure (BP) of this magnitude are sufficient to be of clinical concern.

Sustained BP elevations in the elderly are associated with increases in the risk of both ischemic and hemorrhagic stroke, congestive heart failure, and ischemic cardiac events. [21, 23] For example, in the VALUE trial, differences of approximately 2 to 4 mm Hg in systolic BP control in an older population of hypertensive patients randomly assigned to 2 treatment groups (valsartan or amlodipine) resulted in a clinically and statistically significant relative increase in cardiac events of over 40% in the less-well-controlled group (valsartan recipients) during the first year of the study. [23] Thus, it becomes of substantial importance to understand the relative effects of the various NSAIDs and COX-2 selective inhibitors on BP destabilization in patients with both treated and untreated hypertension.

5. PATHOPHYSIOLOGIC EFFECTS OF NSAIDs AND COX-2 INHIBITORS THAT INDUCE HYPERTENSION

Nonselective COX inhibition can result in inhibition of prostaglandin synthesis and is associated with both anti-natriuretic and vasoconstrictor effects. [24, 27] In some cases, these effects have consequences on BP control and may be of particular relevance in patients with preexisting hypertension, edema, or congestive heart failure.

As shown in Figure 1, inhibition of COX-2 is associated with reductions in both prostaglandin E_2 (PGE_2) and prostaglandin I_2 (PGI_2, or prostacyclin). [27] Inhibition of PGE can cause an acute relative reduction in daily urinary sodium excretion of 30% or more. [28] Within a few days, the kidneys in patients with normal renal function will tend to increase sodium excretion to compensate for the antinatriuretic effects of the COX-2 selective inhibitor or NSAID, to maintain homeostasis of sodium balance (Figure 2). [28] However, in patients with chronic kidney disease this homeostatic process is impaired and, within 1 to 2 weeks of their starting NSAID therapy, a considerable amount of salt and water may accumulate. In such cases, both edema and hypertension commonly develop and, in more severe cases, congestive heart failure. [29, 32]

In addition to causing problems with salt and water balance, the NSAIDs and COX-2 selective inhibitors may impair the vasodilatory benefits of prostacyclin. Loss of this mechanism of vasodilation in the face of numerous vasoconstrictors (eg, angiotensin 2, norepinephrine, and endothelin) may lead to increases in systemic vascular resistance and subsequently to increases in mean arterial pressure (Figure 1).

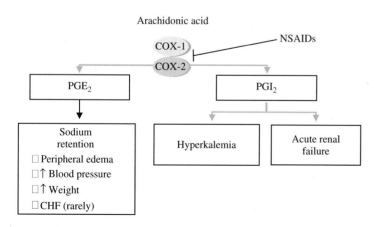

Figure 1. Potential effects of NSAIDs on cardiorenal physiology
Source: From Brater DC. *Am J Med.* 1999;107:65S–70S. Reproduced by permission
Note: COX = cyclooxygenase; PGE_2 = prostaglandin E_2; PGI_2 = prostaglandin I_2; CHF = congestive heart failure

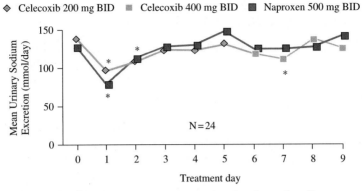

*P<0.05, change from baseline;   P<0.05, change from baseline, celecoxib vs naproxen.

Figure 2. Mean (± standard error) urinary sodium excretion rates after administration of celecoxib and naproxen to older patients with normal renal function. On days 1 and 2, the sodium excretion was significantly reduced by both agents, but on day 3, sodium excretion rates returned towards baseline. *Source:* From Whelton A. *Arch Intern Med.* 2000;160:1465–1470. Reproduced by permission

6.   EFFECTS OF NSAIDs AND COX-2 INHIBITORS IN NORMOTENSIVE PATIENTS

The effects of chronic NSAID and COX-2 selective inhibitor therapies on normotensive patients have not been extensively studied. However, in a pooled analysis of the effects of older NSAIDs on BP, indomethacin induced a slight elevation in BP in normotensive persons. [19] In a fairly recent case-control analysis in a Medicare population, Solomon et al studied the effects of NSAIDs and coxibs on the development of hypertension. [31] The primary finding in this study was that new-onset hypertension developed in 21% of patients for whom celecoxib was prescribed, 23% of those for whom nonselective NSAIDs (ns-NSAIDs) were prescribed, and 27% of those for whom rofecoxib was prescribed. Of note, the background rate of new hypertension in patients not receiving NSAIDs was 22%. [31, 33] Thus, this study demonstrated that rofecoxib was associated with a signifi-cantly higher risk of hypertension than celecoxib and the ns-NSAIDs. Additionally, the risk was higher if patients had a history of congestive heart failure or kidney or liver disease.

7.   EFFECTS OF NSAIDs AND COX-2 INHIBITORS IN TREATED HYPERTENSIVE PATIENTS

A major focus of clinical research during the last several years has been the potential destabilization of BP in hypertensive patients who are receiving angiotensin-converting enzyme (ACE) inhibitors or angiotensin receptor blockers (ARBs), beta-blockers, calcium antagonists, or diuretics. In one of our earlier studies, a placebo-controlled trial, ambulatory BP monitoring was used to assess the effect of high-dose celecoxib (200 mg BID) in 178 patients who were on chronic ACE inhibitor therapy. [32] This study demonstrated that celecoxib (400 mg total daily dose) was associated with a non-significant increase in 24-hour mean BP of 1.6/1.2 mm Hg. Subsequently, a larger trial using the <u>clinic</u> systolic BP as the primary endpoint evaluated the effects of rofecoxib 25 mg/day and celecoxib 200 mg/day in 1,092 patients on chronic, stable doses of antihypertensive therapies. [29] This study showed that rofecoxib induced significant increases in systolic BP in patients who were taking ACE inhibitors and beta-blockers but not in those who were taking calcium antagonists (Figure 3). Patients randomly assigned to receive celecoxib did not show a change in systolic BP regardless of background antihypertensive therapy. These results support the notion that calcium antagonists do not significantly depend on vascular prostacyclin as part of their mechanism of action. [24]

In the most comprehensive randomized, double-blind clinical trial evaluating the effects of NSAIDs in treated hypertensives, entitled the CRESCENT trial, 24-hour ambulatory BP monitoring was performed at baseline and after 6 and 12 weeks of therapy with celecoxib, naproxen, or rofecoxib in nearly 400 patients with diabetes, hypertension, and osteoarthritis. [14] This study demonstrated that at equally effective doses for osteoarthritis, treatment with rofecoxib but not celecoxib or naproxen induced a significant increase in 24-hour systolic BP (Figure 4). In addition, 30% of patients administered rofecoxib had a resultant 24-hour systolic BP of ≥ 135 mm Hg compared with about 16% of patients randomized to celecoxib and 19% to naproxen.

Thus, NSAIDs and COX-2 selective inhibitors do have the potential to destabilize BP in patients who are on chronic antihypertensive regimens, especially drugs

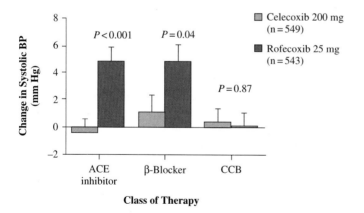

Figure 3. Effects of rofecoxib and celecoxib on clinic systolic BP in patients given ACE inhibitors, beta-blockers, and calcium antagonists. Destabilization occurred after 6 weeks of treatment with rofecoxib in patients taking ACE inhibitors and beta-blockers but not in those taking calcium antagonists. Celecoxib did not affect systolic BP control rates in the antihypertensive drug treatment groups
Source: From Whelton A, et al. *Am J Cardiol.* 2002;90:953–960. Reproduced by permission

24-hr Systolic BP at Baseline and Week 6

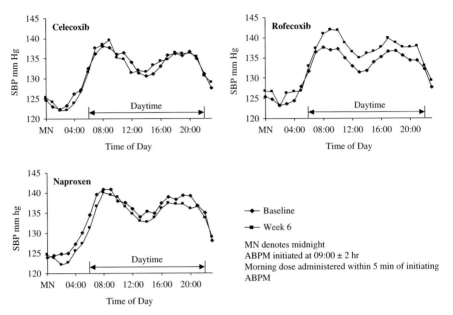

Figure 4. Effects of celecoxib, rofecoxib, and naproxen on hourly mean systolic BP over 24 hours after 6 weeks of therapy. A consistent increase from baseline in ambulatory systolic pressure was observed only in the rofecoxib treatment group

Source: From White WB, et al. *Arch Intern Med.* 2005;165:161–168. Reproduced by permission

affecting the renin-angiotensin system, loop diuretics, and beta-adrenergic blockers. Because NSAIDs and coxibs have an effect within 1 to 2 weeks after the start of therapy, they should be used with caution in hypertensive patients who are taking ACE inhibitors, angiontensin receptor blockers, or beta-blockers, as well as in patients who have diabetes or mild renal disease. These patients should be seen shortly after anti-inflammatory therapy is initiated.

The effects of various agents may vary, as may the responses in different types of patients. Existing data suggest that in patients whose hypertension is being treated, celecoxib and naproxen may destabilize BP less than more potent NSAIDs or COX-2 selective inhibitors such as indomethacin and rofecoxib. In addition, if elevated BP develops in a normotensive patient who is taking NSAIDs or COX-2 selective inhibitors, the physician may not attribute the hypertension to the newly prescribed therapy. The most appropriate way to deal with this potential problem is to interrupt the patient's anti-inflammatory therapy for 2 weeks and then reassess the patient's BP levels carefully in the physician's office.

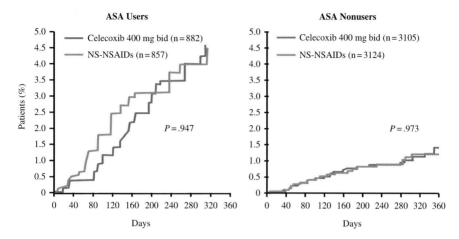

Figure 5. Accumulation of all cardiovascular events in the CLASS trial. Patients were analyzed according to aspirin use. The patients taking aspirin had a nearly 4.5-fold increase in cardiovascular events compared to those who entered the trial not on aspirin. The event rates were similar for celecoxib, 800 mg daily compared to the NSAIDs, ibuprofen (2,400 mg daily) and diclofenac (150 mg daily)
Source: From White WB, et al. *Am J Cardiol.* 2002;89:425–430

8.   EVALUATING CARDIOVASCULAR EVENTS IN CLINICAL TRIALS WITH COX-2 SELECTIVE AGENTS

Cardiovascular event rates among users of NSAIDs, including COX-2 selective inhibitors, have been evaluated in numerous studies. The most robust data come from prospective, randomized clinical trials in which the double-blind was maintained for the entire course of the study. The seminal studies that first examined cardiovascular events in arthritis populations were the VIGOR [2] and CLASS studies. [1, 34] These 2 studies remain highly important with regard to outcomes because they compared supra-therapeutic doses of COX-2 selective inhibitors with maximal therapeutic NSAID doses in the target population with arthritis. Findings were dissimilar because cardiovascular event rates were higher with rofecoxib 50 mg daily than with naproxen 500 mg twice daily in the VIGOR trial, [2] whereas they were similar for celecoxib 800 mg daily, ibuprofen 2,400 mg daily, and diclofenac 150 mg daily in CLASS (Figure 5). [34] The cardiovascular event rates in a meta-analysis of celecoxib and various NSAIDs [35] in the osteoarthritis (OA) and RA populations confirmed that there were similar rates of Anti-Platelet Trialists' Collaboration (APTC) [36] adjudicated endpoints.

Findings from a third study, [37] the Therapeutic Arthritis Research and Gastrointestinal Event Trial (TARGET), were similar to those in CLASS [34] for the investigational COX-2 selective inhibitor lumiracoxib. The cumulative incidence of APTC events in TARGET was relatively low and did not differ between lumiracoxib and naproxen or ibuprofen. However, the effects of placebo could not be studied in that these patients suffered from arthritis and thus these trials also considered efficacy.

9. OBSERVATIONAL STUDIES THAT HAVE ASSESSED THE CARDIOVASCULAR RISK OF NSAIDs AND COX-2 SELECTIVE INHIBITORS

Cardiovascular event rates have been evaluated in numerous databases from health care companies, insurance rosters, and pharmacy benefit management companies. All these studies were retrospective and either nested case-control or cohort analyses based on drug use in the database and, therefore, pose some methodological concerns. However, the large populations and hundreds of cardiovascular events analyzed enhance their value from both clinical and epidemiologic perspectives.

In collaboration with the Food and Drug Administration, Kaiser Permanente in northern California and epidemiologists at the Vanderbilt University School of Medicine reported the results of a case-control study of nearly 1.4 million people, who were observed for 2 years. [38] Nonusers (including those who were remote users) of NSAIDs served as controls, and nonfatal myocardial and cardiovascular death rates associated with various NSAIDs and COX-2 selective agents were then compared. The results showed that use of most nonselective NSAIDs increases the relative risk of a cardiac event (Figure 6). compared with nonuse. High doses (> 25 mg daily) of rofecoxib were associated with a particularly elevated risk of myocardial infarction and sudden death, whereas celecoxib was not.

10. LONGER TERM PLACEBO-CONTROLLED TRIALS WITH NSAIDs AND COX-2 SELECTIVE INHIBITORS

No long-term clinical trials in patients with arthritis have been placebo-controlled because of obvious clinical and ethical issues related to pain management. Thus little, if anything is known about the relative risk of using the nonselective NSAIDs compared with no treatment over time in arthritis or pain management. For the COX-2 selective inhibitors rofecoxib and celecoxib, there are 4 placebo-controlled trials in non-arthritis populations that have received a great deal of attention recently since their safety data were published or announced prior to their efficacy findings.

In one of these trials, the Adenomatous Polyp Prevention on Vioxx (APPROVe) trial, [5] the APTC event rate was 1.50 events/100 patient-years for rofecoxib 25 mg daily versus 0.78 events/100 patient-years for placebo; in the Adenoma Prevention with Celecoxib (APC) trial, [39] the combined APTC and heart failure event rate was approximately 0.4 events/100 patient-years for placebo, 0.86 events/100 patient-years for celecoxib 400 mg daily, and 1.27 events/100 patients-years for celecoxib 800 mg daily.

In these colonic polyp studies, the event rates for the COX-2 selective agents did not appear to increase compared with placebo until after at least 1 year of

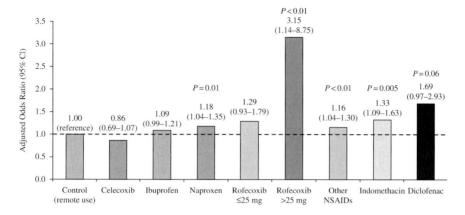

Adjusted for age, gender, health plan region, medical history, smoking, and medication use.

Figure 6. Results of a 2-year observational study in 1.4 million persons administered various NSAIDs in a closed formulary health maintenance organization in California. The relative risk of acute myocardial infarction and sudden cardiovascular death was compared to non-users of NSAIDs and COX-2 inhibitors (control group)
Source: Adapted from Graham D, et al. *Lancet.* 2005;365:475–481

drug exposure. These findings may be of clinical significance in the long-term prevention of various epithelial cell cancers, and further analyses of risk and benefit for those diseases will be warranted. However, the implications of the findings from the APPROVe and APC trials for the chronic treatment of arthritis pain and inflammation in patients for whom placebo is not an option are unclear.

Another important finding from the APPROVe and APC studies [5, 39] pertains to interaction with aspirin. In these studies, aspirin use did not appear to influence the relation of cardiovascular event rates among patients with spontaneous colonic polyps who received COX-2 inhibitors and those who received placebo. Thus, if the hypothesis that COX-2 selective inhibitors are thrombogenic due to imbalance between prostacyclin and thromboxane production is correct, [40] additional suppression of thromboxane synthesis by aspirin should have improved outcomes with the COX-2 inhibitors relative to placebo compared with outcomes for nonusers of aspirin. Additionally, pharmaco-epidemiologic studies have shown that the frequency of cardiovascular events, including MI and sudden cardiac death, is the same with nonselective-NSAIDs that inhibit COX-1 as with COX-2 selective inhibitors. [38]

11.   CONCLUSIONS

The data that have accumulated in recent years underscore the importance of carefully weighing the risks and benefits of traditional NSAIDs and COX-2 selective inhibitors before making therapeutic decisions for the management of chronic arthritis. In clinical practice, the majority of patients with moderate to severe arthritis who might benefit from NSAID or COX-2 therapy are likely to be elderly and, therefore, at higher risk for gastrointestinal and cardiovascular adverse events than younger persons. Thus, these patients are more likely to be taking low-dose aspirin and using over-the-counter NSAIDs for pain.

Selecting a combination of therapies that provides relief from arthritis-related symptoms, minimizes cardiovascular risk, and preserves the gastrointestinal mucosa is complex. Factors to consider include the interference of certain NSAIDs, such as ibuprofen or naproxen, with the antiplatelet effects of aspirin; direct effects of non-selective NSAIDs and of COX-2 selective inhibitors on fluid retention and blood pressure; emerging data about cardiovascular risks associated with these drugs; differences between these agents with regard to associated gastrointestinal adverse event rates; and the feasibility of co-administration of anti-inflammatory therapies with gastro-protective agents.

REFERENCES

1. Silverstein FE, Faich G, Goldstein JL, et al. Gastrointestinal toxicity with celecoxib vs nonsteroidal anti-inflammatory drugs for osteoarthritis and rheumatoid arthritis. The CLASS study: a randomized controlled trial. *JAMA*. 2000;284:1247–1255.
2. Bombardier C, Laine L, Reicin A, et al. Comparison of upper gastrointestinal toxicity of rofecoxib and naproxen in patients with rheumatoid arthritis. *N Engl J Med*. 2000;343:1520–1528.
3. Mukherjee D, Nissen SE, Topol EJ. Risk of cardiovascular events associated with selective COX-2 inhibitors. *JAMA*. 2001;286:954–959.
4. Konstam MA, Weir MR, Reicin A, et al. Cardiovascular thrombotic events in controlled, clinical trials of rofecoxib. *Circulation*. 2001;104:2280–2288.
5. Bresalier RS, Sandler RS, Quan H, et al, for the Adenomatous Polyp Prevention on Vioxx (APPROVe) Trial Investigators. Cardiovascular events associated with rofecoxib in a colorectal adenoma chemoprevention trial. *N Engl J Med*. 2005;352:1092–1102.
6. Nussmeier NA, Whelton AA, Brown MT, et al. Complications of the COX-2 inhibitors parecoxib and valdecoxib after cardiac surgery. *N Engl J Med*. 2005;352:1081–1091.
7. Laine L. Nonsteroidal anti-inflammatory drug gastropathy. *Gastrointest Endosc Clin N Am*. 1996;6:489–504.
8. Wolfe MM, Lichtenstein DR, Singh G. Gastrointestinal toxicity of nonsteroidal anti-inflammatory drugs. *N Engl J Med*. 1999;340:1888–1899.
9. Fries JF, Murtagh KN, Bennett M, Zatarain E, Lingala B, Bruce B. The rise and decline of nonsteroidal antiinflammatory drug-associated gastropathy in rheumatoid arthritis. *Arthritis Rheum*. 2004;50:2433–2440.
10. Meade EA, Smith WL, DeWitt DL. Differential inhibition of prostaglandin endoperoxide synthase (cyclooxygenase) isozymes by aspirin and other non-steroidal anti-inflammatory drugs. *J Biol Chem*. 1993;268:6610–6614.
11. Laine L, Harper S, Simon T, et al, for the Rofecoxib Osteoarthritis Endoscopy Study Group. A randomized trial comparing the effect of rofecoxib, a cyclooxygenase 2-specific inhibitor, with that of ibuprofen on the gastroduodenal mucosa of patients with osteoarthritis. *Gastroenterology*. 1999;117:776–783
12. Simon LS, Weaver AL, Graham DY, et al. Anti-inflammatory and upper gastrointestinal effects of celecoxib in rheumatoid arthritis: a randomized controlled trial. *JAMA*. 1999;282:1921–1928.
13. Laine L, Connors LG, Reicin A, et al. Serious lower gastrointestinal clinical events with nonselective NSAID or coxib use. *Gastroenterology*. 2003;124:288–292.

14. Sowers JR, White WB, Pitt B, et al. for the Celecoxib Rofecoxib Efficacy and Safety in Comorbidities Evaluation Trial (CRESCENT) Investigators. The effects of cyclooxygenase-2 inhibitors and nonsteroidal anti-inflammatory therapy on 24-hour blood pressure in patients with hypertension, osteoarthritis and type 2 diabetes. *Arch Intern Med.* 2005;165:161–168.

15. Edwards JE, McQuay HJ, Moore RA. Efficacy and safety of valdecoxib for treatment of osteoarthritis and rheumatoid arthritis: systematic review of randomised controlled trials. *Pain.* 2004;111:286–296.

16. Hunt RH, Harper S, Watson DJ, et al. The gastrointestinal safety of the COX-2 selective inhibitor etoricoxib assessed by both endoscopy and analysis of upper gastrointestinal events. *Am J Gastroenterol.* 2003;98:1725–1733.

17. Kivitz AJ, Nayiager S, Schimansky T, Gimona A, Thurston HJ, Hawkey C. Reduced incidence of gastroduodenal ulcers associated with lumiracoxib compared with ibuprofen in patients with rheumatoid arthritis. *Aliment Pharmacol Ther.* 2004;19:1189–1198.

18. Schnitzer TJ, Burmester GR, Mysler E, for the TARGET Study Group. Comparison of lumiracoxib with naproxen and ibuprofen in the Therapeutic Arthritis Research and Gastrointestinal Event Trial (TARGET), reduction in ulcer complications: randomised controlled trial. *Lancet.* 2004;364:665–674.

19. Pope JE, Anderson JJ, Felson DT. A meta-analysis of the effects of nonsteroidal anti-inflammatory drugs on blood pressure. *Arch Intern Med.* 1993;153:477–484.

20. Johnson AG, Nguyen TV, Day RO. Do nonsteroidal anti-inflammatory drugs affect blood pressure? A meta-analysis. *Ann Intern Med.* 1994;121:289–300.

21. White WB. Benefits of antihypertensive therapy in older patients with hypertension. *Arch Intern Med.* 2000;160:149–150.

22. ALLHAT Officers and Coordinators for the ALLHAT Collaborative Research Group. Major cardiovascular events in hypertensive patients randomized to doxazosin vs chlorthalidone: the Antihypertensive and Lipid-Lowering Treatment to Prevent Heart Attack Trial (ALLHAT). *JAMA.* 2000;283:1967–1975.

23. Julius S, Kjeldsen SE, Weber M, et al. Outcomes in hypertensive patients at high cardiovascular risk treated with regimens based on valsartan or amlodipine: the VALUE randomised trial. *Lancet.* 2004;19:363:2022–2031.

24. Morgan TO, Anderson A, Bertram D. Effect of indomethacin on blood pressure in elderly people with essential hypertension well controlled on amlodipine or enalapril. *Am J Hypertens.* 2000;13:1161–1167.

25. Schwartz JI, Vandormael K, Malice MP, et al. Comparison of rofecoxib, celecoxib, and naproxen on renal function in elderly subjects receiving a normal-salt diet. *Clin Pharmacol Ther.* 2002;72:50–61.

26. Simon LS, Smolen JS, Abramson SB, et al. Controversies in COX-2 selective inhibition. *J Rheumatol.* 2002;29:1501–1510.

27. Brater DC. Effects of nonsteroidal anti-inflammatory drugs on renal function: focus on cyclooxygenase-2–selective inhibition. *Am J Med.* 1999;107:65S–70S.

28. Whelton A, Schulman G, Wallemark C, et al. Effects of celecoxib and naproxen on renal function in the elderly. *Arch Intern Med.* 2000;160:1465–1470.

29. Whelton A, White WB, Bello AE, Puma JA, Fort JG, and the SUCCESS-VII Investigators. Effects of celecoxib and rofecoxib on blood pressure and edema in patients ≥ 65 years of age with systemic hypertension and osteoarthritis. *Am J Cardiol.* 2002;90:959–963.

30. Whelton A. Nephrotoxicity of nonsteroidal anti-inflammatory drugs: physiologic foundations and clinical implications. *Am J Med.* 1999;106(5B):13S–24S.

31. Solomon DH, Schneeweiss S, Levin R, Avorn J. Relationship between COX-2 specific inhibitors and hypertension. *Hypertension.* 2004;44:140–145.

32. White WB, Kent J, Taylor A, Verburg KM, Lefkowith JB, Whelton A. Effects of celecoxib on ambulatory blood pressure in hypertensive patients on ACE inhibitors. *Hypertension.* 2002;39:929–934.

33. White WB. Hypertension associated with therapies to treat arthritis and pain. *Hypertension.* 2004;44:123–124.

34. White WB, Faich G, Whelton A, et al. Comparison of thromboembolic events in patients treated with celecoxib, a cyclooxygenase-2 specific inhibitor, versus ibuprofen or diclofenac. *Am J Cardiol.* 2002;89:425–430

35. White WB, Faich G, Borer JS, Makuch RW. Cardiovascular thrombotic events in arthritis trials of the cyclooxygenase-2 inhibitor celecoxib. *Am J Cardiol.* 2003;92:411–418.

36. Antiplatelet Trialists Collaboration. Collaborative overview of randomized trials of antiplatelet therapy: I: prevention of death, myocardial infarction, and stroke. *BMJ.* 1994;308:81–106.

37. Farkouh ME, Kirshner H, Harrington RA, et al. Comparison of lumiracoxib with naproxen and ibuprofen in the Therapeutic Arthritis Research and Gastrointestinal Event Trial (TARGET), cardiovascular outcomes: randomised controlled trial. *Lancet.* 2004;364:675–684.

38. Graham DJ, Campen D, Hui R, et al. Risk of acute myocardial infarction and sudden cardiac death in patients treated with cyclo-oxygenase 2 selective and non-selective non-steroidal anti-inflammatory drugs: nested case-control study. *Lancet.* 2005;365:475–481.

39. Solomon SD, McMurray JJV, Pfeffer MA, et al. Cardiovascular risk associated with celecoxib in a clinical trial for colorectal adenoma prevention. *N Engl J Med.* 2005;352:1071–1080.

40. Grosser T, Fries S, FitzGerald GA. Biological basis for the cardiovascular consequences of COX-2 inhibition: therapeutic challenges and opportunities. *J Clin Invest.* 2006;116:4–15

CHAPTER 7

COX-2 INHIBITORS AND CARDIOVASCULAR RISK

DANIEL J. SALZBERG[1,*] AND MATTHEW R. WEIR[2]

[1] *Assistant Professor of Medicine, Program Director, Nephrology Fellowship*
[2] *Professor and Director, Division of Nephrology, University of Maryland School of Medicine, 22 S. Greene Street, Room N3W143 Baltimore, MD 21201*

Abstract: The development of drugs that selectively inhibit cyclooxygenase-2 (COX-2) demonstrates translational research from bench to bedside based on underlying knowledge of micro-cellular structure and function. However, theoretical concerns about potentially prothrombotic effects of selective COX-2 inhibitors coupled with observations of increased cardiovascular risk have produced significant consternation and lead to the withdrawal of two of these agents from the market. A number of questions remain unanswered. It appears clear that both selective and non-selective COX inhibitors are associated with increases in blood pressure. In addition, blood pressure is often increased after starting nonsteroidal therapy, and we know that even small increases in blood pressure in subjects with pre-existing vascular disease are associated with substantial increases in the risk of cardiovascular morbidity. Given this line of reasoning, one might hypothesize that the observed increases in the risk of cardiovascular events associated with COX-inhibitors are largely due to increases in blood pressure in populations of subjects who are already at high risk. But can we generalize that the adverse cardiovascular effects observed for

*University of Maryland Medical System, Division of Nephrology, 22 South Greene Street, Room N3W143, Baltimore, MD 21201-1595.

R. E. Harris (ed.), Inflammation in the Pathogenesis of Chronic Diseases, 159–174.
© 2007 *Springer.*

rofecoxib and valdecoxib are sufficient to indict the entire class of COX-2 inhibitors, or is
this not a class effect, but dependent upon the degree of COX-2 selectivity? In either case,
it seems prudent to recommend that subjects who are at higher risk for a cardiovascular
event and receiving a COX-inhibitor should also be treated with low dose ASA with
close follow up of blood pressure and efficacious use of anti-hypertensive medications.
Finally, modest dietary salt restriction may help lessen the effects of COX-inhibitors on
blood pressure

1.   REVIEW OF PROSTANOID PRODUCTION

Prostaglandins (PGs) are critical mediators of a number of physiological processes
including the regulation of vascular homeostasis and thrombosis, as well as inflammation [1]. Arachidonic acid, which is liberated from membrane-bound phospholipids by phospholipase A_2, is catalyzed by the enzyme cyclooxygenase (COX).
Because COX has two catalytic moieties, a cyclooxygenase and a peroxidase [2], this
enzymatic complex is also referred to as the prostaglandin G/H synthase
(PGHS) [3].

Cyclooxygenase initially generates the unstable endoperoxide intermediate,
prostaglandin $G_2(PGG_2)$, which it then catalyzes to prostaglandin $H_2(PGH_2)$.
Following the production of PGH_2, further enzymatic processes are needed to form
the active prostanoids. Enzymes specific for each tissue (tissue-specific enzymes)
catalyze PGH_2 to biologically active prostanoids [4]: prostaglandin I_2 (PGI_2, or
prostacyclin) synthase produces prostacyclin, thromboxane $A_2(TxA_2)$ synthase
produces thromboxane, and prostaglandin D_2, E_2, and F_2 synthases produce their
respective prostaglandins: PGD_2, PGE_2, and PGF_2 (Figure 1). PGI_2 and TxA_2 are
probably the most important prostanoids in the regulation of vascular homeostasis,
since they have opposing effects on platelet function [3].

Because the rate-limiting step in the production of prostaglandins is the COX
enzyme, COX inhibitors can have potent effects. Although it does not appear that
either PGG_2 or PGH_2 have direct biological effects, inhibition of COX results in a
decrease in the substrate availability for a given tissue's prostanoid synthases.

There are at least two related but distinct gene products that possess cyclooxygenase activity, COX-1 and COX-2. These cyclooxygenase isoforms are differentially expressed and regulated throughout the vascular system. Initial evidence
suggested that COX-1 was constitutively and ubiquitously expressed, and COX-1
was therefore regarded as a housekeeping enzyme. In contrast, COX-2 was thought
to be strictly an inducible enzyme, up- regulated by diverse mitogenic and pro
inflammatory factors, such as bacterial lipopolysaccharides [6], cytokines such as
interleukin-1, and phorbol esters [7]. It is now known that this initial construct
for the COX isoforms was too simplistic. It has been demonstrated that COX-2 is
constitutively expressed in a variety of tissues, including vascular endothelial cells,
renal medullary cells [8, 9], and cells of the macula densa [10]. In addition, there
is evidence that COX-1 is inducible under certain conditions [11]. Of note, a third
enzyme termed COX-3 has been identified and appears to be a variant of COX-1
[12]. COX-3 may be a target for acetaminophen [12].

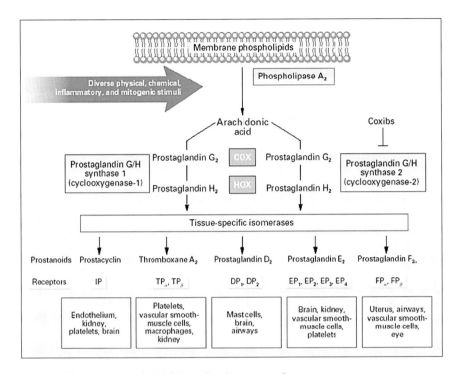

Figure 1. The coxibs, selective inhibitors of cyclooxygenase-2
Source: Reproduced with permission: FitzGerald GA, Patrono C. N Engl J Med. 2001 Aug 9; 345[6]: 433–42 [5]

2. RATIONALE FOR DEVELOPMENT OF COX-2 INHIBITORS

Although NSAIDs are among the most commonly used medications [13, 14], their use is limited by potential GI toxicity (e.g., dyspepsia, peptic ulcer disease, and bleeding). Previous studies have consistently suggested that the constitutively expressed COX-1 isoenzyme contributes to cytoprotective prostanoids that maintain the integrity of the gastric mucosa [15]. As COX-2 was demonstrated to be up-regulated by inflammatory cytokines, it was postulated that the therapeutic effects of conventional NSAIDs were related to inhibition of COX-2 at sites of inflammation whereas the adverse GI effects were attributed to inhibition of COX-1 in the gastric epithelium. This is the basis for the strategy to develop drugs that selectively inhibit the harmful effects of cyclooxygenase without affecting its housekeeping functions, i.e. development of selective COX-2 inhibitors.

It appears that inhibition of COX-2 produces the desired anti-inflammatory response [16]. The first randomized clinical trial showing decreased GI side effects of a selective COX-2 inhibitor was the Vioxx Gastrointestinal Outcome Research (VIGOR) trial. VIGOR compared rofecoxib and naproxen for occurrence of GI toxicity among 8,076 patients with rheumatoid arthritis [13]. However, based on the Adenomatous Polyp Prevention on Vioxx (APPROVe) trial, Merck voluntarily withdrew rofecoxib from the market on September 30, 2004 due to an observed increase in cardiovascular risk among patients taking the drug for more than 18 months [17].

Four selective COX-2 inhibitors, celecoxib (*Celebrex*; Pfizer), rofecoxib (*Vioxx*; Merck), valdecoxib (*Bextra*; Pfizer), and meloxicam (*Mobic*; Boehringer Ingelheim Pharmaceuticals), have been approved for use by the FDA [19]. Celecoxib was approved in December, 1998, rofecoxib in May, 1999, valdecoxib in November, 2001, and meloxicam in April, 2004. A fifth drug, etoricoxib (*Arcoxia*, Merck), has been approved by the European regulatory authority (19)⁻and a sixth drug, lumiracoxib (*Prexige*; Novartis), was recently approved in England and Mexico [18, 19, 20]. On April 7, 2005, Pfizer voluntarily withdrew Valdecoxib from the market due to concerns about cardiovascular risk and hypersensitivity reactions [21].

Chemical structures of first and second generation COX-2 inhibitors are shown below.

Celecoxib   Rofecoxib   Valdecoxib   Meloxicam

- First generation compounds: celecoxib (sulfonamide) & rofecoxib (sulfone)
- Second generation compounds: valdecoxib (sulfonamide), etoricoxib (sulfone), meloxicam (oxicam) & lumiracoxib (which contains no sulfonamide or sulfone group)

Selective COX-2 inhibitors such as lumiracoxib, etoricoxib, meloxicam, valdecoxib, rofecoxib and celecoxib differ in terms of their relative selectivity for COX-2 versus COX-1. Lumiracoxib is the most selective COX-2 inhibitor [18], whereas celecoxib has relatively low selectivity for COX-2 [22]. Theoretically, high selectivity of COX-2 inhibition could produce important cardiovascular side effects by upsetting the balance between TxA_2 and PGI_2

3.   BALANCE BETWEEN PGI_2 AND TXA_2: THEORETICAL EXPLANATION FOR THROMBOPHILIA

It is important to understand the interactions of TxA_2 and PGI_2 in platelets and the vascular epithelium, and the major role they play in the regulation of vascular homeostasis. Of note, the only isoform of cyclooxygenase that platelets contain is COX-1 [23], and the major prostanoid produced by platelets is TxA_2 [23]. Thromboxane A_2 is a potent stimulator of platelet activation [24], platelet aggregation, and to a lesser extent, vasoconstriction [25]. As noted above, nonspecific

COX-inhibitors, typified by the nonsteroidal anti-inflammatory drugs (NSAIDs), do not directly inhibit TxA_2 synthase, but rather they work upstream by inhibiting cyclooxygenase to potentially decrease TxA_2 production. Aspirin (ASA), unlike other NSAIDs, is unique in its ability to bind irreversibly to COX [26]. The antithrombotic effect of ASA is likely due to its ability to inhibit platelet TxA_2 synthesis [26]. Aspirin irreversibly inhibits platelet COX-1 by acetylating a serine residue at position 529 [27]. Since platelets lack nuclei, they are unable to reconstitute irreversibly inhibited cyclooxygenase, and the effects of ASA are prolonged. Other NSAIDs also block platelet TxA_2 synthesis, but they do so in a non-irreversible manner.

As opposed to TxA_2, PGI_2 is a potent inhibitor of platelet aggregation and induces vasodilation [26]. PGI_2 is formed by vascular endothelium, and since intact vascular endothelium can reconstitute COX after exposure to ASA, low dose ASA has little effect on PGI_2 production [1]. Therefore, a possible mechanism for the antithrombotic effect of low dose ASA is that it tips the balance of prostaglandins away from pro-thrombotic TxA_2. However, high doses of ASA also decrease PGI_2, which may diminish its anti-thrombotic effects. Traditional NSAIDs tend to inhibit both TxA_2 and PGI_2, in a manner similar to high dose ASA.

4.   COX-2 INHIBITORS AND CARDIOVASCULAR EVENTS

4.1.   Risk of Myocardial Infarction

According to one theory, all drugs that selectively block COX-2 may have an adverse cardiovascular profile because they upset the balance between pro-thrombotic TxA_2 and anti-thrombotic PGI_2. Aspirin and traditional NSAIDs inhibit both TxA_2 and PGI_2, whereas COX-2 inhibitors decrease PGI_2 production without affecting TxA_2. Suppression of COX-2 dependent formation of PGI_2 by coxibs may thus predispose subjects to MI and thrombotic stroke [28]. To better assess the clinical risk of COX-2 inhibitors, it is important to review the recent studies. Nevertheless, it should be noted that many of these studies did not have cardiovascular outcome as a primary endpoint, and may not have been powered to detect differences in the rates of these events [29].

One of the first randomized prospective studies examining the clinical effectiveness of COX-2 inhibitors was the Celecoxib Long-term Arthritis Safety Study (CLASS), published in September, 2000 [30]. In this prospective, randomized, double-blind, multicenter, international study, subjects with rheumatoid arthritis (RA) or osteoarthritis (OA) were treated with the COX-2 inhibitor, celecoxib, or a traditional NSAID, either ibuprofen or diclofenac. Of note, the dose of celecoxib studied (400 mg twice a day) was two to four times the maximum FDA-approved effective dosage for RA and OA, respectively. All other NSAIDs were prohibited, except for doses of ASA up to 325 mg per day. A total of 8,059 subjects were randomized, of whom 3,987 received celecoxib. Of this group, 833 subjects were on ASA (20.9% compared to 20.4% among those receiving traditional NSAID therapy). Treatment with celecoxib was associated with a trend toward a decrease in the incidence of complicated GI ulcers and erosions (2.08% vs 3.54%, P = 0.09). There was no difference noted in the incidence of cardiovascular events, irrespective of ASA use [30]. However, the initial published report had selected time-censored data, reporting on only the first 6 months of the study [31]. Examination of the later data suggested that by week 65, celecoxib was associated with a similar number of ulcer complications [32].

The second major clinical trial was the Vioxx Gastrointestinal Outcome Research (VIGOR) trial, published in November, 2000 [13]. In this prospective, randomized, non-blinded, multicenter, international study, subjects with rheumatoid arthritis (RA) were treated with the COX-2 inhibitor, rofecoxib, or the traditional NSAID, naproxen. As in the CLASS study, the dose of the COX-2 inhibitor was at twice the maximum FDA-approved effective dosage for RA (50 mg once daily). All other NSAIDs were prohibited, including ASA. Exclusion criteria included morbid obesity or a history of myocardial infarction/coronary artery bypass (CABG) or cerebrovascular events within 1 and 2 years, respectively, of enrollment in the study. A total of 8,076 subjects were randomized, of whom 4,047 received rofecoxib, with a median follow up of 9 months. Both drugs had similar efficacy against RA, but rofecoxib resulted in significantly lower rates of upper GI e/vents compared to naproxen. The overall mortality rates (0.5% vs 0.4%) and the death rates from cardiovascular causes (0.2% vs 0.2%), and ischemic cerebrovascular events (0.2% vs 0.2%) were similar in both groups, rofecoxib vs naproxen, respectively. However, there were more myocardial infarctions in the rofecoxib group (0.4% vs 0.1%), and in addition, the composite endpoint of non-fatal MI, non-fatal stroke, and sudden death was higher in the rofecoxib group (0.8% vs 0.4%, P < 0.05) [33] Given these results, Merck changed the exclusion criteria of other rofecoxib studies (in May, 2000) to allow subjects to use low-dose ASA [13].

Both the CLASS and VIGOR trials were designed to assess GI tolerability and safety for COX-2 inhibitors relative to traditional NSAIDs. Neither trial was designed or powered to assess possible pro-thrombotic effects of these agents [29]. Therefore, larger outcome trials or meta-analyses were needed to better define this potential risk.

The results of the Therapeutic Arthritis Research and Gastrointestinal Event Trial (TARGET) were published in August, 2004 [33]. As in the CLASS and VIGOR trials, TARGET was a prospective, randomized, multicenter, international study. In this large outcome study, subjects with OA were randomized to one of two sub-studies, lumiracoxib (400 mg once daily) versus naproxen (500 mg twice daily) or ibuprofen (800 mg thrice daily). Since naproxen and ibuprofen may have differential cardioprotective effects due to their inhibition of platelet function [34, 35], both drugs were used as traditional NSAID "active" controls. Subjects with a history of cardiovascular disease (MI, stroke, CABG, percutaneous coronary intervention) were excluded if they were not on low-dose ASA. Additional exclusion criteria included use of any other NSAIDs or anticoagulation therapy other than low dose ASA. A total of 18,325 subjects were randomized of whom 9,117 received lumiracoxib. Randomization was stratified by ASA use, with a target and achieved total of 24% of participants taking low dose ASA. Observed rates of GI ulcer complications did not differ between lumiracoxib and either NSAID group. The primary cardiovascular endpoint was a composite of non-fatal MI, non-fatal stroke, or cardiovascular death. Overall, no significant differences were noted in the rates of MI between the lumiracoxib and combined NSAID treatment groups (Figure 2). However, in the naproxen sub-study, more subjects who were not on low-dose ASA had an MI in the lumiracoxib vs the naproxen group (0.28% vs 0.11%), although the difference was not significant The incidence of stroke and CV deaths was comparable across treatment groups, and the combined endpoint of non-fatal MI,

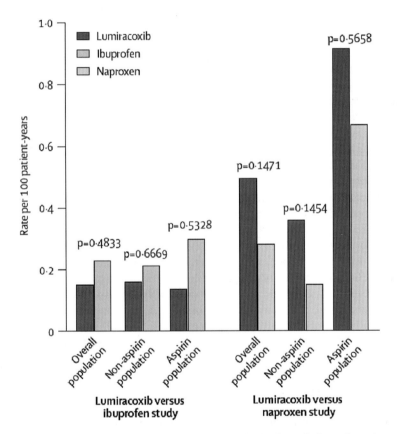

Figure 2. Incidence of myocardial infarction comparing lumiracoxib, ibuprofen and naproxen
Source: Reproduced with permission: Farkouh ME, Kirshner H, Harrington RA, Ruland S, Verheugt FW, Schnitzer TJ, Burmester GR, Mysler E, Hochberg MC, Doherty M, Ehrsam E, Gitton X, Krammer G, Mellein B, Gimona A, Matchaba P, Hawkey CJ, Chesebro JH; TARGET Study Group. Comparison of lumiracoxib with naproxen and ibuprofen in the Therapeutic Arthritis Research and Gastro- intestinal Event Trial (TARGET), cardiovascular outcomes: randomised controlled trial. Lancet. 2004 Aug 21–27;364(9435):675–84. PMID: 15325832 (33)

non-fatal stroke, or CV death did not differ between treatment groups (0.65% vs 0.55%, lumiracoxib vs traditional NSAID, respectively). Of note, the incidence of congestive heart failure occurred less frequently in the lumiracoxib group compared to the combined traditional NSAID group (0.24% vs 0.34%) although the difference was not significant.

The Adenomatous Polyp Prevention on Vioxx (APPROVe) trial was designed to evaluate the chemopreventive effect of rofecoxib among subjects with a history of colorectal adenomas over three years of therapy [36]. Subjects were initially excluded if they were taking low dose ASA, but the protocol was amended after May, 2000, based on the VIGOR trial results. Additional exclusion criteria included uncontrolled HTN, angina or congestive heart failure, or a history of myocardial infarction/coronary artery bypass (CABG) or cerebrovascular events within 1 and 2 years, respectively, of enrollment in the study (similar to the VIGOR trial). A total of 2,586 subjects were randomized, of whom 1,287 received rofecoxib. On September 30, 2004, the study was terminated about two months before the planned completion date, at the recommendation of the external safety-monitoring board, at which time a total of 1,857 subjects had completed the planned 3 years of treatment (877 subjects in the rofecoxib group).

At this time, Merck voluntarily withdrew rofecoxib from the market due to a significant increase in the rate of cardiovascular outcomes in patients taking the drug for more than 18 months. There were 10 deaths in each group, but the rofecoxib group had an increased number of adjudicated cardiac events (2.4% vs 0.9%) and confirmed cerebrovascular events (1.2% vs 0.5%, rofecoxib vs placebo, respectively). In addition to adjudicated events, there were higher percentages of subjects with hypertension and edema-related events, which included congestive heart failure, pulmonary edema, and cardiac failure. The rates of cardiovascular events were similar for the rofecoxib and placebo groups during the first 18 months of the study, but differences became evident after 18 months (Figure 3).

In December 2004, a meta-analysis was published examining 18 randomized controlled trials and 11 observational studies comparing rofecoxib with other NSAIDs, or placebo, using a primary endpoint of MI. The combined relative risk for an MI on rofecoxib vs placebo was 2.24 (Figure 4).

Building on data suggesting that COX-2 acts as a promoter of intestinal tumorigenesis [38], and that celecoxib treatment (400 mg twice daily for six months) decreased the number of colorectal polyps in subjects with familial adenomatous polyposis [39], the Adenoma Prevention with Celecoxib (APC) study was undertaken. In this prospective, randomized, double-blind, multicenter, international study, subjects who had undergone endoscopic polypectomy for adenomas were treated with either celecoxib 200 mg twice daily, celecoxib 400 mg twice daily, or placebo. In light of the APPROVe data demonstrating an increased number of cardiac events in the COX-2 inhibitor group, the APC drug and safety monitoring board requested a focused reassessment of cardiovascular safety [40]. At the time of this analysis, a total of 2,035 subjects had undergone randomization, of which 685 were in the celecoxib 200 mg twice-daily group and 671 in the celecoxib 400 mg

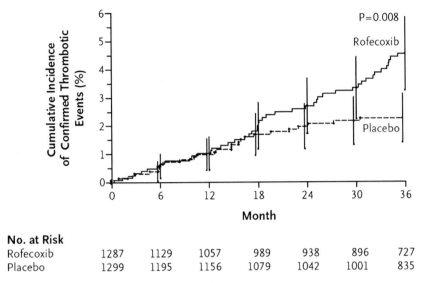

Figure 3. Estimates of the cumulative incidence of confirmed serious thrombotic events comparing rofecoxib and placebo

Source: Reproduced with permission: Bresalier RS, Sandler RS, Quan H, Bolognese JA, Oxenius B, Horgan K, Lines C, Riddell R, Morton D, Lanas A, Konstam MA, Baron JA; Adenomatous Polyp Prevention on Vioxx (APPROVe) Trial Investigators. Cardiovascular events associated with rofecoxib in a colorectal adenoma chemoprevention trial. N Engl J Med. 2005 Mar 17;352(11):1092–102. Epub 2005 Feb 15. PMID: 15713943. [36]

twice-daily group. For the composite endpoint of death from cardiovascular causes, MI, stroke or heart failure, compared to placebo, the hazard ratio was 2.3 and 3.4 for the 200 and 400 mg twice-daily groups, respectively (Figure 5). On the basis of the results that celecoxib led to a dose-related increase in the risk of serious cardiovascular events, on December 16, 2004, the steering committee stopped the use of celecoxib in this study.

The cardiovascular safety committee also completed a preliminary review of cardiovascular safety in another study, the Prevention of Spontaneous Adenomatous Polyps (PreSAP) trial, which randomly assigned patients with a history of colorectal adenomas to receive either 400 mg of celecoxib once daily or placebo. The preliminary analysis did not show an increase in risk at this dose. [40] The authors suggested that "differences in the dosing regimens between the APC study and the PreSAP trial, twice daily compared with once daily, support the hypothesis that sustained inhibition of prostacyclin (PGI_2) may contribute to the increase in cardiovascular risk." [40]

Two studies examined the use of valdecoxib, and or its intravenous prodrug, parecoxib, in subjects who had just undergone coronary artery bypass grafting (CABG) surgery. The first study, published in June, 2003, was a multicenter, phase III, placebo-controlled, double blind, randomized, parallel-group trial. Four

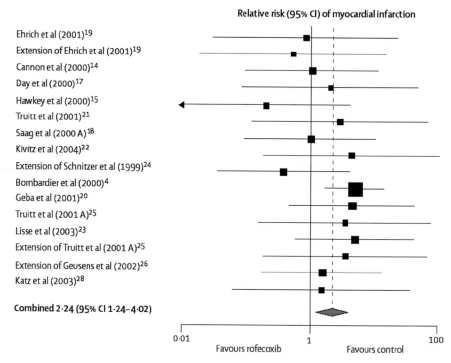

Figure 4. Relative risk of MI comparing rofecoxib with control
Source: Reproduced with permission: Juni P, Nartey L, Reichenbach S, Sterchi R, Dieppe PA, Egger M. Risk of cardiovascular events and rofecoxib: cumulative meta-analysis. Lancet. 2004 Dec 4–10;364(9450):2021–9. PMID: 15582059. [37]

hundred and sixty two subjects were randomized to either parecoxib/valdecoxib (311 subjects) or placebo. Although the treatment group had higher incidence of deaths [4 (0.9%) vs 0 (0%), P = 0.309], MI [5 (1.6%) vs 1 (0.7%), P = 0.669] and cardiovascular complications [9 (2.9%) vs 1 (0.7%), P = 0.177], these differences did not reach statistical significance [41]. Given these results, another trial with increased power was undertaken to clarify the safety of these COX-2 inhibitors after CAGB. Unlike the first study, there were three groups. Group 1 received intravenous parecoxib (first dose 40 mg IV, then 20 mg IV twice daily for 3 days) followed by valdecoxib (20 mg twice daily through day 10). Group 2 received intravenous placebo (twice daily for 3 days) followed by valdecoxib (20 mg twice daily through day 10). The third group received placebo throughout the study. Of the 1,671 subjects randomized, 555 where assigned to group 1,556 to group 2, and 560 to placebo. Cardiovascular events occurred significantly more frequently in group 1 vs placebo (2.0% vs 0.5%, P = 0.03). Both treatment groups had a higher rate of adverse events (7.4% vs 4.0%, P = 0.02) when compared to the placebo group (Figure 6). On April 7, 2005, Pfizer voluntarily withdrew Valdecoxib from the market due to concerns about cardiovascular risk and hypersensitivity reactions.

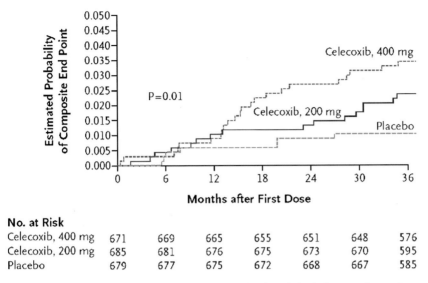

Figure 5. Estimates of the risk of the composite end point of death from cardiovascular causes, myocardial infarction, stroke, or heart failure among subjects who received celecoxib (200 mg twice daily or 400 mg twice daily) or placebo

Source: Reproduced with permission: Solomon SD, McMurray JJ, Pfeffer MA, Wittes J, Fowler R, Finn P, Anderson WF, Zauber A, Hawk E, Bertagnolli M; Adenoma Prevention with Celecoxib (APC) Study Investigators. Cardiovascular risk associated with celecoxib in a clinical trial for colorectal adenoma prevention. N Engl J Med. 2005 Mar 17;352(11):1071–80. Epub 2005 Feb 15. PMID: 15713944. [40]

4.2.　　Effects on Blood Pressure

Traditional NSAIDs have been observed to increase blood pressure [43], as well as increase the risk of development of hypertension [44]. Animal models suggest that selective COX-2 inhibitors may have similar hemodynamic effects [45].

The Celecoxib Rofecoxib Efficacy and Safety in Co-morbidities Evaluation Trial (CRESCENT) was designed to investigate the effects of COX-2 inhibitors on 24-hour blood pressure. In this prospective, randomized, double blind, multicenter, international study, subjects with OA and type 2 diabetes were treated with celecoxib (200 mg daily), rofecoxib (25 mg daily), or naproxen (500 mg twice daily) for 12 weeks [46]. After 6 weeks of therapy, the mean systolic BP was significantly increased by rofecoxib, but not by celecoxib or naproxen.

In a multicenter, parallel-group, double blind, randomized, controlled trial examining the effects of COX-2 inhibitors on blood pressure and edema, subjects greater than 64-years old with hypertension and OA were randomized to either celecoxib (200 mg daily) or rofecoxib (25 mg daily) for 6 weeks [47]. Subjects in the rofecoxib group had a higher incidence of clinically significant elevation in systolic BP vs the celecoxib group, defined as a > 20 mmHg increase from baseline and absolute value $\geq$ 140 mmHg (14.9% vs 6.9%, P < 0.001) (Figure 7).

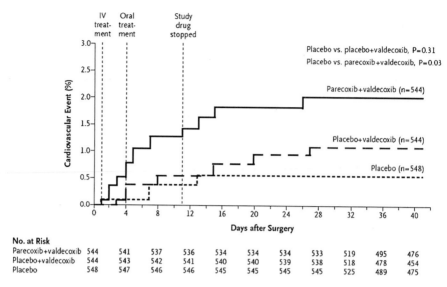

Figure 6. Kaplan-Meier estimates of the time to a cardiovascular event
Source: Reproduced with permission: Nussmeier NA, Whelton AA, Brown MT, Langford RM, Hoeft A, Parlow JL, Boyce SW, Verburg KM. Complications of the COX-2 inhibitors parecoxib and valdecoxib after cardiac surgery. N Engl J Med. 2005 Mar 17;352(11):1081–91. Epub 2005 Feb 15. PMID: 15713945. [42]

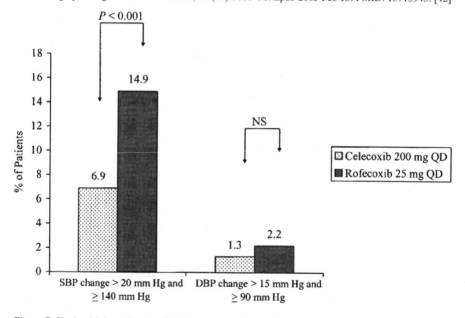

Figure 7. Kaplan-Meier estimates of the time to a cardiovascular event
Source: Reproduced with permission: Whelton A, White WB, Bello AE, Puma JA, Fort JG; SUCCESS-VII Investigators. Effects of celecoxib and rofecoxib on blood pressure and edema in patients > or = 65 years of age with systemic hypertension and osteoarthritis. Am J Cardiol. 2002 Nov 1;90(9):959–63. PMID: 12398962. [47]

In addition, edema occurred more often in the rofecoxib group than in the celecoxib group (7.7% vs 4.7%, P = 0.045).

A meta-analysis examining 19 randomized trials using COX-2 inhibitors attempted to better define their effect on blood pressure [48]. The COX-2 inhibitors studied were celecoxib, rofecoxib, and etoricoxib. The COX-2 inhibitors caused a weighted mean increase in systolic blood pressure when compared to placebo (3.85 vs 1.06 mm Hg, respectively) and traditional NSAID (2.83 vs 1.34 mm Hg, respectively).

5.   CONCLUSION

In summary, the development of drugs that selectively inhibit cyclooxygenase-2 (COX-2) demonstrates translational research from bench to bedside based on underlying knowledge of micro-cellular structure and function. However, theoretical concerns about potentially pro-thrombotic effects of selective COX-2 inhibitors coupled with observations of increased cardiovascular risk have produced significant consternation and lead to the withdrawal of two of these agents from the market. A number of questions remain unanswered. It appears clear that both selective and non-selective COX inhibitors are associated with increases in blood pressure. In addition, blood pressure is often increased after starting nonsteroidal therapy, and we know that even small increases in blood pressure in subjects with pre-existing vascular disease (e.g., hypertension, diabetes mellitus) are associated with substantial increases in the risk of cardiovascular morbidity [46]. Given this line of reasoning, one might hypothesize that the observed increases in the risk of cardiovascular events associated with COX-inhibitors may be largely due to increases in blood pressure in populations of subjects who are already at high risk. But can we generalize that the adverse cardiovascular effects observed for rofecoxib and valdecoxib are sufficient to indict the entire class of COX-2 inhibitors, or is this not a class effect, but dependent upon the degree of COX-2 selectivity? In either case, it seems prudent to recommend that subjects who are at higher risk for a cardiovascular event and receiving a COX-inhibitor should also be treated with low dose ASA [5] with close follow up of blood pressure and efficacious use of anti-hypertensive medications. Finally, modest dietary salt restriction may help lessen the effects of COX-inhibitors on blood pressure [49].

REFERENCES

1. Krotz F, Schiele TM, Klauss V, Sohn HY. J Vasc Res. Epub 2005 Jun 20. Selective COX-2 inhibitors and risk of myocardial infarction. 2005 Jul-Aug;42(4):312–24. PMID: 15976506
2. Funk CD, Funk LB, Kennedy ME, Pong AS, Fitzgerald GA. Human platelet/erythroleukemia cell prostaglandin G/H synthase: cDNA cloning, expression, and gene chromosomal assignment. FASEB J. 1991 Jun;5(9):2304–12. PMID: 1907252
3. Davidge ST. Circ Res. Prostaglandin H synthase and vascular function. 2001 Oct 12;89(8):650–60. PMID: 11597987

4. Helliwell RJ, Adams LF, Mitchell MD. Prostaglandin synthases: recent developments and a novel hypothesis. Prostaglandins Leukot Essent Fatty Acids. 2004 Feb;70(2):101–13. PMID: 14683687

5. FitzGerald GA, Patrono C. N Engl J Med. The coxibs, selective inhibitors of cyclooxygenase-2. 2001 Aug 9;345(6):433–42. PMID: 11496855

6. O'Sullivan MG, Huggins EM Jr, Meade EA, DeWitt DL, McCall CE. Lipopolysaccharide induces prostaglandin H synthase-2 in alveolar macrophages. Biochem Biophys Res Commun. 1992 Sep 16;187(2):1123–7. PMID: 1382414

7. Crofford LJ, Wilder RL, Ristimaki AP, Sano H, Remmers EF, Epps HR, Hla T. Cyclooxygenase-1 and -2 expression in rheumatoid synovial tissues. Effects of interleukin-1 beta, phorbol ester, and corticosteroids. J Clin Invest. 1994 Mar;93(3):1095–101. PMID: 8132748

8. Vio CP, Cespedes C, Gallardo P, Masferrer JL. Renal identification of cyclooxygenase-2 in a subset of thick ascending limb cells. Hypertension. 1997 Sep;30(3 Pt 2):687–92. PMID: 9323006

9. Harris RC, Breyer MD. Physiological regulation of cyclooxygenase-2 in the kidney. Am J Physiol Renal Physiol. 2001 Jul;281(1):F1–11. PMID: 11399641

10. Harris RC, McKanna JA, Akai Y, Jacobson HR, Dubois RN, Breyer MD. Cyclooxygenase-2 is associated with the macula densa of rat kidney and increases with salt restriction. J Clin Invest. 1994 Dec;94(6):2504–10. PMID: 7989609

11. Murphy JF, Steele C, Belton O, Fitzgerald DJ. Induction of cyclooxygenase-1 and -2 modulates angiogenic responses to engagement of alphavbeta3. Br J Haematol. 2003 Apr;121(1):157–64. PMID: 12670347

12. Chandrasekharan NV, Dai H, Roos KL, Evanson NK, Tomsik J, Elton TS, Simmons DL. COX-3, a cyclooxygenase-1 variant inhibited by acetaminophen and other analgesic/antipyretic drugs: cloning, structure, and expression. Proc Natl Acad Sci U S A. 2002 Oct 15;99(21):13926–31. Epub 2002 Sep 19. PMID: 12242329

13. Bombardier C, Laine L, Reicin A, Shapiro D, Burgos-Vargas R, Davis B, Day R, Ferraz MB, Hawkey CJ, Hochberg MC, Kvien TK, Schnitzer TJ. VIGOR Study Group. Comparison of upper gastrointestinal toxicity of rofecoxib and naproxen in patients with rheumatoid arthritis. VIGOR Study Group. N Engl J Med. 2000 Nov 23;343(21):1520–8, 2 p following 1528. PMID: 11087881

14. Manoria P, Manoria PC. COX-2 inhibitors and heart. Indian Heart J. 2005 Nov-Dec;57(6):772–7. PMID: 16521658

15. Crofford LJ, Lipsky PE, Brooks P, Abramson SB, Simon LS, van de Putte LB. Basic biology and clinical application of specific cyclooxygenase-2 inhibitors. Arthritis Rheum. 2000 Jan;43(1):4–13. PMID: 10643694

16. Marnett LJ, Rowlinson SW, Goodwin DC, Kalgutkar AS, Lanzo CA. Arachidonic acid oxygenation by COX-1 and COX-2. Mechanisms of catalysis and inhibition. J Biol Chem. 1999 Aug 13;274(33):22903–6. PMID: 10438452

17. http://www.vioxx.com/vioxx/documents/english/vioxx press release.pdf

18. Mangold JB, Gu H, Rodriguez LC, Bonner J, Dickson J, Rordorf C. Pharmacokinetics and metabolism of lumiracoxib in healthy male subjects. Drug Metab Dispos. 2004 May;32(5):566–71. PMID: 15100180

19. Fitzgerald GA. Coxibs and cardiovascular disease. N Engl J Med. 2004 Oct 21;351(17):1709–11. Epub 2004 Oct 6. PMID: 15470192

20. Topol EJ. Failing the public health–rofecoxib, Merck, and the FDA. N Engl J Med. 2004 Oct 21;351(17):1707–9. Epub 2004 Oct 6. PMID: 15470193

21. Brophy JM. Celecoxib and cardiovascular risks. Expert Opin Drug Saf. 2005 Nov;4(6):1005–15. PMID: 16255660

22. FitzGerald GA. COX-2 and beyond: Approaches to prostaglandin inhibition in human disease. Nat Rev Drug Discov. 2003 Nov;2(11):879–90. PMID: 14668809

23. Smith WL. The eicosanoids and their biochemical mechanisms of action. Biochem J. 1989 Apr 15;259(2):315–24. PMID: 2655580

24. Paul BZ, Jin J, Kunapuli SP. Molecular mechanism of thromboxane A(2)-induced platelet aggregation. Essential role for p2t(ac) and alpha(2a) receptors. J Biol Chem. 1999 Oct 8;274(41):

29108–14. PMID: 10506165

25. Armstrong RA. Platelet prostanoid receptors. Pharmacol Ther. 1996;72(3):171–91. PMID: 9364574

26. Patrono C, Coller B, Dalen JE, FitzGerald GA, Fuster V, Gent M, Hirsh J, Roth G. Platelet-active drugs : the relationships among dose, effectiveness, and side effects. Chest. 2001 Jan;119(1):39S–63S. PMID: 11157642

27. Loll PJ, Picot D, Garavito RM. The structural basis of aspirin activity inferred from the crystal structure of inactivated prostaglandin H2 synthase. Nat Struct Biol. 1995 Aug;2(8):637–43. PMID: 7552725

28. Belton O, Byrne D, Kearney D, Leahy A, Fitzgerald DJ. Cyclooxygenase-1 and -2-dependent prostacyclin formation in patients with atherosclerosis. Circulation. 2000 Aug 22;102(8):840–5. PMID: 10952950

29. Strand V, Hochberg MC. The risk of cardiovascular thrombotic events with selective cyclooxygenase-2 inhibitors. Arthritis Rheum. 2002 Aug;47(4):349–55. PMID: 12209478

30. Silverstein FE, Faich G, Goldstein JL, Simon LS, Pincus T, Whelton A, Makuch R, Eisen G, Agrawal NM, Stenson WF, Burr AM, Zhao WW, Kent JD, Lefkowith JB, Verburg KM, Geis GS. Gastrointestinal toxicity with celecoxib vs nonsteroidal anti-inflammatory drugs for osteoarthritis and rheumatoid arthritis: the CLASS study: A randomized controlled trial. Celecoxib Long-term Arthritis Safety Study. JAMA. 2000 Sep 13;284(10):1247–55. PMID: 10979111

31. Hawkey CJ, Farkouh M, Gitton X, Ehrsam E, Huels J, Richardson P. Therapeutic arthritis research and gastrointestinal event trial of lumiracoxib – study design and patient demographics. Aliment Pharmacol Ther. 2004 Jul 1;20(1):51–63. PMID: 15225171

32. Hrachovec JB, Mora M. Reporting of 6-month vs 12-month data in a clinical trial of celecoxib. JAMA. 2001 Nov 21;286(19):2398; author reply 2399–400. PMID: 11712924

33. Farkouh ME, Kirshner H, Harrington RA, Ruland S, Verheugt FW, Schnitzer TJ, Burmester GR, Mysler E, Hochberg MC, Doherty M, Ehrsam E, Gitton X, Krammer G, Mellein B, Gimona A, Matchaba P, Hawkey CJ, Chesebro JH. TARGET Study Group. Comparison of lumiracoxib with naproxen and ibuprofen in the Therapeutic Arthritis Research and Gastrointestinal Event Trial (TARGET), cardiovascular outcomes: randomised controlled trial. Lancet. 2004 Aug 21–27;364(9435):675–84. PMID: 15325832

34. Capone ML, Tacconelli S, Sciulli MG, Grana M, Ricciotti E, Minuz P, Di Gregorio P, Merciaro G, Patrono C, Patrignani P. Clinical pharmacology of platelet, monocyte, and vascular cyclooxygenase inhibition by naproxen and low-dose aspirin in healthy subjects. Circulation. 2004 Mar 30;109(12):1468–71. Epub 2004 Mar 22. PMID: 15037526

35. McIntyre BA, Philp RB, Inwood MJ. Effect of ibuprofen on platelet function in normal subjects and hemophiliac patients. Clin Pharmacol Ther. 1978 Nov;24(5):616–21. PMID: 699486

36. Bresalier RS, Sandler RS, Quan H, Bolognese JA, Oxenius B, Horgan K, Lines C, Riddell R, Morton D, Lanas A, Konstam MA, Baron JA. Adenomatous Polyp Prevention on Vioxx (APPROVe) Trial Investigators. Cardiovascular events associated with rofecoxib in a colorectal adenoma chemoprevention trial. N Engl J Med. 2005 Mar 17;352(11):1092–102. Epub 2005 Feb 15. PMID: 15713943

37. Juni P, Nartey L, Reichenbach S, Sterchi R, Dieppe PA, Egger M. Risk of cardiovascular events and rofecoxib: cumulative meta-analysis. Lancet. 2004 Dec 4–10;364(9450):2021–9. PMID: 15582059

38. Liu CH, Chang SH, Narko K, Trifan OC, Wu MT, Smith E, Haudenschild C, Lane TF, Hla T. Overexpression of cyclooxygenase-2 is sufficient to induce tumorigenesis in transgenic mice. J Biol Chem. 2001 May 25;276(21):18563–9. Epub 2001 Mar 7. PMID: 11278747

39. Steinbach G, Lynch PM, Phillips RK, Wallace MH, Hawk E, Gordon GB, Wakabayashi N, Saunders B, Shen Y, Fujimura T, Su LK, Levin B. The effect of celecoxib, a cyclooxygenase-2 inhibitor, in familial adenomatous polyposis. N Engl J Med. 2000 Jun 29;342(26):1946–52. PMID: 10874062

40. Solomon SD, McMurray JJ, Pfeffer MA, Wittes J, Fowler R, Finn P, Anderson WF, Zauber A, Hawk E, Bertagnolli M. Adenoma Prevention with Celecoxib (APC) Study Investigators. Cardiovascular risk associated with celecoxib in a clinical trial for colorectal adenoma prevention. N Engl J Med. 2005 Mar 17;352(11):1071–80. Epub 2005 Feb 15. PMID: 15713944

41. Ott E, Nussmeier NA, Duke PC, Feneck RO, Alston RP, Snabes MC, Hubbard RC, Hsu PH, Saidman LJ, Mangano DT. Multicenter Study of Perioperative Ischemia (McSPI) Research Group; Ischemia Research and Education Foundation (IREF) Investigators. Efficacy and safety of the cyclooxygenase 2 inhibitors parecoxib and valdecoxib in patients undergoing coronary artery bypass surgery. J Thorac Cardiovasc Surg. 2003 Jun;125(6):1481–92. PMID: 12830070

42. Nussmeier NA, Whelton AA, Brown MT, Langford RM, Hoeft A, Parlow JL, Boyce SW, Verburg KM. Complications of the COX-2 inhibitors parecoxib and valdecoxib after cardiac surgery. N Engl J Med. 2005 Mar 17;352(11):1081–91. Epub 2005 Feb 15. PMID: 15713945

43. Pope JE, Anderson JJ, Felson DT. A meta-analysis of the effects of nonsteroidal anti-inflammatory drugs on blood pressure. Arch Intern Med. 1993 Feb 22;153(4):477–84. PMID: 8435027

44. Curhan GC, Willett WC, Rosner B, Stampfer MJ. Frequency of analgesic use and risk of hypertension in younger women. Arch Intern Med. 2002 Oct 28;162(19):2204–8. PMID: 12390063

45. Muscara MN, Vergnolle N, Lovren F, Triggle CR, Elliott SN, Asfaha S, Wallace JL. Selective cyclo-oxygenase-2 inhibition with celecoxib elevates blood pressure and promotes leukocyte adherence. Br J Pharmacol. 2000 Apr;129(7):1423–30. PMID: 10742298

46. Sowers JR, White WB, Pitt B, Whelton A, Simon LS, Winer N, Kivitz A, van Ingen H, Brabant T, Fort JG. Celecoxib Rofecoxib Efficacy and Safety in Comorbidities Evaluation Trial (CRESCENT) Investigators. The Effects of cyclooxygenase-2 inhibitors and nonsteroidal anti-inflammatory therapy on 24-hour blood pressure in patients with hypertension, osteoarthritis, and type 2 diabetes mellitus. Arch Intern Med. 2005 Jan 24;165(2):161–8. Erratum in: Arch Intern Med. 2005 Mar 14;165(5):551. PMID: 15668361

47. Whelton A, White WB, Bello AE, Puma JA, Fort JG. SUCCESS-VII Investigators. Effects of celecoxib and rofecoxib on blood pressure and edema in patients > or = 65 years of age with systemic hypertension and osteoarthritis. Am J Cardiol. 2002 Nov 1;90(9):959–63. PMID: 12398962

48. Aw TJ, Haas SJ, Liew D, Krum H. Meta-analysis of cyclooxygenase-2 inhibitors and their effects on blood pressure. Arch Intern Med. 2005 Mar 14;165(5):490–6. Epub 2005 Feb 14. PMID: 15710786

49. Vaneckova I, Cahova M, Kramer HJ, Huskova Z, Skaroupkova P, Komers R, Bader M, Ganten D, Cervenka L. Acute effects of cyclooxygenase-2 inhibition on renal function in heterozygous ren-2-transgenic rats on normal or low sodium intake. Kidney Blood Press Res. 2004;27(4):203–10. Epub 2004 Jul 20. PMID: 15273422

CHAPTER 8

A BIOLOGICAL RATIONALE FOR THE CARDIOTOXIC EFFECTS OF ROFECOXIB

Comparative analysis with other COX-2 selective agents and NSAIDs

R. PRESTON MASON[1,2], MARY F. WALTER[2,3],
CHARLES A. DAY[2] AND ROBERT F. JACOB[2]

[1]*Cardiovascular Division, Brigham and Women's Hospital, Harvard Medical School, Boston, MA;*
[2]*Elucida Research LLC, Beverly, MA;*
[3]*Atlanta VA Medical Center, Atlanta, GA*

Abstract: Clinical investigations have demonstrated a relationship between the extended use of rofecoxib and increased risk for atherothrombotic events. This has led to the removal of rofecoxib from the market and explicit cardiovascular safety warnings for other COX-2 selective and non-selective agents that remain on the market. Early explanations for the cardiotoxicity of rofecoxib, such as the relative cardioprotective effect of comparator agents (naproxen) or an "imbalance" between thromboxane and

R. E. Harris (ed.), Inflammation in the Pathogenesis of Chronic Diseases, 175–190.
© 2007 *Springer.*

prostacyclin biosynthesis due to an absence of concomitant aspirin use, have not been substantiated by the evidence. New experimental findings indicate that the cardiotoxicity of rofecoxib is not a general class effect but may be due to its intrinsic chemical structure and unique primary metabolism. Specifically, rofecoxib has been shown to increase the susceptibility of human LDL and cell membrane lipids to oxidative modification, a hallmark feature of atherosclerosis. Rofecoxib was also found to promote the non-enzymatic formation of isoprostanes from biological lipids, which act as important mediators of inflammation in the atherosclerotic plaque. The explanation for such cardiotoxicity is that rofecoxib forms a reactive maleic anhydride in the presence of oxygen due to its chemical structure and primary metabolism (cytoplasmic reductase). By contrast, adverse effects on rates of LDL and membrane lipid oxidation were not observed with other chemically distinct (sulfonamide) COX-2 inhibitors under identical conditions. These findings provide a compelling rationale for distinguishing the differences in cardiovascular risk among COX-selective inhibitors on the basis of their intrinsic physico-chemical properties

1.   INTRODUCTION

Cyclooxygenase (COX) enzyme inhibitors block the rate-limiting step in the synthesis of prostaglandins. Two isoforms of COX, designated as COX-1 and COX-2, have been identified, both of which are inhibited by nonsteroidal anti-inflammatory drugs (NSAIDs). The advantage of COX-2-selective inhibitors is attributed to the observation that the COX-2 enzyme is expressed in limited fashion throughout most tissues unless induced by inflammatory stimuli or mitogens. Clinical investigations confirm that these agents produce fewer gastrointestinal complications than NSAIDs that block both isoforms of COX. [1, 2] The expression of COX-2 has also been specifically linked to cardiovascular disease, as levels of this protein are elevated in atherosclerotic lesions. [3, 4] The use of these agents has been proposed in the treatment of atherosclerosis, a disease characterized by widespread inflammation. [5]

2.   EVIDENCE FOR THE CARDIOTOXIC EFFECTS
OF ROFECOXIB: COMPARISON TO OTHER COX
INHIBITORS

Despite their therapeutic advantages, the widespread use of selective COX inhibitors has been questioned over concern for their cardiovascular safety. Prospective, randomized clinical trials demonstrated a deleterious relationship between the extended use of rofecoxib and risk for atherothrombotic events. [1, 6] In The Adenomatous Polyp Prevention on Vioxx (APPROVe) Trial, rofecoxib use was associated with an unacceptable increase in cardiovascular events. [6] This study, conducted in collaboration with the National Cancer Institute, evaluated a novel pharmacologic benefit for rofecoxib in preventing the recurrence of colorectal polyps among 2,600 patients with a history of colorectal adenomas. However, the study was terminated early when it was discovered that patients receiving 25 mg/day rofecoxib had twice the risk of thromboembolic events compared with those receiving placebo (15 versus 7 per 1000 patients annually). The increased risk of serious thrombotic events became statistically significant after 18 months.

The adverse effects with rofecoxib in APPROVe were observed despite the concomitant use of aspirin, an inhibitor of both COX isoforms. This directly contradicted the so-called "imbalance hypothesis" which had argued that relatively unopposed COX-2 inhibition leads to increased thromboxane A_2 levels and enhanced thrombotic risk. [7–9] In fact, the use of aspirin among patients receiving rofecoxib had no influence on their risk for an atherothrombotic event. Additionally, while COX-2 is involved with production of the vasodilator prostacyclin, the increased risk with rofecoxib use was unrelated to blood pressure changes. Beyond APPROVe, an enhanced risk of cardiovascular disease among users of rofecoxib has also been reported in large case-control and cohort studies. [10–12]

The findings from APPROVe confirmed earlier concerns of a relationship between use of rofecoxib and cardiovascular risk that had been reported several years earlier. In 2000, the results of the Vioxx Gastrointestinal Outcomes Research (VIGOR) trial revealed unexpected evidence of increased myocardial infarction and stroke among patients on rofecoxib, despite the exclusion of patients with known and significant preexisting coronary artery disease. [1] This study, conducted as a double-blind, randomized, prospective clinical trial, included 8,076 patients with rheumatoid arthritis. The study compared the occurrence of gastrointestinal toxicity of rofecoxib (50 mg/day) and another nonsteroidal anti-inflammatory drug (NSAID), naproxen (1000 mg/day). As expected, there was a greater than 50% reduction in risk of serious gastrointestinal events among those receiving rofecoxib, as compared to naproxen. But what was unexpected at the time was a significant five-fold increase in the incidence of myocardial infarction in the rofecoxib group, as compared to naproxen. It was initially hypothesized that the increased cardiovascular risks were due to potential cardioprotection with naproxen, as opposed to a cardiotoxic effect of rofecoxib. However, a meta-analysis of naproxen studies and a later independent study conducted among 1.39 million Kaiser Permanente members by David Graham of the FDA have since revealed that the cardioprotective effect of this agent is small, at best, and could not account for these findings in VIGOR. [13, 14]

A single trial called into question the safety of celecoxib, another COX-2 selective agent, when administered at higher doses (up to 400 twice daily) for an extended period, [15] but a consistent adverse effect has not been observed. [10–12] This trial known as the Prevention of Sporadic Colorectal Adenomas with Celecoxib (APC) trial used doses in excess of those recommended for patients with osteoarthritis (100 to 200 mg) and rheumatoid arthritis (200 to 400 mg). At the time of the release of this trial, another cancer study called Prevention of Spontaneous Adenomatous Polyps (PreSAP) failed to show an increase risk at these elevated levels while yet a third trial involving patients with Alzheimer's disease patients (ADAPT) showed increased risk with naproxen, but not celecoxib. Based on the preponderance of the evidence, the FDA in early 2005 decided that celecoxib should remain on the market (valdecoxib was removed due to its link to a rare skin disorder). In an independent analysis of cardiovascular events of over one million subjects, 26,748 of whom took rofecoxib and 40,405 of whom took celecoxib, higher doses (50 mg/day) of rofecoxib tripled the risk for heart attack and sudden cardiac death. [14] Remarkably, these results showed that naproxen failed to offer any cardioprotection compared to the expected rates of cardiovascular events, and celecoxib did not significantly alter the cardiovascular risk. [14] Thus, the apparent differences in thrombotic risk among these agents cannot be simply attributed to their selective or even non-selective COX inhibition.

Despite the controversy surrounding NSAIDs and COX-2 inhibitors, the benefit of aspirin for secondary prevention in patients at high risk for cardiovascular disease remains well established due to inhibition of platelet aggregation. COX-1 and thromboxane synthase are both constitutively expressed in platelets and have an essential role in regulating aggregation. The COX-2 enzyme, in particular, is responsible for oxygenation of arachidonic acid into prostaglandin endoperoxide H_2 followed by enzymatic conversion into thromboxane A_2 (TXA_2), a potent inducer of vasoconstriction and platelet aggregation. Platelet-derived TXA_2 can also work through a paracrine pathway to upregulate endothelial COX-2 expression and prostacyclin synthesis. [16] These features of the COX system explain why low dose aspirin preferentially inhibits COX-1 in platelets, resulting in a reduction in TXA_2 while sparing COX-2–derived prostacyclin biosynthesis. On the other hand, nonspecific NSAIDs block both COX isoforms and thereby reduce both the prothrombotic actions of TXA_2 and the antithrombotic properties of prostacyclin. Despite an apparent balance in their effects on these two pathways, NSAIDs have been linked to increased cardiovascular risk at higher doses. [17]

3.   COX-2 INHIBITORS HAVE DISTINCT PHARMACOLOGIC PROPERTIES

A compelling explanation for the differences in cardiovascular safety among COX-2 selective inhibitors is their distinct pharmacokinetic properties. While these agents share a common pharmacologic target, they otherwise possess different pharmacokinetic and pharmacodynamic properties that contribute directly to their overall efficacy and safety. These agents vary significantly in their rates of absorption, amount of protein binding, membrane locations, metabolism and selectivity for their enzymatic target (Table 1). Such pharmacokinetic differences also influence efficacy, tolerance, tissue distribution, safety, and drug interactions. As postulated by Nobel laureate John Vane in 2002, such fundamental differences in the physico-chemical properties and metabolism of the COX-2 inhibitors should be considered as an explanation for the increased cardiovascular risk associated with use of rofecoxib, as had already been reported by that time in the VIGOR trial. [18, 19]

Table 1. Chemical and Pharmacologic Comparison of Celecoxib and Rofecoxib

	Celecoxib	Rofecoxib
Chemical structure		
Chemical family	Sulfonamide	Methylsulfone
COX-2 selectivity*	9	> 50
Charge at physiologic pH	Charged	Neutral
Membrane location	Hydrocarbon core	Headgroup region
Oral bioavailability, %	22–40	92–93
Elimination half-life, h	6–12	15–18
Volume of distribution, L	400	90
Plasma protein binding, %	> 97	86
Primary liver metabolism (cytochrome P450 enzymes)	Oxidation by CYP2C9, 3A4	Cytosolic reductase

(Table was modified from Chang IJ and Harris RC. *Hypertension.* 2005; 45:178–180.)

* COX-2 selectivity based on the IC_{80} (80% inhibitory concentration) of COX-2 relative to COX-1 using the William Harvey human modified whole blood assay. [20]

COX-2 inhibitors can be classified by their chemical properties as belonging to either the *methylsulfone* or *phospholipid* class groups. These chemical differences influence the drugs' chemical charge at physiologic pH, thereby affecting their lipophilicity, tissue penetration, volume of distribution and even susceptibility to oxidative modification. These chemical properties also contribute to other *non*-COX related actions of these agents, such as endothelial-dependent nitric oxide release, vasodilation, and renal function preservation, as demonstrated in animal models under well controlled conditions. [18, 19, 21] These direct comparator studies showed a consistently different effect for rofecoxib with respect to cardiovascular disease surrogate biomarkers, as compared to other COX-selective and non-selective agents. [18, 19] These studies also support the earlier hypothesis [22] that basic chemical differences among COX-2 agents can be manifest in their biological actions, some of which are entirely independent of COX-2 inhibition *per se*.

4.   ROFECOXIB FORMS A HIGHLY REACTIVE METABOLITE THAT HAS POTENT PRO-OXIDANT ACTIVITY

Direct support for cardiotoxicity with rofecoxib, as opposed to other agents in this class, has been provided by E.J. Corey (Nobel laureate in chemistry, 1990). To understand the basis for this finding, it is important to note that the metabolism of rofecoxib is unique among these agents. While the metabolism of all coxibs is oxidative and involves cytochrome P450 enzymes, rofecoxib is first metabolized by a cytoplasmic reductase (5-α-reductase) to form potential reactive metabolites, as will be discussed. [23] By contrast, agents like celecoxib have an additional methyl group on their primary structure which leads to inactivation via the high-capacity hepatic cytochrome P450 enzyme system. [24] This results in more predictable metabolism of these compounds compared to rofecoxib which is processed into a variety of metabolites. [25] Indeed, Reddy and Corey reported that rofecoxib readily formed a reactive metabolite, a maleic anhydride derivative (see Figure 1). in the presence of oxygen. [26] This metabolite is capable of reactions with nucleophilic groups of various biological molecules, especially amine groups, to cause disruption in essential cellular structure-function relationships. It is noteworthy that this reactive metabolite could not be derived from other COX-2 selective agents, including celecoxib, valdecoxib and lumaricoxib due to their inability to form analogous chemical metabolites. [26]

The formation of a reactive metabolite from rofecoxib may contribute specifically to mechanisms of atherothrombotic disease. In particular, the maleic anhydride can form highly reactive peroxyl radicals, thereby promoting lipid oxidation. As evidence for such a mechanism, we observed that rofecoxib, but not sulfonamide-type COX-2 inhibitors (celecoxib and valdecoxib), caused an increase in susceptibility of human LDL and membrane lipids to oxidative modification. [27] The formation of isoprostanes and aldehydes with rofecoxib was non-enzymatic and may be mediated by its reactive metabolite. In addition to a biochemical mechanism mediated by its metabolite, we observed that rofecoxib (and etoricoxib) altered

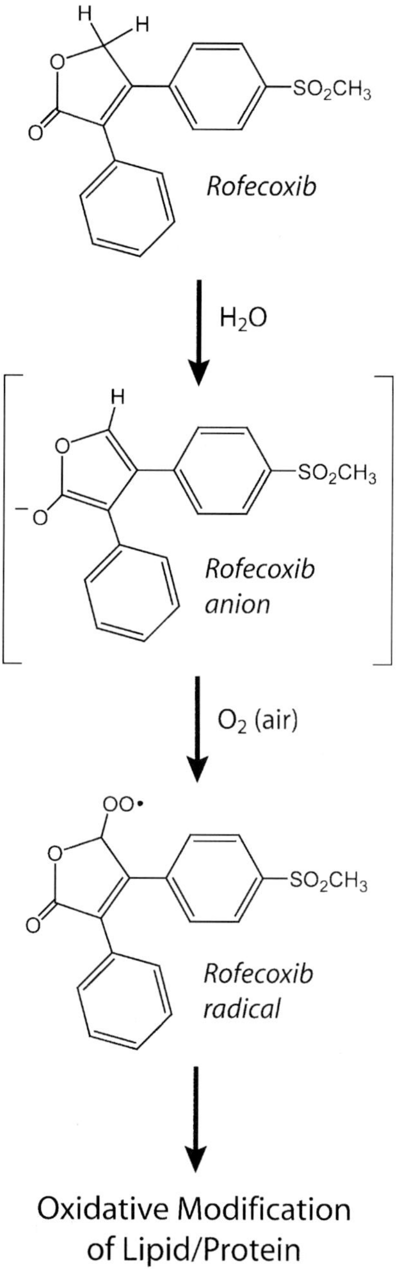

Figure 1. Chemical steps involved in the formation of a reactive metabolite for rofecoxib. Under physiologic conditions, rofecoxib readily ionizes to an anion that then forms a reactive maleic anhydride in the presence of oxygen. [26] the metabolite is capable of reacting with PUFAs associated with membrane phospholipid or LDL to form toxic lipid peroxyl groups. The metabolite may also react with amine groups in proteins, thereby altering essential aspects of cellular structure and function

the three-dimensional structure of the lipid molecules, a process that could further accelerate the rate of lipid peroxidation. [27] Again, these toxic effects of rofecoxib were not reproduced by other COX-selective or non-selective agents, including naproxen, ibuprofen, diclofenac or meloxicam.

5.   **ROFECOXIB INCREASES THE SUSCEPTIBILIY OF HUMAN**
      LDL TO OXIDATIVE MODIFICATION: COMPARISON
      TO OTHER COX-2 INHIBITORS AND NSAIDs

Minimally modified or oxidized LDL has an essential role in atherosclerotic plaque instability by contributing to mechanisms of endothelial dysfunction and inflammation. [28, 29] Oxidative LDL contributes directly to foam cell formation, endothelial dysfunction and destructive inflammatory processes associated with plaque instability and thrombus formation. [30, 31] *In vivo* studies show that levels of oxidized LDL strongly correlate with the severity of acute coronary syndromes and plaque instability. [32, 33] In a prospective study of over 600 patients, we observed that levels of lipid oxidation markers were highly predictive of coronary events over a three year period, independent of traditional risk factors and markers of inflammation. [34] Thus, a pro-oxidant effect with rofecoxib may be an important clue for understanding the basis for its toxicity and developing pharmacologic approaches to block this activity.

We evaluated the effects of rofecoxib on rates of lipid peroxidation in isolated human LDL and lipid vesicles enriched with polyunsaturated fatty acids (*e.g.*, arachidonic acid), the substrate for lipid peroxidation. Oxidative changes in these various biological preparations were monitored and compared to another selective COX-2 inhibitor (celecoxib) and non-selective COX inhibitors (naproxen, diclofenac) under identical conditions. The activity of rofecoxib was also compared to sulfone analogs, including methyl phenyl sulfone and dimethyl sulfone. Following incubation with human LDL, rofecoxib significantly ($p < 0.001$) *decreased* the lag time for human LDL conjugated diene formation by $42.8 \pm 1.5\%$ at 100 nM (Figure 2). This pronounced effect on the rate of conjugated diene formation indicates that rofecoxib has potent pro-oxidant activity, as evidenced by depleted LDL antioxidant capacity.

In addition to measuring conjugated diene formation, we also measured the effects of these agents on the formation of reactive aldehydes, especially malondialdehyde (MDA). Consistent with its effect on conjugated diene formation, rofecoxib and etoricoxib also caused marked increases in MDA levels. The comparative effects of these agents on MDA formation from human LDL (measured as TBARS) are reported in Figure 2. Compared to celecoxib, naproxen and diclofenac, only rofecoxib caused a significant increase in MDA levels, even at a concentration (50 nM) that was 10-fold lower (50 nM) than that used for comparison drugs. Pro-oxidant changes in conjugated diene formation or MDA levels were not observed following treatment with other COX selective or non-selective inhibitors under identical conditions. Additionally, other sulfone-containing compounds (methyl

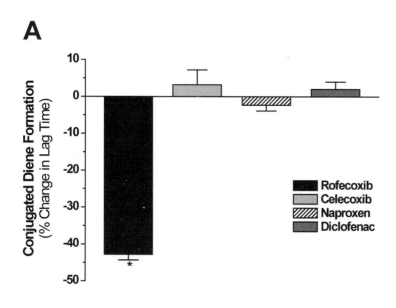

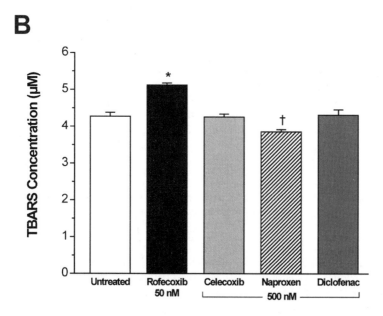

Figure 2. (Continued)

phenyl sulfone, dimethyl sulfone) had no effect on LDL oxidation (data not shown). As compared to vehicle treated LDL samples (MDA level of $3.23 \pm 0.28\,\mu M$), there were no significant changes in LDL oxidation for samples treated with either dimethyl sulfone ($3.32 \pm 0.19\,\mu M$, $p = 0.9$) or methyl phenyl sulfone ($3.25 \pm 0.13\,\mu M$, $p = 0.7$) at a concentration of $1\,\mu M$. [27]

6. EFFECT OF COX-2 INHIBITORS AND NSAIDs ON ISOPROSTANE FORMATION FROM MEMBRANE SULFONAMIDE

Isoprostanes are prostaglandin isomers that can be generated non-enzymatically by free radical modification of arachidonic acid associated with phospholipids in LDL and cellular membranes. F_2-isoprostanes have been specifically identified in atherosclerotic plaques where they are mediators of inflammation. [35] We tested the effects of these agents on peroxidation of lipid vesicles containing arachidonic acid, the substrate for non-enzymatic formation of isoprostanes. Using mass spectroscopy, we observed pronounced differences in isoprostane generation among the COX-2 inhibitors. [27] Levels of isoprostanes were shown to increase from $140 \pm 25\,ng/ml$ (mean $\pm$ S.D.) in vehicle-treated samples to $190 \pm 18\,ng/ml$ ($p < 0.0025$) and $224 \pm 22\,ng/ml$ ($p < 0.0001$) in the presence of $100\,nM$ rofecoxib and etoricoxib, respectively (Figure 3A). By contrast, celecoxib had no significant effect on peroxidation of arachidonic acid-enriched vesicles, even at higher concentrations.

7. EFFECT OF ROFECOXIB AND CELECOXIB ON THE OXYGEN RADICAL ANTIOXIDANT CAPACITY (ORAC) OF HUMAN PLASMA

As reported in the *Physicians Desk Reference* (2003), the maximum plasma concentration (C_{max}) for celecoxib at an approved $200\,mg$ dose is $1.85\,\mu M$ ($705\,ng/ml$). In the case of rofecoxib, an approved dose of $25\,mg$ results in a plasma concentration of $658\,nM$ ($207\,ng/ml$). The comparative effects of rofecoxib and celecoxib

---

Figure 2. (A) Comparative effects of NSAIDs on rates of conjugated diene formation in human LDL ($100\,\mu g$ protein/ml) following incubation with COX-2 selective (celecoxib, rofecoxib) and non-selective inhibitors (diclofenac, naproxen). Diene formation in the presence of each agent at a concentration of $100\,nM$ was monitored at $234\,nm$ and compared to vehicle (control). The lag time was calculated from the intercept of the lines drawn through the linear portions of the lag phase and propagation phase. LDL oxidation was initiated with $CuSO_4$ at $37\,°C$. Values are mean $\pm$ S.D. of experiments done in triplicate. $^*p < 0.001$, different from vehicle-treated LDL samples. (B) Comparative effects of NSAIDs on formation of TBARS in human LDL ($100\,\mu g$ protein/ml) following incubation with COX-2 selective (celecoxib, rofecoxib) and non-selective inhibitors (diclofenac, naproxen, ibuprofen) at $500\,nM$. Oxidation was initiated with $CuSO_4$ at $37\,°C$. The effects of the drugs on LDL oxidation were compared to vehicle (control) based on TBARS formation measured at an absorbance of $532\,nm$. $^*p < 0.001$ and $^†p < 0.01$ versus vehicle treated samples. (Figure reproduced from an earlier article. [27])

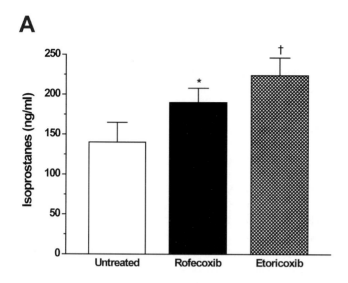

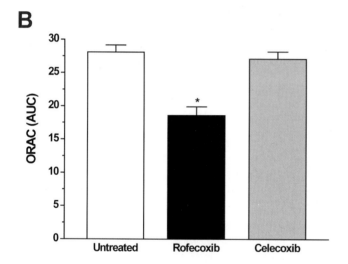

Figure 3. (A) Effects of rofecoxib and etoricoxib (100 nM) versus vehicle-treatment on isoprostane formation from lipid vesicles enriched with arachidonic acid (0.25 mg/ml). Peroxidation of lipids occurred over time in the absence of any exogenous initiators at 37 °C. Total levels of F_2-isoprostanes were measured by GC-MS with negative chemical ionization in DAPC lipid vesicles prepared in the presence of vehicle or drug. Values are mean ± S.D. (n = 4), *$p < 0.01$ and †$p < 0.0001$ versus vehicle treated samples. (B) Comparative effects of COX-2 inhibitors rofecoxib and celecoxib on the antioxidant capacity of human plasma were assessed using the Oxygen Radical Absorption Capacity (ORAC) assay. The area under the curve (AUC) from the analysis was reported as a function of treatment at 1.0 μM. Plasma oxidation was initiated with AAPH at 37 °C. The effects of the drug were compared to vehicle (control). *$p < 0.0001$, rofecoxib versus either vehicle or celecoxib treated samples. (Figure reproduced from an earlier article. [27])

on the antioxidant capacity of human plasma were assessed using the Oxygen Radical Absorption Capacity or ORAC assay. [36] The area under the curve (AUC) from the ORAC analysis is reported in Figure 3B. Consistent with a pro-oxidant effect, rofecoxib significantly ($p < 0.001$) reduced the ORAC value by 34% (28.1 ± 1.2 in vehicle-treated samples to 18.6 ± 1.3) at $1.0\,\mu M$. In parallel experiments, celecoxib did not significantly change this value, even at the highest concentration tested ($10.0\,\mu M$), in which the ORAC value was 28.5 ± 0.1. [27]

8.   EFFECT OF COX-2 INHIBITORS ON LIPID STRUCTURE

To further understand how the distinct properties of the COX-2 inhibitors influence the susceptibility of LDL and membrane lipids to oxidative modification, we used small-angle x-ray diffraction approaches to measure their interaction with biological membranes. [37] The addition of rofecoxib produced a change in electron density consistent with a location in the phospholipids headgroup. [27] At the same time, rofecoxib caused disordering in the hydrocarbon core, similar to thermal heating or oxidative damage to the membrane. [38, 39] Thus, the pro-oxidant activity of rofecoxib may be related, in part, to physico-chemical changes in lipid structure. By contrast, the addition of celecoxib to the phospholipids bilayer was associated with the hydrocarbon core, a location attributed to its greater lipophilicity. These

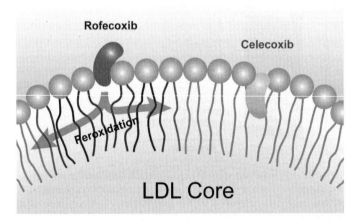

Figure 4. Schematic illustration of structural changes in membrane lipids with rofecoxib, based on small angle x-ray diffraction analysis. The location of rofecoxib in the phospholipid headgroup region caused a disordering of the phospholipid acyl chains. The alteration in the intermolecular packing of the lipid molecules may facilitate the diffusion of free radicals. By contrast, celecoxib had a well-defined location in the membrane hydrocarbon core; a position consistent with its highly lipophilic properties. The equilibrium position of the celecoxib molecule did not cause a disordering in the lipid molecules

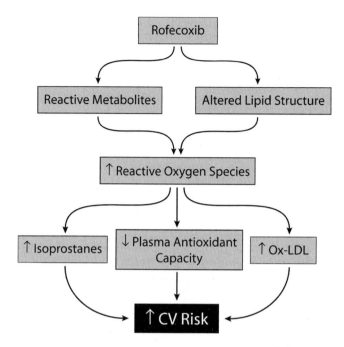

Figure 5. A summary of the cardiotoxic mechanism for rofecoxib based on experimental findings. [26, 27] The rofecoxib molecule alters lipid structure and undergoes conversion to a reactive metabolite that may stimulate formation of reactive oxygen species, such as lipid peroxyl groups. As evidence of this pro-oxidant activity, rofecoxib increased levels of isoprostanes, oxidized LDL, and reduced plasma antioxidant capacity. These oxidized lipids contribute to endothelial dysfunction and inflammation, thereby contributing to mechanisms of atherothrombosis

differences in the molecular membrane interactions of the COX-2 inhibitors may contribute to their distinct physico-chemical effects on lipid peroxidation (Figure 4).

9. CONCLUSION

We have reviewed a mechanistic basis for cardiotoxicity with rofecoxib that can be attributed to its distinct chemical properties, unique primary metabolism and potent pro-oxidant activity. These findings are summarized in Figure 5. Following primary metabolism, rofecoxib readily forms a highly reactive maleic anhydride derivative that causes oxidative damage in various biological targets, including human LDL and arachidonic acid, to form atherogenic aldehydes and isoprostanes. The toxic effects of rofecoxib could not be reproduced by sulfonamide COX-2 inhibitors, such as celecoxib, or NSAIDs when tested under identical conditions. Collectively, these findings indicate that rofecoxib is cardiotoxic due to inherent chemical properties that are unrelated to COX-2 inhibition.

REFERENCES

1. Bombardier C, Laine L, Reicin A, Group. fTVS. Comparison of upper gastrointestinal toxicity of rofecoxib and naproxen in patients with rheumatoid arthritis. *N. Engl. J. Med.* 2000;343:1520–1528.
2. Silverstein FE, Faich G, Goldstein JL, Simon LS, Pincus T, Whelton A, Makuch R, Eisen G, Agrawal NM, Stenson WF, Burr AM, Zhao WW, Kent JD, Lefkowith JB, Verburg KM, Geis GS. Gastrointestinal toxicity with celecoxib vs nonsteroidal anti-inflammatory drugs for osteoarthritis and rheumatoid arthritis: the Celecoxib Long-Term Arthritis Safety Study (CLASS): a randomized control trial. *JAMA.* 2000;284:1247–1255.
3. Schoenbeck U, Sukhova GK, Graber P, Coulter S, Libby P. Augmented expression of cyclo-oxygenase-2 in human atherosclerotic lesions. *Am. J. Pathol.* 1999;155:1281–1291.
4. Baker CS, Hall RJ, Evans TJ, Pomerance A, Maclouf J, Creminon C, Yacoub MH, Polak JM. Cyclooxygenase-2 is widely expressed in atherosclerotic lesions affecting native and transplanted human coronary arteries and colocalizes with inducible nitric oxide synthase and nitrotryrosine particularly in macrophages. *Arterioscler. Thromb. Vasc. Biol.* 1999;19:646–655.
5. Pitt B, Pepine CJ, Willerson JT. Cyclooxygenase-2 inhibition and cardiovascular events. *Circulation.* 2002;106:167–169.
6. Bresalier RS, Sandler RS, Quan H, Bolognese JA, Oxenius B, Horgan K, Lines C, Riddell R, Morton D, Lanas A, Konstam MA, Baron JA. Cardiovascular events associated with rofecoxib in a colorectal adenoma chemoprevention trial. *N. Engl. J. Med.* 2005;352:1092–1102.
7. FitzGerald GA, Smith B, Pedersen AK, Brash AR. Increased prostacylin biosynthesis in patients with severe atherosclerosis and platelet activation. *N. Engl. J. Med.* 1984;310:1065–1068.
8. Cheng Y, Austin SC, Rocca B, Koller BH, Coffman TM, Grosser T, Lawson JA, FitzGerald GA. Role of prostacyclin in the cardiovascular response to thromboxane A2. *Science.* 2002;296:539–541.
9. Mukherjee D, Nissen ST, Topol EJ. Risk of cardiovascular events associated with selective COX-2 inhibitors. *JAMA.* 2000;286:954–959.
10. Ray WA, Stein CM, Daugherty JR, Hall K, Arbogast PG, Griffin MR. COX-2 selective non-steroidal anti-inflammatory drugs and risk of serious coronary heart disease. *Lancet.* 2002;360:1071–1073.
11. Solomon DH, Schneeweiss S, Glynn RJ, Kiyota Y, Levin R, Mogun H, Avorn J. Relationship between selective cyclooxygenase-2 inhibitors and acute myocardial infarction in older adults. *Circulation.* 2004;109:2068–2073.
12. Mamdani M, Juurlink DN, Lee DS, Rochon PA, Kopp A, Nagile G, Austin PC, Laupacis A, Stukel TA. Cyclo-oxygenase-2 inhibitors versus non-selective non-steroidal anti-inflammatory drugs and congestive heart failure outcomes in elderly patients: A population-based cohort study. *The Lancet.* 2004;363:1751–1756.
13. Juni P, Nartey L, Reichenbach S, Sterchi R, Dieppe PA, Egger M. Risk of cardiovascular events and rofecoxib: cumulative meta-analysis. *Lancet.* 2004;364:2021–2029.
14. Graham DJ, Campen D, Hui R, Spence M, Cheetham C, Levy G, Shoor S, Ray WA. Risk of acute myocardial infarction and sudden cardiac death in patients treated with cyclo-oxygenase 2 selective and non-selective non-steroidal anti-inflammatory drugs: nested case-control study. *Lancet.* 2005;365:475–481.
15. Solomon SD, McMurray JJV, Pfeffer MA, Wittes J, Fowler R, Finn P, Anderson WF, Zauber A, Hawk E, Bertagnolli M. Cardiovascular risk associated with celecoxib in a clinical trial for colorectal adenoma prevention. *N. Engl. J. Med.* 2005;352:1071–1080.
16. Caughey GE, Cleland LG, Gamble JR, James MJ. Up-regulation of endothelial cyclooxygenase-2 and prostanoid synthesis by platelets: role of thromboxane A2. *J. Biol. Chem.* 2001;276:37839–37845.
17. Chan AT, Manson JE, Albert CM, Chae CU, Rexrode KM, Curhan GC, Rimm EB, Willett WC, Fuchs CS. Nonsteroidal antiinflammatory drugs, acetaminophen, and the risk of cardiovascular events. *Circulation.* 2006;113:1578–1587.

18. Hermann M, Shaw S, Kiss E, Camici G, Buhler N, Chenevard R, Luscher TF, Grone HJ, Ruschitzka F. Selective COX-2 inhibitors and renal injury in salt-sensitive hypertension. *Hypertension*. 2005;45:193–197.

19. Hermann M, Camici G, Fratton A, Hurlimann D, Tanner FC, Hellermann JP, Fiedler M, Thiery J, Neidhart M, Gay RE, Gay S, Lüscher TF, Ruschitzka F. Differential effects of selective cyclooxygenase-2 inhibitors on endothelial function in salt-induced hypertension. *Circulation*. 2003;108:2308–2311.

20. Warner TD, Giuliano F, Vojnovic I, Bukasa A, Mitchell JA, Vane JR. Nonsteroid drug selectivities for cyclo-oxygenase-1 rather than cyclo-oxygenase-2 are associated with human gastrointestinal toxicity: A full in vitro analysis. *Proc Natl Acad Sci U S A*. 1999;96:7563–7568.

21. Chenevard R, Hurlimann D, Bechir M, Enseleit F, Spieker L, Hermann M, Riesen W, Gay S, Gay RE, Neidhart M, Michel B, Luscher TF, Noll G, Ruschitzka F. Selective COX-2 inhibition improves endothelial function in coronary artery disease. *Circulation*. 2003;107:405–409.

22. Vane JR. Back to an aspirin a day? *Science*. 2002;296:474–475.

23. Brune K, Hinz B. Selective cyclooxygenase-2 inhibitors: similarities and differences. *Scand. J. Rheumatol*. 2004;33:1–6.

24. Tang C, Shou M, Mei Q, Rushmore TH, Rodrigues AD. Major role of human liver microsomal cytochrome P450 2C9 (CYP2C9) in the oxidative metabolism of celecoxib, a novel cyclooxygenase-II inhibitor. *J. Pharmacol. Exp. Ther*. 2000;293:453–459.

25. Slaughter D, Takenaga N, Lu P, Assang C, Walsh DJ, Arison BH, Cui D, Halpin RA, Geer LA, Vyas KP, Baillie TA. Metabolism of rofecoxib in vitro using human liver subcellular fractions. *Drug Metab Dipos*. 2003;31:1398–1408.

26. Reddy LR, Corey EJ. Facile air oxidation of the conjugate base of rofecoxib (Vioxx), a possible contributor to human toxicity. *Tetrahedron Letters*. 2005;46:927–929.

27. Walter MF, Jacob RF, Day CA, Dahlborg R, Weng Y, Mason RP. Sulfone COX-2 inhibitors increase susceptibility of human LDL and plasma to oxidative modification: Comparison to sulfonamide COX-2 inhibitors and NSAIDs. *Atherosclerosis*. 2004;177:235–243.

28. Steinberg D, Parthasarathy S, Carew TE, Khoo JC, Witztum JL. Beyond cholesterol. Modifications of low-density lipoprotein that incease its atherogenicity. *N. Engl. J. Med*. 1989;320:915–924.

29. Steinbrecher UP, Lougheed M, Kwan WC, Dirks M. Recognition of oxidized low density lipoprotein by the scavenger receptor of macrophages results from derivatization of apolipoprotein B by products of fatty acid peroxidation. *J. Biol. Chem*. 1989;264:15216–15223.

30. Witztum JL, Berliner JA. Oxidized phospholipids and isoprostanes in atherosclerosis. *Curr. Opin. Lipidol*. 1998;9:441–448.

31. Steinberg D. Low density lipoprotein oxidation and its pathobiological significance. *J. Biol. Chem*. 1997;272:20963–20966.

32. Nishi K, Itabe H, Uno M, Kitazato KT, Horiguchi H, Shinno K, Nagahiro S. Oxidized LDL in carotid plaques and plasma associates with plaque instability. *Arterioscler. Thromb. Vasc. Biol*. 2002;22:1649–1654.

33. Ehara S, Ueda M, Naruko T, Haze K, Itoh A, Otsuka M, Komatsu R, Matsuo T, Itabe H, Takano T, Tsukamoto Y, Yoshiyama M, Takeuchi K, Yoshikawa J, Becker AE. Elevated levels of oxidized low density lipoprotein show a positive relationship with the severity of acute coronary syndromes. *Circulation*. 2001;103:1955.

34. Walter MF, Jacob RF, Jeffers B, Ghadanfar MM, Preston GM, Buch J, Mason RP. Serum levels of TBARS predict cardiovascular events in patients with stable coronary artery disease: A longitudinal analysis of the PREVENT study. *J. Am. Coll. Cardiol*. 2004;44:1996–2002.

35. Pratico D, Iuliano L, Mauriello A, Spagnoli L, Lawson JA, Rokach J, Maclouf J, Violi F, FitzGerald GA. Localization of distinct F_2-isoprostanes in human atherosclerotic lesions. *J. Clin. Invest*. 1997;100:2028–2034.

36. Huang D, Ou B, Hampsch-Woodill M, Flanagan JA, Prior RL. High-throughput assay of oxygen radical absorbance capacity (ORAC) using a multichannel liquid handling system coupled with a microplate fluorescence reader in 96-well format. *J Agric Food Chem*. 2002;50:1815–1821.

37. Mason RP, Jacob RF. X-ray diffraction analysis of membrane structure changes with oxidative stress. In: Armstrong D, ed. *Methods in Molecular Biology: Ultrastructural and Molecular Biology Protocols*. Totowa, NJ: Humana Press Inc.; 2002:71–80.

38. Tulenko TN, Chen M, Mason PE, Mason RP. Physical effects of cholesterol on arterial smooth muscle membranes: Evidence of immiscible cholesterol domains and alterations in bilayer width during atherogenesis. *J. Lipid. Res.* 1998;39:947–956.

39. Mason RP, Walter MF, Mason PE. Effect of oxidative stress on membrane structure: Small angle x-ray diffraction analysis. *Free Radic. Biol. Med.* 1997;23:419–425.

SECTION IV

**COX-2 BLOCKADE IN CANCER PREVENTION
AND THERAPY**

CHAPTER 9

CANCER CHEMOPREVENTION BY CYCLOOXYGENASE 2 (COX-2) BLOCKADE
Results of case control studies

RANDALL E. HARRIS*, JOANNE BEEBE-DONK
AND GALAL A. ALSHAFIE

The Ohio State University College of Medicine & School of Public Health, A150B Starling-Loving Hall, 320 W. 10th Avenue, Columbus, OH 43210

* E-mail: Harris.44@osu.edu

R. E. Harris (ed.), Inflammation in the Pathogenesis of Chronic Diseases, 193–212.
© 2007 *Springer.*

Abstract: Significant use of selective cyclooxygenase-2 (COX-2) blocking agents prescribed for the treatment of arthritis during 1999 to 2005 facilitates epidemiologic investigations to illuminate their chemopreventive effects against human cancer. We therefore conducted a set of case control studies of selective COX-2 blocking agents to determine their chemopreventive potential for the four major cancers: breast, prostate, colon, and lung. Newly diagnosed cases (323 breast cancer patients, 229 prostate cancer patients, 326 colon cancer patients, and 486 lung cancer patients) were ascertained during 2002 to September 30, 2004, at The James Cancer Hospital and Solove Research Institute, The Ohio State University Medical Center, Columbus, Ohio. All cases of invasive cancer were confirmed by examination of the pathology report. Healthy controls without cancer were ascertained from hospital screening clinics during the same time period. Controls were frequency matched at a rate of 2:1 to the cases by age, gender, and county of residence. We collected information on type, frequency, and duration of use of selective COX-2 inhibitors and nonselective nonsteroidal anti-inflammatory drugs (NSAIDs). Other potentially important risk factors (smoking, drinking, body mass, medical history, blood pressure and cholesterol medications, family history of cancer, occupational history, and reproductive history for women) were also recorded for each subject. Estimates of odds ratios were obtained with adjustment for age and other potential confounders using logistic regression analysis. Use of selective COX-2 inhibitors resulted in a significant risk reduction for each type of cancer (71% for breast cancer, 55% for prostate cancer, 70% for colon cancer, and 79% for lung cancer) and an overall 68% risk reduction for all four cancers. This investigation demonstrates that COX-2 blocking agents have strong potential for the chemoprevention of cancers of the breast, prostate, colon and lung

1. INTRODUCTION

1.1. Burden of Cancer

The American Cancer Society estimates that more than 1.4 million new cases of invasive cancer will be diagnosed during 2006 in the United States, and more than 564,000 Americans will die from cancer [1]. When age-adjusted death rates are considered, cancer has surpassed heart disease and is now the leading cause of death among American women and men under age 85. The majority (about 60%) of cancer deaths are attributable to four major cancer types: lung, breast, prostate, and colon. Among women, cancers of the lung and bronchus, breast, and colon account for more than half of the deaths. Among men, the majority of deaths are due to cancers of the lung and bronchus, prostate, and colon. Lung cancer is the leading cause of cancer death in both men and women, causing nearly 93,000 deaths in men and 82,000 deaths in women every year. Breast cancer is the most common malignancy among American women and the second leading cause of cancer death. In 2006, 213,000 women are expected to develop invasive breast cancer and nearly 41,000 will die from the disease. Prostate cancer is the most common malignancy among American men and the second leading cause of death. In 2006, 234,000 men are expected to develop invasive prostate cancer and 27,000 will die from the disease. Colon cancer is the third leading cause of death in both men and women and will cause nearly 55,000 deaths in 2006. Despite intensive efforts aimed primarily at early detection and therapy, the high mortality rates of these malignancies have persisted for several decades. Innovative research efforts must therefore be redirected towards chemoprevention of the early stages of carcinogenesis.

1.2.   Nonsteroidal Anti-inflammatory Drugs (NSAIDs) and Cancer

Epidemiologic studies indicate that nonsteroidal anti-inflammatory drugs (NSAIDs) reduce the risk of virtually all cancers [2]. Recently, we comprehensively reviewed the published scientific literature on non-steroidal anti-inflammatory drugs (NSAIDs) and cancer and evaluated results based upon epidemiologic criteria of judgment: consistency of results, strength of association, dose response, molecular specificity, and biological plausibility [3]. Sufficient data from 91 epidemiologic studies were available to examine the association of relative risk and NSAID intake for ten human malignancies. Results showed a significant decrease in the risk with intake of NSAIDs (primarily aspirin or ibuprofen) for 7 of 10 malignancies including the four major types: colon, breast, lung, and prostate cancer. Daily intake of NSAIDs (325 mg aspirin or 200 mg ibuprofen) produced risk reductions of 63% for colon cancer, 39% for breast cancer, 36% for lung cancer, and 39% for prostate cancer. Significant risk reductions were also observed for esophageal cancer (73%), stomach cancer (62%), and ovarian cancer (47%). NSAID effects became apparent after five or more years of use and were stronger with longer duration. Observed protective effects were also consistently stronger for gastrointestinal malignancies (esophagus, stomach, and colon). Results for pancreatic cancer, urinary bladder cancer, and renal cancer were inconsistent. Initial epidemiologic studies of malignant melanoma, Hodgkin's disease, and adult leukemia also found that NSAIDs are protective.

The epidemiologic literature therefore provides compelling evidence that regular intake of NSAIDs with non-selective activity against cyclooxygenase-2 (COX-2) protects against the development of many types of cancer. When results are combined according to the relative incidence of these malignancies, it is estimated that regular NSAID intake is associated with a 36% reduction in overall cancer risk. This estimate is in close agreement with the findings of Gonzalez-Perez and colleagues [4] who reported a similar reduction in overall cancer risk with NSAID use.

1.3.   Antineoplastic Effects of NSAIDs

The anti-inflammatory effects of NSAIDs stem primarily from inhibition of cyclooxygenase, the rate limiting enzyme of the prostaglandin cascade [5]. Two primary genes are responsible for the genetic control of cyclooxygenase, a constitutive gene (COX-1) and its inducible isoform (COX-2) [6, 7]. Molecular studies show that the inducible cyclooxygenase-2 gene (COX-2) is over-expressed in virtually every type of human cancer that has been studied including colon cancer, breast cancer, prostate cancer, lung cancer [8–14], see also Chapter 10.

Metabolism of arachidonic acid via the cyclooxygenase pathway produces various prostaglandins, prostacyclins and thromboxanes, and increased levels have been shown in malignant tumors in comparison to benign tumors and normal tissues [15–19]. Certain prostaglandins, for example PGE2, PGF2-alpha and 6-keto-PGF-1-alpha, are upregulated in association with tumor formation [20]. Both in vitro and in vivo studies have demonstrated that inhibition of the cyclooxygenase pathway, and particularly COX-2, results in the inhibition of tumor growth and development [21–28].

In the past quarter century, scores of independent investigations employing animal models of carcinogenesis have generated compelling evidence that NSAIDs have significant and consistent effects against cancer development at several anatomic sites. Early investigations in the 1980's by Pollard and Luckert [29, 30] and Reddy et al. [31, 32] showed that administration of indomethacin and piroxicam significantly inhibited colon carcinogenesis. Karmali et al. [33, 34] discovered similar effects of NSAIDs against breast cancer, and also elucidated differential effects of essential dietary fatty acids in prostaglandin biosynthesis and tumor promotion. Her studies showed that dietary supplementation with the n-6 fatty acid, linoleic acid, promoted tumor growth and development via enhanced arachidonic acid metabolism and elevated levels of PG activity, whereas the n-3 essential fatty acid, linolenic acid, had the opposite effect. Subsequent investigations have confirmed these early findings not only for colon and breast cancer, but also for lung cancer [35], prostate cancer [36], and a variety of other tumors that have been investigated in animal models [37]. In these studies of chemically induced tumors, supplemental administration of general NSAIDs such as aspirin, ibuprofen, piroxicam, sulindac, and others, in the diet or drinking water consistently reduced the growth and development of malignant neoplasms by 25 to 75%. It is important to note that recent preclinical studies have demonstrated even stronger antineoplastic effects of selective COX-2 inhibitors such as celecoxib, rofecoxib, valdecoxib, and nimesulide against colon cancer [38, 39] and breast cancer [40, 41], as well as other malignancies. Animal models of carcinogenesis therefore provide compelling evidence that NSAIDs inhibit tumor growth and development.

Various physiologic mechanisms may be responsible for the observed anti-tumor effects of NSAIDs. Inhibition of cyclooxygenase and blockade of the prostaglandin cascade may impact upon neoplastic growth and development by reducing key features of carcinogenesis, vis a vis, mutagenesis, angiogenesis, and mitosis, and also by stimulating apoptosis of malignant cells [42, 43, 44]. It has recently been discovered that up-regulation of COX-2 and correlative production of prostaglandin E2 (PGE2) effectively and specifically induces the promoter II region of the cytochrome P-450 gene (CYP-19) which is transcribed and translated into aromatase, the chief enzyme in the biosynthesis of estrogen [45, 46]. It is well known that estrogen has strong proliferative effects and mitogenic potential, and procedures which reduce estrogen levels or estrogen activity have been associated with decreased risk of breast cancer as well as other malignancies. The COX blocking agents have also been found to activate the peroxisome proliferator-activated receptors (PPAR), ligands which modulate neoplastic transcription in conjunction with upregulation of the prostaglandin cascade [47]. Recent investigations of cell lines of adenocarcinoma of the lung reveal the presence of acetylcholine receptors which modulate arachidonic acid release and stimulate carcinogenesis; notably, these effects are blocked by administration of NSAIDs [48, 49]. These multiple lines of evidence suggest that aberrant induction and upregulation of the prostaglandin cascade play a significant role in carcinogenesis, and that blockade of this process has strong potential for intervention.

1.4.   Breast Cancer and NSAIDs

Karmali's early work on breast cancer development in animals provided unequivocal proof that dietary supplementation with the essential n-6 fatty acid, linoleic acid, heightens prostaglandin biosynthesis and promotes breast cancer development, whereas the n-3 fatty acid linolenic acid has the opposite effect [33, 34]. Independent studies by many investigators have consistently demonstrated that aspirin, indomethacin, ibuprofen, and other NSAIDs significant reduce the incidence of chemically induced breast cancer in animals [50–56]. A recent report by Harris, Alshafie, Abou-Issa, and Seibert provides the first evidence that the selective COX-2 blocker, celecoxib, has striking chemopreventive and therapeutic effects against mammary carcinogenesis in vivo, vis a vis., in the Sprague-Dawley rat model of breast cancer, celecoxib is a dramatically effective inhibitor of tumor initiation, multiplicity, growth, and development [40].

   Harris and colleagues have reported the results of four separate epidemiologic investigations, each suggesting that NSAIDs such as ibuprofen and aspirin significantly reduce the risk of breast cancer [57–61]. Perhaps the most notable of these studies is the Women's Health Initiative national sample of 81,000 postmenopausal women, wherein long term regular use of over the counter NSAIDs reduced the risk of breast cancer by 28% and the use of ibuprofen per se reduced the risk by 49%, whereas acetaminophen, an analgesic without COX-2 activity, had no effect on the risk [61]. Our recent meta-analysis of seventeen independent epidemiologic studies found that regular use of over the counter NSAIDs produced a 39% reduction in breast cancer risk [3]. Most recently, the final results of a large multi-center epidemiologic investigation of more than 7,000 breast cancer cases found that aspirin and other NSAIDs significantly decreased breast cancer risk [62]. In molecular studies of breast tissues, over-expression of the COX-2 gene is a feature of most human breast cancers [11], and COX-2 levels in malignant cells are correlated with upregulation of aromatase and heightened estrogen biosynthesis in adjacent breast adipose [46]. Overall, the evidence shows consistency of chemopreventive effects of non-selective NSAIDs against breast cancer plus molecular specificity of COX-2 over-expression in mammary carcinogenesis, thus setting the stage for studies of the selective COX-2 inhibitors.

1.5.   Prostate Cancer and NSAIDs

An early animal study by Pollard and luckert [63] demonstrated that the NSAID, piroxicam, produced significant inhibition of the metastatic spread of transplanted prostate cancer. Subsequently, molecular studies showed that most prostate tumors over-express COX-2 [64, 65], and in vitro studies found that the growth of prostate cancer cell lines is enhanced by arachadonic acid and inhibited by NSAIDs [36, 66].

Nelson and Harris [67] first reported that common over the counter NSAIDs such as aspirin and ibuprofen significantly reduce the risk of prostate cancer. Our recent meta-analysis of thirteen published epidemiology investigations found evidence of heterogeneity among studies; nevertheless, regular intake of non-selective NSAIDs reduced the risk of prostate cancer by 39% [3].

1.6.   Colon Cancer, Colon Polyps and NSAIDs

The greatest concentration of effort in cancer research on NSAIDs and COX-2 blockade has focused on colon carcinogenesis. Pollard and Luckert [29, 30], and Reddy and colleagues [31, 32, 38, Chapter 13] first published the results of animal investigations which show that NSAIDs block the development of colon cancer; these findings have been confirmed by many independent investigations [38]. Preclinical studies also provide convincing evidence that selective COX-2 blockade by celecoxib and other COX-2 inhibitors markedly reduces the incidence of colon cancer in vivo [39].

Human clinical and epidemiologic studies of sporadic adenomatous polyps have consistently shown that intake of aspirin, ibuprofen, or other NSAIDs reduces the risk of colonic polyp development [68–75]. Thun et al. [76], initially published the results of an epidemiologic study showing that intake of aspirin is protective against fatal colon cancer. Subsequent independent epidemiologic studies provide good corroborative evidence that NSAIDs have antineoplastic effects against colon carcinogenesis [77]. Our recent meta-analysis of twenty-one epidemiologic studies found that regular intake of over the counter NSAIDs, primarily aspirin, produced a 63% reduction in the risk of colon cancer [3].

Molecular studies tend to substantiate these observations in revealing marked over-expression of COX-2 by the vast majority of malignant colonic tumors [12, 13, 14, 78, 79]. Randomized clinical trials have established that regular and continuing intake of celecoxib suppresses the formation of preneoplastic adeno-matous polyps and causes regression of existing polyps in patients with Familial Adenomatous Polyposis [80], and that regular intake of aspirin reduces the incidence of colon polyps in patients with prior colorectal cancer [81]. These studies which are thoroughly reviewed elsewhere [77, 82] provide convincing evidence that sustained intake of compounds with COX-2 blocking activity not only inhibits the development of colon cancer per se, but also interrupts the evolution of preneoplastic lesions of the colonic mucosa.

1.7. Lung Cancer and NSAIDs

The early preclinical studies of Schuller et al. [35] and Castonguay and Rioux [83, 84] provide convincing evidence that inhibition of prostaglandin biosynthesis by various NSAIDs reduces the development of chemically induced pulmonary adeno-carcinoma. Wolf et al. [8], Hida et al. [9], Koki et al. [14], and other investigators have observed that COX-2 is over-expressed in 70–90% of human pulmonary adeno-carcinomas and other non-small cell lung cancers. Additional molecular studies by Schuller and colleagues [48, 49] determined that lung carcinogenesis is linked to the stimulation of beta-adrenergic receptors by nitrosamines and possibly other tobacco carcinogens. They have identified a novel mechanism by which the nitrosamine, NNK, modulates the arachidonic acid cascade and DNA synthesis through signal transduction involving both beta-1 and beta-2 adrenergic receptors. Notably, this effect is inhibited by administration of NSAIDs [85].

Early prospective epidemiologic investigations by Peto et al. [86] and Schreinemachers and Everson [87] suggested that regular aspirin intake produced a significant reduction in lung cancer risk. Subsequently, other investigators have also observed protective effects of aspirin and other NSAIDs against the development of lung cancer; our meta-analysis of eleven published epidemiologic studies found that regular intake of NSAIDs produced a 36% reduction in the risk of lung cancer [3].

Since cigarette smoking is the predominant risk factor for lung cancer, we conducted a case control study to specifically compare the use of NSAIDs between smokers who developed lung cancer (smoking cases) and control subjects who also smoked. The important design feature of this study was that cigarette smoking was matched out in the analysis in order to focus specifically on potential effects of NSAIDs in preventing tobacco carcinogenesis. We observed that regular intake of NSAIDs with COX-2 activity (primarily aspirin and ibuprofen) produced a 69% reduction in the relative risk of lung cancer [88]. In contrast, acetaminophen, the comparator analgesic without COX-2 activity, had no effect on the risk of lung cancer. These findings clearly suggest that COX-2 blockade inhibits lung carcino-genesis among smokers.

1.8. Rationale for Epidemiologic Investigation of Selective COX-2 Inhibitors

Taken together, the above results provide the background and significance to conduct further epidemiologic studies to examine the chemopreventive potential of selective COX-2 blockade against common solid tumors. Significant use of selective cyclooxygenase-2 (COX-2) blocking agents such as celecoxib (Celebrex) and rofecoxib (Vioxx) prescribed for the treatment of arthritis during 1999 to September 30, 2004 (the date of the recall of Vioxx from the worldwide marketplace by its manufacturer, Merck) facilitates epidemiologic investigations to illuminate their chemopreventive effects against major cancers.

We therefore designed a case control investigation to estimate and test odds ratios as measures of preventive effects of selective COX-2 agents against the four major types of cancer in the United States. Specifically, we examined the chemo-preventive effects of selective COX-2 inhibitors (celecoxib, valdecoxib, rofecoxib, and meloxicam) against invasive carcinomas of the breast, prostate, colon, and lung utilizing a case control epidemiological design. Effects of COX-2 blockade were quantified in comparisons of cancer cases with healthy controls. This investigation was designed to collect initial critical evidence on the relative potential of selective COX-2 blocking agents in the chemoprevention of cancers of the breast, prostate, colon and lung.

2. RESEARCH DESIGN AND METHODS

2.1. Experimental Design and Population Studied

The experimental design is a retrospective case control study of breast cancer, prostate cancer, colon cancer, and lung cancer with frequency matching of cases and control subjects for age, gender, and location of residence. Our ultimate goal is to study 500–600 cases of each type of cancer with histological verification based upon review of the pathology records, and cancer-free controls frequency matched to the cases at a 2:1 ratio [89]. The current report provides an interim analysis of the available cases and controls for which data has been collected, validated, and computerized.

All cases were ascertained from the James Cancer Hospital and Research Institute (CHRI) at The Ohio State University Medical Center, Columbus, Ohio. Selected ambulatory clinics and services were utilized to ascertain suitable control subjects without cancer. Specifically, we utilized the mammography screening service and the prostate screening service for ascertainment of healthy control subjects. The controls were frequency matched to the cases at a rate of 2:1 on age, gender, race, place (county) of residence. The protocol was approved by the Internal Review Board of The Ohio State University Medical Center.

2.2. Data Collection

Critical information on exposure to selective COX-2 inhibitors, non-selective NSAIDs, and other factors was obtained by trained medical personnel at the time of cancer diagnosis for cases or screening visit for controls. We collected accurate and comprehensive information on the type, frequency of use, dose, and duration of use of both prescription and non-prescription drugs. Other data variables collected consisted of demographic characteristics, height, weight, menstrual and pregnancy history for women, family history of cancer, comprehensive information on cigarette smoking, alcohol intake, pre-existing medical conditions (arthritis, chronic headache, cardiovascular conditions including hypertension, angina, ischemic attacks, stroke, and myocardial infarction, lung disease, and diabetes mellitus), and medication history including over the counter and prescription NSAIDs, and exogenous hormones. Regarding selective COX-2 inhibitors and other NSAIDs, the use pattern (frequency, dose, and duration), the type, such as celecoxib, valdecoxib, rofecoxib, meloxicam, aspirin, ibuprofen, naproxen, indomethacin, etc, were recorded. Data on the related analgesic, acetaminophen were collected for comparison with selective COX-2 inhibitors and other NSAIDs.

2.3.   Biostatistical Analysis

Effects of the selective COX-2 inhibitors as a group were quantified by estimating odds ratios and their 95% confidence intervals. Odds ratios were adjusted for age and other factors by logistic regression analysis [90, 91]. Estimates were obtained for each type of cancer (breast, prostate, colon, and lung) and tested for heterogeneity by chi square tests. Data were stratified by gender (for lung and colon cancer), ethnicity, and by cancer risk factors (e.g., smokers and non-smokers) and odds ratios estimated within subgroups and checked (by chi square tests) for internal consistency, effect modification, and confounding. Adjusted estimates were obtained for specific types of compounds, e.g, celecoxib and rofecoxib. Homogeneous data were pooled for examination of adjusted effects across risk factors and across all malignancies combined. Similar methods were applied for the non-selective NSAIDs, low dose $< 80\,$mg) aspirin. We also estimated the effects of acetaminophen (an analgesic that has no COX-2 blocking activity) for comparison with selective COX-2 inhibitors and other NSAIDs.

3.   RESULTS

3.1.   Breast Cancer Results

Results for breast cancer are presented in Table 1. Daily intake of selective COX-2 inhibitors for two years or more produced a significant reduction in the risk of breast cancer (OR $= 0.29$, 95% CI $= 0.14$–0.59). Risk reductions were similar for individual COX-2 inhibitors (OR $= 0.17$ for celecoxib and OR $= 0.36$ for rofecoxib). Significant risk reductions were also observed for the intake of two or more pills per week of regular aspirin (OR $= 0.49$, 95% CI $= 0.26$–0.95), and ibuprofen or naproxen (OR $= 0.37$, 95% CI $= 0.18$–0.72). Neither acetaminophen nor baby aspirin (81 mg) had any effect on the relative risk of breast cancer.

3.2.   Prostate Cancer Results

Results for prostate cancer are presented in Table 2. Daily intake of selective COX-2 inhibitors for two years or more produced a significant reduction in the risk of prostate cancer (OR $= 0.45$, 95% CI $= 0.20$–1.00). Estimated risk reductions were

Table 1. Odds ratios with 95% confidence intervals for breast cancer and selective cyclooxygenase-2 (COX-2) inhibitors and over the counter nonsteroidal anti-inflammatory drugs (OTC NSAIDs)

Compound	Number of cases	Number of controls	Multivariate OR[d] (95% CI)
None/Infrequent Use[a]	262	453	1.00
COX-2 Inhibitors[b]	10	52	0.29 (0.14–0.59)
OTC NSAIDs[c]			
Aspirin	15	40	0.49 (0.26–0.94)
Ibuprofen/Naproxen	11	52	0.37 (0.18–0.72)
Acetaminophen	8	16	1.02 (0.39–2.20)
Baby Aspirin	17	36	0.77 (0.42–1.41)

[a] No use of any NSAID or analgesic or infrequent use of no more than one pill per week for less than one year;

[b] COX-2 inhibitors include celecoxib, rofecoxib, valdecoxib, and meloxicam used daily for two years or more.

[c] Over the counter (OTC) NSAIDs/analgesics used at least two times per week for two years or more.

[d] Multivariate odds ratios are adjusted for continuous variables (age and body mass) and categorical variables (parity, menopausal status, family history, smoking, and alcohol intake).

Table 2. Odds ratios with 95% confidence intervals for prostate cancer and selective cyclooxygenase-2 (COX-2) inhibitors, and over the counter nonsteroidal anti-inflammatory drugs (OTC NSAIDs)

Compound	Number of cases	Number of controls	Multivariate OR[d] (95% CI)
None/Infrequent Use[a]	158	175	1.00
COX-2 Inhibitors[b]	12	20	0.45 (0.20–1.00)
OTC NSAIDs[c]			
Aspirin	24	39	0.52 (0.29–0.93)
Ibuprofen	12	16	0.62 (0.27–1.42)
Acetaminophen	7	8	1.05 (0.37–3.03)
Baby Aspirin	16	27	0.61 (0.31–1.17)

[a] No use of any NSAID or analgesic or infrequent use of no more than one pill per week for less than one year;

[b] COX-2 inhibitors include celecoxib, rofecoxib, valdecoxib, and meloxicam used daily for two years or more.

[c] Over the counter (OTC) NSAIDs/analgesics used at least two times per week for two years or more.

[d] Multivariate odds ratios are adjusted for continuous variables (age and body mass) and categorical variables (family history, smoking, and alcohol intake).

similar for individual COX-2 inhibitors (OR = 0.51 for celecoxib and OR = 0.27 for rofecoxib). A significant risk reduction was also observed for the intake of two or more pills per week of regular aspirin (OR = 0.52, 95% CI = 0.29–0.93), and a non-significant risk reduction was observed for intake of ibuprofen (OR = 0.62, 95% CI = 0.27–1.42). Neither acetaminophen nor baby aspirin (81 mg) had a significant effect on the relative risk of prostate cancer.

3.3. Colon Cancer Results

Results for colon cancer are presented in Table 3. Daily intake of selective COX-2 inhibitors for two years or more produced a significant reduction in the risk of colon cancer (OR = 0.30, 95% CI = 0.16–0.55). Estimated risk reductions were similar for women (OR = 0.25) and men (OR = 0.42), as well as for the individual COX-2 inhibitors, celecoxib (OR = 0.37) and rofecoxib (OR = 0.23). Significant risk reductions were also observed for the intake of two or more pills per week of regular aspirin (OR = 0.27, 95% CI = 0.16–0.48), and ibuprofen or naproxen (OR = 0.18, 95% CI = 0.08–0.39). The effect of baby (81 mg) aspirin was marginally significant (OR = 0.61, P < 0.05) whereas acetaminophen use did not significantly influence the relative risk of colon cancer.

3.4. Lung Cancer Results

Results for lung cancer are presented in Table 4. It is important to note that all estimates are adjusted for a measure of the predominant risk factor for lung cancer, pack years of cigarette smoking. Daily intake of selective COX-2 inhibitors for two years or more produced a significant reduction in the risk of lung cancer (OR = 0.21, 95% CI = 0.11–0.44). Estimated risk reductions were similar for women (OR = 0.43) and men (OR = 0.09), as well as for the individual COX-2 inhibitors, celecoxib (OR = 0.23) and rofecoxib (OR = 0.19). Significant risk reductions were also observed for the intake of two or more pills per week of regular aspirin (OR = 0.30, 95% CI = 0.17–0.52), and ibuprofen or naproxen (OR = 0.36, 95% CI = 0.20–0.69). The effect of baby (81 mg) aspirin was marginally

Table 3. Odds ratios with 95% confidence intervals for colon cancer and selective cyclooxygenase-2 (COX-2) inhibitors, and over the counter nonsteroidal anti-inflammatory drugs (OTC NSAIDs)

Compound	Number of cases	Number of controls	Multivariate OR[d] (95% CI)
None/Infrequent Use[a]	248	616	1.00
COX-2 Inhibitors[b]	15	96	0.30 (0.16–0.55)
OTC NSAIDs[c]			
Aspirin	19	96	0.27 (0.16–0.48)
Ibuprofen/Naproxen	7	112	0.18 (0.08–0.39)
Acetaminophen	8	37	0.66 (0.28–1.55)
Baby Aspirin	29	104	0.63 (0.38–1.00)

[a] No use of any NSAID or analgesic or infrequent use of no more than one pill per week for less than one year;

[b] COX-2 inhibitors include celecoxib, rofecoxib, valdecoxib, and meloxicam used daily for two years or more.

[c] Over the counter (OTC) NSAIDs/analgesics used at least two times per week for two years or more.

[d] Multivariate odds ratios are adjusted for continuous variables (age and body mass) and categorical variables (family history, smoking, and alcohol intake).

Table 4. Odds ratios with 95% confidence intervals for lung cancer and selective cyclooxygenase-2 (COX-2) inhibitors, and over the counter nonsteroidal anti-inflammatory drugs (OTC NSAIDs)

Compound	Number of cases	Number of controls	Multivariate OR[d] (95% CI)
None/Infrequent Use[a]	355	628	1.00
COX-2 Inhibitors[b]	20	76	0.21 (0.11–0.44)
OTC NSAIDs[c]			
Aspirin	32	97	0.30 (0.17–0.52)
Ibuprofen/Naproxen	21	116	0.36 (0.20–0.69)
Acetaminophen	20	38	1.21 (0.58–2.54)
Baby Aspirin	38	107	0.59 (0.35–0.99)

[a] No use of any NSAID or analgesic or infrequent use of no more than one pill per week for less than one year;

[b] COX-2 inhibitors include celecoxib, rofecoxib, valdecoxib, and meloxicam used daily for two years or more.

[c] Over the counter (OTC) NSAIDs/analgesics used at least two times per week for two years or more.

[d] Multivariate odds ratios are adjusted for continuous variables (pack years of cigarette smoking, age and body mass) and categorical variables (family history and alcohol intake).

significant (OR = 0.63, P < 0.05) whereas acetaminophen use did not significantly influence the relative risk of lung cancer.

4.   DISCUSSION

This is the first epidemiologic investigation to observe significant risk reductions in human breast cancer, prostate cancer, colon cancer, and lung cancer due to intake of selective COX-2 inhibitors. Standard daily dosages of celecoxib (200 mg) or rofecoxib (25 mg) taken for two or more years produced a statistically significant risk reduction for each type of cancer (71% for breast cancer, 55% for prostate cancer, 70% for colon cancer, and 79% for lung cancer). The composite estimate across all four cancers shows a 70% decrease in cancer risk (OR = 0.30, 95% CI = 0.21–0.42) (Figure 1). Comparator NSAIDs with non-selective COX-2 activity (325 mg aspirin, 200 mg ibuprofen or 250 mg naproxen) also produced significant risk reductions, although their observed effects were not as strong as selective compounds. In contrast, acetaminophen, a compound with negligible COX-2 activity, produced no significant change in the risk of any of the cancers under study. These results coupled with existing preclinical, molecular, and epidemiologic evidence suggest that aberrant induction of COX-2 and up-regulation of the prostaglandin cascade play a significant role in human carcinogenesis, and that blockade of this process has strong potential for intervention.

Celecoxib (Celebrex) and rofecoxib (Vioxx) were approved for the treatment of arthritis by the FDA in 1999. In randomized clinical trials, both compounds demonstrated better gastrointestinal safety and efficacy profiles than their NSAID predecessors [92, 93, 94, 95, 96]. Following FDA approval, each of these drugs was

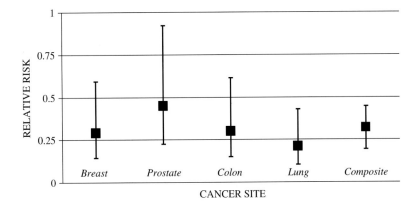

Figure 1. Composite results for COX-2 Inhibitors and cancer

routinely prescribed to millions of individuals who suffered from arthritis and other inflammatory conditions. It was thus unsettling to both patients and prescribing physicians alike when Merck recalled Vioxx from the market due to concerns regarding cardiovascular outcomes [97]. Subsequently, the cardiovascular safety of all selective COX-2 inhibitors has come under scrutiny [98].

Randomized clinical trials (RCTs) have traditionally been the gold standard for unbiased assessment of the risks versus benefits of therapeutic and chemopreventive medications. Extraordinary media coverage has been given to the two RCTs wherein increases were observed in the risk of adverse cardiovascular outcomes with long term intake of well-known selective COX-2-inhibiting agents (rofecoxib and celecoxib) [99, 100, 101]. Unfortunately, several potential pitfalls in these investigations have not been explored. These include the following:

1. Dosages of both rofecoxib (Vioxx) and celecoxib (Celebrex) administered in these RCTs were above the standard recommended doses (2 and 4 times, respectively, the typical dose used in the treatment of arthritis).
2. Only fixed doses were tested without adjustment according to body size as recommended by the drug manufacturers. Because the therapeutic window of smaller individuals is usually reduced, their dose should have been lowered and safety tolerance checked by measuring individual blood levels.
3. Data of both RCTs were examined by "intention to treat" analysis which assumes that all individuals who were enrolled for study completed the full course of treatment. Since there was substantial loss of subjects to follow-up in both RCTs, this method may have led to unreliable results pertaining to etiologic effects of the compounds.
4. Cox regression analysis was applied in the examination of data; however, the Cox model used incorporated only treatment effects without adjustment for individual cardiovascular risk factors. As a consequence, results may have been influenced by confounding, interaction (effect modification), or both.

5. Since neither RCT was designed to examine cardiovascular outcomes, inclusion of only such outcomes (as opposed to all adverse events) may have compromised probability levels in tests of significance.

Furthermore, focus on these two studies at the exclusion of others has produced misinformation about the cardiovascular safety of individual COX-2 inhibitors. For example, recent analyses of studies of celecoxib reflect a slight protective effect of standard daily 400 mg dosage in the cardiovascular system [102, 103].

Clearly, future chemopreventive studies should attempt to eliminate sources of bias and accurately elucidate risk versus benefit of the selective COX-2 inhibitors. Comparative studies should be designed to determine the appropriate dose, duration, side effects, and cost-effectiveness of individual compounds. Continued exploration of selective COX-2 inhibitors should be considered a top cancer research priority. Our findings of marked decreases in cancer risk with COX-2 blockade underscores the critical need for human clinical investigations of these compounds in order to expedite their efficacious application in the chemoprevention and therapy of cancer. Furthermore, experimental designs of chemopreventive clinical trials should embellish rather than ignore two golden rules of medicine: the dose makes the poison and first do no harm [104].

5.   CONCLUSIONS

We conducted a set of case control studies to examine the effects of selective COX-2 inhibitors on the four major human cancers (breast, prostate, colon, and lung). Results are summarized below:

1. Daily intake of selective COX-2 inhibitors produced a significant reduction in the risk for each type of cancer (71% for breast cancer, 55% for prostate cancer, 70% for colon cancer, and 79% for lung cancer).
2. Similar risk reductions were observed for individual COX-2 inhibitors, celecoxib and rofecoxib.
3. The observed chemopreventive effects were associated with recommended daily doses of celecoxib (median dose = 200 mg) or rofecoxib (median dose = 25 mg).
4. Significant risk reductions of lesser magnitude were observed for over the counter NSAIDs with non-selective COX-2 activity, such as regular (325mg) aspirin and (200 mg) ibuprofen.
5. Daily intake of baby (81 mg) aspirin produced marginally significant risk reductions for colon cancer and lung cancer, but did not significantly reduce the risk of breast cancer or prostate cancer.
6. Acetaminophen, an analgesic without COX-2 activity, did not produce a significant change in the risk of any of the cancers studied.

Notably, selective COX-2 inhibitors (celecoxib and rofecoxib) were only recently approved for use in 1999, and rofecoxib (Vioxx) was withdrawn from the marketplace in 2004. Nevertheless, even in the short window of exposure to these compounds, the selective COX-2 inhibitors produced significant reductions in the risk of the four major human cancers (breast, prostate, colon, and lung). These early results tend to substantiate the important role of COX-2 in carcinogenesis, and reciprocally, the strong potential for selective COX-2 blockade in cancer chemoprevention [105]. Further studies will be required to determine the appropriate dose, frequency of intake, duration, side effects and cost effectiveness of COX-2 inhibitors in the chemoprevention of cancer.

REFERENCES

1. Ahmedin J, Siegel R, Ward E, Murray T, Xu J, Smigal C, Thun MJ. Cancer Statistics, 2006. CA Cancer J Clin 56 (2): 106–130, 2006.
2. Harris RE. COX-2 blockade in cancer prevention and therapy: widening the scope of impact. In: RE Harris (ed), COX-2 Blockade in Cancer Prevention and Therapy, pp 341–365, Humana Press, Totowa, NJ, 2002.
3. Harris RE, Beebe-Donk J, Doss H, Burr-Doss D. Aspirin, ibuprofen, and other non-steroidal anti-inflammatory drugs in cancer prevention: a critical review of non-selective COX-2 blockade (review). Oncology Reports 13: 559–583, 2005.
4. Gonzalez-Perez A, Garcia Rodriquez LA, Lopez-Ridaura R. Effects of non-steroidal anti-inflammatory drugs on cancer sites other than the colon and rectum: a meta-analysis. BMC Cancer 3: 1–12, 2003.
5. Vane JR. Inhibition of prostaglandin synthesis as a mechanism of action for aspirin-like drugs. Nature 231: 323–235, 1971.
6. Herschman HR. Regulation of prostaglandin synthase-1 and prostaglandin synthase-2. Cancer and Metas Rev 13: 241–256, 1994.
7. Hla T, Neilson K. Human cyclooxygenase-2 cDNA. Proc Natl Acad Sci USA 89: 7384–7388, 1992.
8. Wolff H, Saukkonen K, Anttila S, Karjalainen A, Vainio H, Ristimaki A. Expression of cyclooxygenase-2 in human lung carcinoma. Cancer Res 58 (22): 4997–50, 1998.
9. Hida T, Yatabe Y, Achiwa H, Muramatsu H, Kozaki K, Nakamura S, Ogawa M, Mitsudomi T, Sugiura T, Takahashi T. Increased expression of cylcooxygenase 2 occurs frequently in human lung cancers, specifically in adenocarcinomas. Cancer Res 59: 198–204, 1999.
10. Eberhart CE, Coffey RJ, Radhika A, Giardiello FM, Ferrenbach S, Dubois RN. Up-regulation of cyclooxygenase-2 gene expression in human colorectal adenomas and adenocarcinomas. Gastroenterology 107: 1183–1188, l994.
11. Parrett ML, Harris RE, Joarder FS, Ross MS, Clausen KP, Robertson FM. Cyclooxygenase-2 gene expression in human breast cancer. International Journal of Oncology 10: 503–507, 1997.
12. Masferrer JL, Leahy KM, Koki AT, Aweifel BS, Settle SL, Woerner BM, Edwards DA, Flickinger AG, Moore RJ, Seibert K. Antiangiogenic and antitumor activities of cyclooxygenase-2 inhibitors. Cancer Res 60 (5): 1306–1311, 2000.
13. Sano H, Kawahito Y, Wilder R, Hashiramoto A, Mukai S, Asai K, Kimura S, Kato H, Kondo M, Hla T. Expression of cyclooxygenase-1 and -2 in human colorectal cancer. Cancer Res 55: 3785–3789, 1995.
14. Koki AT, Leahy KM, Harmon JM, Masferrer JL. Cyclooxygenase-2 and cancer. In: RE Harris (ed), COX-2 Blockade in Cancer Prevention and Therapy, pp 185–204, Humana Press, Totowa, NJ, 2002.
15. El-Bayoumy K. Evaluation of chemoprevention agents against breast cancer and proposed strategies for future clinical intervention trials. Carcinogenesis 15 (11): 2395–2420, 1994.
16. Bennett A, Tacca MD, Stamford IF, Zebro T. Prostaglandins from tumors of human large bowel. Br J Cancer 35: 881–4, 1977.
17. Bennett A, Civier A, Hensby CN, et al. Measurement of arachidonate and its metabolites extracted from human normal and malignant gastrointestinal tissues. Gut 28: 315–8, 1987.
18. Narisawa T, Kusaka H, Yamazaki Y, Takahashi M, Koyama H, Koyama K, et al. Relationship between blood plasma prostaglandin E_2 and liver and lung metastases in colorectal cancer. Dis Colon Rectum 33: 840–5, 1990.

19. Rolland PH, Martin PM, Jacquemier J, Rolland AM, Toga M. Prostaglandins in human breast cancer: evidence suggesting that an elevated prostaglandin production is a marker of high metastatic potential for neoplastic cells. J Natl Cancer Inst 64 (5): 1061–70, 1980.

20. Kort WJ, Bijma AM, van Dam JJ, vd Ham AC, Hekking JM, Ingh HF, Meijer WS, van Wilgenburg MGM, Zijlstra FJ. Eicosanoids in breast cancer patients before and after mastectomy. Prostaglandins Leukotrienes and Essential Fatty Acids, 45: 319–327, 1991.

21. Ara G, Teicher BA. Cyclooxygenase and lipoxygenase inhibitors in cancer therapy. Prostagland, Leuk and Essent Fatty Acids 54: 3–16, 1996.

22. Kelloff GJ, Johnson JR, Crowell JA, Boone CW, DeGeorge JJ, Steele VE, Mehta MU, Temeck JW, Schmidt WJ, Burke G, Greenwald P, Temple RJ. Guidance for development of chemopreventive agents, Clinical Development Plan: Aspirin, J Cellular Biochemistry, Suppl. 20: 74–83, 1994.

23. Greenwald P. Chemoprevention of cancer. Scientific American 275 (3): 96–100, 1996.

24. Greenwald P, Kelloff G, Burch-Whitman C, Kramer BS. Chemoprevention. CA Cancer Journal for Clinicians 45 (1): 31–49, 1995.

25. Boone CW, Kelloff GJ, Steele VE. Natural history of intraepithelial neoplasia in humans with implications for cancer chemopreventive strategy. Cancer Res 52 (7): 1651–1659, 1992.

26. Eberhart CE, Dubois RN. Eicosanids and the gastrointestinal gract. Gastroenterology 109: 285–301, 1995.

27. Mitchell JA, Akarasereenont P, Thiemermann C, Flower RJ, Vane JR. Selectivity of nonsteroidal anti-inflammatory drugs as inhibitors of constitutive and inducible cyclooxygenase. Proc Natl Acad Sci USA 90: 11693–11697, Dec 1994.

28. Marnett LJ. Aspirin and the potential role of prostaglandins in colon cancer. Cancer Res 52: 5575–5589, 1992.

29. Pollard M, Luckert PH. Prolonged antitumor effect of indomethacin on autochthonous intestinal tumors in rats. J Natl Cancer Inst 70: 1103–5, 1983.

30. Pollard M, Luckert PH. Prevention and treatment of primary intestinal tumors in rats by piroxicam. Cancer Res 49: 6471–3, 1989.

31. Reddy BS, Maruyama H, Kelloff G. Dose related inhibition of colon carcinogenisis by dietary piroxicam, a nonsteroidal antiinflammatory drug, during different stages of rat colon tumor development. Cancer Res 47: 5340–6, 1987.

32. Reddy BS, Tokumo K, Kulkarni N, Aligia C, Kelloff G. Inhibition of colon carcinogenesis by prostaglandin synthesis inhibitors and related compounds. Carcinogenesis 13: 1019–23, 1992.

33. Karmali RA, Marsh J, Fuchs C. Effect of omega-3 fatty acids on growth of a rat mammary tumor. J Natl Cancer Inst 73: 457–461, 1984.

34. Karmali RA. Dietary fatty acids, COX-2 blockade, and carcinogenesis. In: RE Harris (ed), COX-2 Blockade in Cancer Prevention and Therapy, pp 3–12, Humana Press, Totowa, NJ, 2002.

35. Schuller HM. The role of cyclooxygenase-2 in the prevention and therapy of lung cancer. In: RE Harris (ed), COX-2 Blockade in Cancer Prevention and Therapy, pp 99–116, Humana Press, Totowa, NJ, 2002.

36. Rose DP, Connolly JM. Effects of fatty acids and eicosanoid synthesis inhibitors on the growth of two human prostate cancer cell lines. Prostate 18: 243–254, 1991.

37. Kelloff GJ, Steele VE, Sigman CC. Chemoprevention of cancer by NSAIDs and selective COX-2 blockade. In: RE Harris (ed), COX-2 Blockade in Cancer Prevention and Therapy, pp 279–300, Humana Press, Totowa, NJ, 2002.

38. Reddy BS, Rao CV. Role of synthetic and naturally occurring cyclooxygenase inhibitors in colon cancer prevention. In: RE Harris (ed), COX-2 Blockade in Cancer Prevention and Therapy, pp 71–83, Humana Press, Totowa, NJ, 2002.

39. Kawamori T, Rao CV, Siebert K, Reddy BS. Chemopreventive activity of celecoxib, a specific cyclooxygenase 2 inhibitor, against colon carcinogenesis. Cancer Res 58: 409–412, 1998.

40. Harris RE, Alshafie GA, Abou-Issa H, Seibert K. Chemoprevention of breast cancer in rats by celecoxib, a specific cyclooygenase-2 (COX-2) inhibitor. Cancer Res 60: 2101–2103, 2000.

41. Abou-Issa HM, Alshafie GA, Harris RE. Chemoprevention of breast cancer by nonsteroidal anti-inflammatory drugs and selective COX-2 blockade in animals. In: RE Harris (ed), COX-2 Blockade in Cancer Prevention and Therapy, pp 85–98, Humana Press, Totowa, NJ, 2002.

42. Shiff SJ, Rigas B. The role of cyclooxygenase inhibition in the antineoplastic effects of nonsteroidal anti-inflammatory drugs (NSAIDs). J Exp Med 190: 445–450, 1999.

43. Howe LR, Subbaramaiah K, Brown AMC, Dannenberg AJ. Cyclooxygenase-2: a target for the prevention and treatment of breast cancer. Endocrine-Related Cancer 8: 97–114, 2001.

44. Harris RE, Robertson FM, Farrar WB, Brueggemeier RW. Genetic induction and upregulation of cyclooxygenase (COX) and aromatase (CYP-19): an extension of the dietary fat hypothesis of breast cancer. Medical Hypotheses 52 (4): 292–293, 1999.

45. Zhao Y, Agarwal VR, Mendelson CR, Simpson ER. Estrogen biosynthesis proximal to a breast tumor is stimulated by PGE2 via cyclic AMP, leading to activation of promoter II of the CYP19(aromatase) gene. Endocrinology 137 (12): 5739–5742, 1996.

46. Brueggemeier RW, Quinn AL, Parrett ML, Joarder FS, Harris RE, Robertson FM. Correlation of aromatase and cyclooxygenase gene expression in human breast cancer specimens. Cancer Letters 140 (1–2): 27–35, 1999.

47. Lehmann JM, Lenhard Jm, Oliver BB, Ringold GM, Kliewer SA. Perioxisome proliferator-activated receptors alpha and gamma are activated by indomethacin and other nonsteroidal anti-inflammatory drugs. J Biol Chem 272 (6): 3406–3410, 1997.

48. Schuller HM, Orloff M. Tobacco-specific carcinogenic nitrosamines. Ligands for nicotinic acetyl-choline receptors in human lung cancer cells. Biochem Pharmacol 55 (9): 1377–1384, 1998.

49. Schuller HM. Cell type specific, receptor-mediated modulation of growth kinetics in human lung cancer cell lines by nicotine and tobacco-related nitrosamines. Biochem Pharmacol 38 (20): 3439–3442, 1989.

50. Joarder FS, Abou-Issa H, Robertson FM, Parrett ML, Alshafie G, Harris RE. Growth arrest of DMBA-induced mammary carcinogenesis with ibuprofen treatment in female Sprague-Dawley rats, Proc Amer Assoc Cancer Res 38 (2480): 370, 1997.

51. Alshafie GA, Harris RE, Robertson FM, Parrett ML, Ross M, Abou-Issa H. Comparative chemo-preventive activity of ibuprofen and N-(4-hydroxyphenyl) retinamide against the development and growth of rat mammary adenocarcinomas. Anticancer Research 19: 3031–3036, 1999.

52. Carter CA, Milholland RJ, Shea W, Ip MM. Effect of prostaglandin synthetase inhibitor indomethacin on 7,12-dimethylbenz[a]anthracene-induced mammary tumorigenesis in rats fed different levels of fat. Cancer Res 43: 3559–3562, 1983.

53. Fulton AM. In vivo effects of indomethacin on the growth of murine mammary tumors. Cancer Res 44: 2416–2420, 1984.

54. Ip MM, Mazzer C, Watson D, Ip C. The effect of eicosanoid synthesis inhibitors on DMBA-induced rat mammary carcinogenesis. Proc Amer Assoc Cancer Res, 30 (721): 182, 1989.

55. Lee PP, Ip MM. Regulation of proliferation of rat mammary tumor cells by inhibitors of cyclooxy-genase and lipoxygenase. Prostalgand Leuk Essent Fatty Acids 45 (1): 21–31, 1992.

56. Steele VE, Moon RC, Lubet RA, Grubbs CJ, Reddy BS, Wargovich M, McCormick DK, Pereira MA, Crowell JA, Bagheri D. Sigman CC, Boone CS, Kelloff G Jr. Preclinical efficacy evaluation of potential chemopreventive agents in animal carcinogenesis models: methods and results from the NCI drug chemoprevention drug development program. J Cell Biol Suppl 20: 32–53, 1994.

57. Harris RE, Namboodiri KK, Stellman SD, Wynder EL. Breast cancer and NSAID use: Hetero-geneity of effect in a case-control study. Preventive Medicine 24: 119–120, 1995.

58. Harris RE, Namboodiri KK, Farrar WB. Epidemiologic study of non-steroidal anti-inflammatory drugs and breast cancer. Oncology Reports 2: 591–592, 1995.

59. Harris RE, Namboodiri KK, Farrar WB. Nonsteroidal anti-inflammatory drugs and breast cancer. Epidemiology 7: 203–205, 1996.

60. Harris RE, Kasbari S, Farrar WB. Prospective study of nonsteroidal anti-inflammatory drugs and breast cancer. Oncology Reports 6: 71–73, 1999.

61. Harris RE, Chlebowski RT, Jackson RD, Frid DJ, Ascensco JL, Anderson G, Loar A, Rodabough RJ, White E, McTiernan A. Breast cancer and nonsteroidal anti-inflammatory drugs: prospective results from the Women's Health Initiative. Cancer Research 63: 6096–6101, 2003.

62. Zhang Y, Coogan PF, Palmer JR, Strom BL, Rosenberg L. Use of nonsteroidal anti-inflammatory drugs and risk of breast cancer, the Case-Control Surveillance Study revisited. Am J Epidemiol 162 (2): 165–170, 2005.

63. Pollard M, Luckert PH. The beneficial effects of diphosphonate and piroxicam on the osteolytic and metastatic spread of rat prostate carcinoma cells. Prostate 8: 81–86, 1986.

64. Gupta S, Srivastava M, Ahmad N, Bostwick DG, Mukhtar H. Over-expression of cyclooxygenase-2 in human prostate adenocarcinoma. Prostate 42: 73–78, 2000.

65. Yoshimura R, Sano H, Masuda C, Kawamura M, Tsubouchi Y, Charui J, Yoshimura N, Hla T, Wada S. Expression of cyclooxygenease-2 in prostate carcinoma. Cancer 89: 589–596, 2000.

66. Ghosh J, Myers CE. Arachidonic acid stimulates prostate cancer cell growth: critical role of 5-lipoxygenase. Biochemical and Biophysiological Research Community 235 (2): 418–423, 1997.

67. Nelson JE, Harris RE. Inverse association of prostate cancer and nonsteroidal anti-inflammatory drugs (NSAIDs): results of a case control study. Oncology Reports 7: 169–170, 2000.

68. Labayle D, Fischer D, Vielh P, Drouhin F, Pariente A, Bories C, Duhamel O, Troussett M, Attali P. Sulindac causes regression of rectal polyps in familial adenomatous polyposis. Gastroenterology 101: 635–639, 1991.

69. Giardiello FM, Hamilton SR, Krush AJ, Piantadosi S, Hylind LM, Celano P, Booker SV, Robinson CR, Offerhaus JA. Treatment of colonic and rectal adenomas with sulindac in familial adenomatous polyposis. N Engl J Med 328: 1313–6, 1993.

70. Nugent KP, Farmer KC, Spigelman AD, Williams CB, Phillips RK. Randomized controlled trial of the effect of sulindac on duodenal and rectal polyposis and cell proliferation in patients with familial adenomatous polyposis. Br J Surg 80: 1618–9, 1993.

71. Greenberg ER, Baron JA, Freeman DH Jr, Mandel JS, Haile R. Reduced risk of large bowel adenomas among aspirin users. The Polyp Prevention Study Group. J Natl Cancer Inst 85: 912–916, 1993.

72. Logan RF, Litte J, Hawtin PG, Hardcastle JD. Effect of aspirin and nonsteroidal anti-inflammatory drugs on colorectal adenomas: case-control study of subjects participating in the Nottingham faecal occult blood screening program. BMJ 307: 285–289, 1993.

73. Martinez M, McPherson RS, Levin B, Annegers JF. Aspirin and other nonsteroidal anti-inflammatory drugs and risk of colorectal adenomatous polyps among endoscoped individuals. Cancer Epidemiol Biomarkers Prev 4: 703–707, 1995.

74. Sandler RS, Galanko JC, Murray SC, Helm JF, Woosley JT. Aspirin and nonsteroidal anti-inflammatory agents and risk for colorectal adenomas. Gastroenterology 114: 441–448, 1998.

75. Breuer-Katschinski B, Nemes K, Rump B, Leiendecker B, Marr A, Breuer N, et al. Long-term use of nonsteroidal anti-inflammatory drugs and the risk of colorectal adenomas. The Colorectal Adenoma Study Group. Digestion 61: 129–134, 2000.

76. Thun M, Namboodiri MM, Heath CW. Aspirin use and reduced risk of fatal colon cancer. N Eng J Med 325: 1593–1596, 1991.

77. Thun M, Henley SJ. Epidemiology of nonsteroidal anti-inflammatory drugs and colorectal cancer. In: RE Harris (ed), COX-2 Blockade in Cancer Prevention and Therapy, pp 35–55, Humana Press, Totowa, NJ, 2002.

78. Eberhart CE, Coffey RJ, Radhika A, Giardiello FM, Ferrenbach S, Dubois RN. Up-regulation of cycloxygenase-2 gene expression in human colorectal adenomas and adenocarcinomas. Gastroenterology 107: 1183–1188, 1994.

79. Eberhart CE, Dubois RN. Eicosanids and the gastrointestinal gract. Gastroenterology 109: 285–301, 1995.

80. Steinbach G, Lynch PM, Phillips RK, Wallace MB, Hawk E, Gordon G, et al. The effect of celecoxib, a cyclooxygenase-2 inhibitor, in familial adenomatous polyposis. New Engl J Med 342: 1946–52. 2000.

81. Sandler RS, Halabi S, Baron JA, Budinger S, Paskett E, Keresztes R, Petrelli N, Pipas JM, Karp DD, Loprinzi CL, Steinbach G, Schilsky R. A randomized trial of aspirin to prevent colorectal adenomas in patients with previous colorectal cancer. New Engl J Med 348 (19): 883–390, 2003.

82. Thun MJ, Henley SJ, Patrono C. Nonsteroidal anti-inflammatory drugs as anticancer agents: mechanistic, pharmacologic, and clinical issues. J Natl Cancer Inst 94 (20): 252–266, 2002.

83. Castonguay A, Rioux N. Inhibition of lung tumorigenesis by sulindac: comparison of two experimental protocols. Carcinogenesis 19: 1393–1400, 1997.

84. Rioux N, Castonguay A. Prevention of NNK-induced lung tumorigeneis in A/J mice by acteylsalicaylic acid and NS-398. Cancer Res 58: 5354–5360, 1998.

85. Schuller HM, Plummer HK III, Bochsler PN, Dudric P, Bell JL, Harris RE. Co-expression of beta-adrenergic receptors and cyclooxygenase-2 in pulmonary adenocarcinoma. Int J Oncol 19(3): 445–449, 2001.

86. Peto R, Gray R, Collins R, Wheatley K, Hennekens C, Jamrozik K, Warlow C, Hafner B, Thompson E, Norton S. Randomised trial of prophylactic daily aspirin in British male doctors. Br Med J (Clin Res Ed): 296 (6618): 313–316, 1988.

87. Schreinemachers DM, Everson RB. Aspirin use and lung, colon, and breast cancer incidence in a prospective study. Epidemiology 5: 138–146, 1994.

88. Harris RE, Beebe-Donk J, Schuller HM. Chemoprevention of lung cancer by nonsteroidal anti-inflammatory drugs among cigarette smokers. Oncology Reports 9: 693–695, 2002.

89. Walter SD. Determination of significant relative risks and optimal sampling procedures in prospective and retrospective comparative studies of various sample sizes. Am J Epidemiol 105: 387–397, 1977.

90. Schlesselman JJ. Case Control Studies: Design, Conduct, Analysis. Oxford University Press, New York, NY, 1982.

91. Harrell F. Logistic Regression Procedure. Statistical Analysis System (SAS), 2005.

92. Bombardier C, Laine L, Reicin A, Shapiro D. Burgo-Vargas R, Davis B, Day R, Ferraz MB, Hawkey CJ, Hochberg MC, Kvien TK, Schuitzer TJ. VIGOR Study Group. Comparison of upper gastrointestinal toxicity of rofecoxib and naproxen in patients with rheumatoid arthritis. N Engl J Med 343 (21): 1520–1528, 2000.

93. Silverstein FE, Faich G, Goldstein JL, Simon LS, Pincus T, Whelton A, Makuch R, Eisen G, Agrawal NM, Stenson WF, Burr AM, Zhao WW, Kent JD, Lefkowith JB, Verburg KM, Geis GS. Gastrointestinal toxicity with celecoxib vs nonsteroidal anti-inflammatory drugs for osteoarthritis and rheumatoid arthritis: the CLASS study: a randomized controlled trial. Celecoxib Long-term Arthritis Safety Study. JAMA 284 (10): 1247–1255, 2000.

94. Simon LS, Weaver AL, Graham DY, Kivitz AJ, Kipsky PE, Hubbard RC, Isakson PC, Verburg KM, Yu SS, Zhao WW, Geis GS. Anti-inflammatory and upper gastrointestinal effects of celecoxib in rheumatoid arthritis. Journal of the American Medical Association 282: 1921–1928, 1999.

95. Langman MJ, Jensen DM, Watson DJ, Harper SE, Zhao PL, Quan H, Bolognese JA, Simon TJ. Adverse upper gastrointestinal effects of rofecoxib compared with NSAIDs. Journal of the American Medical Association 282: 1929–1933, 1999.

96. Shah AA, Thjodleifsson B, Murray FE, Kay E, Barry M, Sigthorsson G, Gudjonsson H, Oddsson E, Price AB, Fitzgerald DJ, Bjarnason I. Selective inhibition of COX-2 in humans is associated with less gastrointestinal injury: a comparison of nimesulide and naproxen. Gut 48 (3): 339–346, 2001.

97. Mukherjee D, Nissen SE, Topol EJ. Risk of cardiovascular events associated with selective COX-2 inhibitors. JAMA 286 (8): 954–959, 2001.

98. Couzin J. Withdrawal of Vioxx casts a shadow over COX-2 inhibitors. Science, 306: 384–385, 2004.

99. Bresalier RS, Sandler RS, Quan H, Bolognese JA, Oxenius B, Horgan K, Lines C, Riddell R, Morton D, Lanas A, Konstam MA, Baron JA. Cardiovascular events associated with rofecoxib in a colorectal adenoma chemoprevention trial. N Engl J Med 2005, 352 (11): 1092–1102.

100. Solomon SD, McMurray JJ, Pfeffer MA, Wittes J, Fowler R, Finn P, Anderson WF, Zauber A, Hawk E, Bertagnolli M. Cardiovascular risk associated with celecoxib in a clinical trial for colorectal adenoma prevention. N Engl J Med, 352 (11), 1071–1080, 2005.

101. Couzin J. Clinical Trials: Nail-biting time for trials of drugs. Science, 306: 1673–1675, 2004.

102. White WB, Faich G, Whelton A, Maurath C, Ridge NJ, Verburg KM, Geis GS, Lefkowith JB. Comparison of thromboembolic events in patients treated with celecoxib, a cyclooxygenase-2 specific inhibitor, versus ibuprofen or diclofenac. Am J Cardiol 89 (4): 425–430, 2002.
103. White WB, Faich G, Borer JS, Makuch RW. Cardiovascular thrombotic events in arthritis trials of the cyclooxygenase-2 inhibitor, celecoxib. Am J Cardiol 92 (4): 411–418, 2003.
104. Harris RE. Does the dose make the poison? Science 308, 203, 2005.
105. Harris RE, Beebe-Donk J, Alshafie GA. Reduction in the risk of human breast cancer by selective cyclooxygenase-2 (COX-2) inhibitors. BMC Cancer 6: 27, 2006.

CHAPTER 10

STRATEGIES FOR COLON CANCER PREVENTION
Combination of chemopreventive agents

BANDARU S. REDDY[1,*]

[1] *Susan Lehman Cullman Laboratory for Cancer Research*

Abstract: Large bowel cancer is one of the most common human malignancies in western countries, including North America. Several epidemiological studies have detected decreases in the risk of colorectal cancer in individuals who regularly use aspirin or other nonsteroidal anti-inflammatory drugs (NSAIDs). Clinical trials with NSAIDs in patients with familial adenomatous polyposis have demonstrated that treatment with NSAIDs causes regression of pre-existing adenomas. Preclinical efficacy studies using realistic laboratory animal models have provided scientifically sound evidence as to how NSAIDs act to

* Department of Chemical Biology, Rutgers, The State University of New Jersey, Piscataway, New Jersey 08854
Bandaru S. Reddy, Department of Chemical Biology, Ernest Mario School of Pharmacy, Rutgers, The State University of New Jersey, 164 Frelinghuysen Road, Piscataway, New Jersey 08854. E-mail: breddy@rci.rutgers.edu

R. E. Harris (ed.), Inflammation in the Pathogenesis of Chronic Diseases, 213–225.
© 2007 *Springer.*

retard, block, and reverse colonic carcinogenesis. Selective COX-2 inhibitors (celecoxib) as well as naturally occurring anti-inflammatory agents (curcumin) have proven to be effective chemopreventive agents against colonic carcinogenesis. There is growing optimism for the view that realization of preventive concepts in large bowel cancer will also serve as a model for preventing malignancies of the prostate, the breast, and many other types of cancer. There is increasing interest in the use of combinations of low doses of chemopreventive agents that differ in their modes of action in order to increase their efficacy and minimize toxicity. Preclinical studies conducted in our laboratory provide strong evidence that the administration of combinations of chemopreventive agents (NSAIDs, COX-2 inhibitors, DFMO, statins) at low dosages inhibit carcinogenesis more effectively and with less toxicity than when these agents are given alone

1.   INTRODUCTION

Cancer of the colon is one of the leading causes of cancer death in men and women in Western countries, including the United States [1]. Therefore, it is a major public health problem. The limited success of current treatment for advanced colon cancer has provided the impetus for increased emphasis on prevention. An expert panel assembled by the American Institute for Cancer Research and World Cancer Research Fund concluded that certain dietary factors, particularly caloric intake, modulate the risk for colorectal cancer development [2]. This finding is supported by experimental evidence from preclinical studies using well-established colon cancer models. Dietary epidemiologic studies have led to the identification of naturally-occurring chemopreventive agents present in fruits, vegetables, and grains. These natural products are principal sources of anti-inflammatory agents and antioxidants [2, 3].

An impressive body of evidence supports the concept that chemoprevention has the potential to be a major component of colorectal cancer control. Chemoprevention refers to the administration of chemical agents, those naturally occurring in foods as well as synthetic analogues that may block the tumor initiation (mutation) and promotion events that form the sequential stages of cancer development [4, 5]. Inhibition of these processes before the occurrence of clinically detectable tumors is receiving increasing attention as an attractive and plausible approach for cancer control [4, 5]. Reduced exposure to the underlying risk factors or use of chemopreventive agents that retard, block, or reverse the process of carcinogenesis, can be applied for patients with pre-cancerous lesions and for those diagnosed with early-stage cancer [5]. The potential benefits of chemoprevention are very substantial because the goals are to reduce cancer incidence and mortality. In the past 25 years, much progress has been achieved in the chemoprevention of colorectal cancer by naturally-occurring agents and their synthetic analogs, and particularly with anti-inflammatory pharmacologic agents [4–6]. This review briefly summarizes our current knowledge of the preventive effects of several naturally-occurring and pharmacological anti-inflammatory agents administered individually and in combination in modulating the pathogenesis of colon carcinogenesis in preclinical models.

2.   NONSTEROIDAL ANTI-INFLAMMATORY DRUGS (NSAIDs)

Coussens and Werb [7] reviewed the literature and concluded that inflammation is a critical component of tumor progression. These authors emphasized that the tumor microenvironment is orchestrated by inflammatory cells contributing to the neoplastic process. There is strong evidence that inflammatory cytokines and chemokines which are produced by the tumor cells may contribute directly to malignant progression [8]. These insights have fostered new approaches to cancer development and its prevention by NSAIDs.

In recent years attention has been drawn to the potential chemopreventive properties of NSAIDs. An effective preventive strategy for colon cancer could be envisioned on the basis of recent epidemiological, clinical, and laboratory investigations that combine to present an inverse relationship between the use of NSAIDs and colorectal cancer development [5, 6, 9–12]. These studies have consistently reinforced the evidence that NSAIDs are indeed effective chemopreventive agents against colon cancer development.

2.1.   Epidemiologic Evidence

Combined evidence from epidemiologic studies supports the notion that NSAID use, specifically aspirin, prevents colorectal cancer [9–12]. Case-control and prospective studies consistently show that aspirin use reduces colorectal cancer risk by about 30–50% [9–12]. The results of a large American Cancer Society cohort study of more than 650,000 subjects indicated that taking aspirin at least 16 times/month produced a risk reduction of approximately 40% compared to subjects who reported not taking aspirin [9, 10]. Thus, the available data from human epidemiologic studies clearly suggest that aspirin intake protects against colorectal cancer in both men and women.

2.2.   Evidence from Preclinical Studies

Developmental strategies for colorectal cancer prevention in humans by chemopreventive agents, including NSAIDs, have been facilitated by the relevant laboratory animal models, including azoxmethane (AOM)-induced colon cancer in various strains of rats [13–23]. Pioneering studies by Narisawa et al [14, 15] and Pollard and Luckert [16] demonstrated that indomethacin and piroxicam administered to rodents in drinking water or in the diet inhibited colon tumors induced by a variety of carcinogens. Since that time, a number of investigators have evaluated the chemopreventive effects of these agents [17–23]. Of particular interest is that aspirin, piroxicam, and sulindac reduced spontaneous intestinal tumorigenesis in APC^{Min} mice that are genetically predisposed to develop intestinal tumors due to a germline mutation in the *APC* gene [24–26]. Irrespective of the type of NSAID tested (indomethacin, aspirin, ibuprofen, piroxicam, ketoprofen, or sulindac) and variations in the timing of treatment (initiation/post-initiation, or promotion and progression phase), these agents suppressed the incidence and multiplicity of colon tumors.

In our laboratory experiments, nonselective NSAIDs (aspirin, ibuprofen, ketoprofen, piroxicam, and sulindac) reduced colon tumorigenesis by 40% to 70% in a dose-dependent manner when administered at up to 80% of the tolerable dose levels (Figure 1). [6, 17–19]. Thus, epidemiological, clinical, and laboratory animal model studies together have provide compelling evidence that the use of NSAIDs is effective in reducing the risk of colon cancer.

The mechanisms by which NSAIDs act to reduce the risk of colon carcinogenesis are not yet clearly understood. Accumulating evidence points to inhibition of arachidonic acid metabolism via blockade of cyclooxygenase enzymes, which in turn modulates the synthesis of prostaglandins that affect cell proliferation, tumor growth, and immune responsiveness [5, 6, 26–28]. Two mammalian isozymes, cyclooxygenase-1 (COX-1) and cyclooxygenase-2 (COX-2), encoded by different genes, are known to be present in colon tumors of humans and rodents, and to catalyze the conversion of arachidonic acid to prostaglandins [27–30]. Increased levels of COX-2 have been found in both human and chemically induced colon tumors in F-344 rats and intestinal adenomas from APC^{Min} and $APC^{\Delta 716}$ mice [29–33].

Genetic evidence also supports a role for COX-2 in the development of intestinal neoplasia. Oshima et al [29] assessed the development of intestinal adenomas in $APC^{\Delta 716}$ mice (a model in which a targeted truncation deletion in the tumor

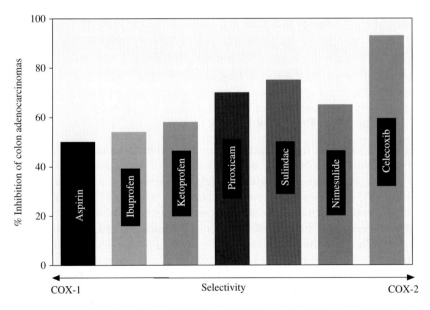

Figure 1. Chemopreventive efficacy of NSAIDs and COX-2 selective inhibitors on AOM-induced colon adenocarcinoma formation. Aspirin, ibuprofen, ketoprofen, piroxicam and sulindac were given at 80% tolerable dose and nimesulide and celecoxib were given at $\sim$ 35–40% tolerable dose during initiation and postinitiation stages of colon carcinogenesis

suppressor gene *APC* causes intestinal polyposis) in a wild-type and homogenous null COX-2 genetic background. The number and size of intestinal tumors were reduced by 6- to 8-fold in the COX-2 null mice compared with COX-2 wild type mice. This finding led to the hypothesis that COX-2 may play a key role in colon cancer growth and progression. While both isozymes carry out essentially the same catalytic reaction, many of the inflammatory, inducible effects of cyclooxygenase appear to be mediated by COX-2, whereas the normal physiological functions of cyclooxygenase are mediated by COX-1 [29–33]. The expression of COX-1 does not fluctuate due to stimuli, whereas cytokines, mitogens, growth factors and tumor promoters induce COX-2 expression. In addition, intestinal epithelial cells over-expressing the COX-2 gene develop adhesion properties and they resist apoptosis [6]. Therefore, over-expression of COX-2 may alter the tumorigenic potential of intestinal epithelial cells. However, it has also been shown that prolonged administration of NSAIDs can cause unwanted adverse effects, such as gastrointestinal bleeding, ulceration and renal toxicity, which are manifested mainly by the inhibition of COX-1 activity.

Several selective COX-2 inhibitors have been identified and tested for their efficacy in preclinical studies [6, 25, 32–34, 36]. We have extensively examined celecoxib in the AOM-induced colon tumor rat model. High doses of celecoxib (1500 ppm in food) reduced the incidence of colon tumors by 90% and were better tolerated ($\sim 35\%$ of tolerable dose) than comparable (80% tolerable) doses of nonselective NSAIDs [6, 30, 32, 33]. It is noteworthy that the degree of inhibition of colon carcinogenesis by celecoxib markedly exceeded the observed inhibition with NSAIDs, including aspirin, ibuprofen, sulindac and piroxicam, which we tested previously for their chemopreventive potency in similar experimental designs [6, 30] (Figure 1).

Selective COX-2 inhibitors such as celecoxib also inhibit tumor development in *APC*[Min] mice [29, 31]. These models mimic the rapid development of adenomatous polyps that affect humans with germline inactivation of one *APC* gene but differ from FAP in that the mouse tumors occur predominantly (>95%) in the small intestine and rarely in the colon.

2.3. Phytochemicals with Anti-inflammatory Activities

Certain natural dietary components exhibit biochemical and physiologic properties analogous to those of NSAIDs. This observation has fostered increased research on the potential of natural dietary agents possessing anti-inflammatory activities in reducing the risk of cancer. Agents such as curcumin, phenylethyl methyl-caffeate, ursolic acid, and oleanolic acid have been shown to possess anti-inflammatory activities [34–39]. Importantly, most of these phytochemicals induce anti-inflammatory activities by modulating inducible nitric oxide synthase (iNOS) and COX expression, similar to the effects induced by synthetic NSAIDs. Nevertheless, these natural compounds are less toxic than the NSAIDs. Among naturally occurring anti-inflammatory agents, curcumin (diferuloylmethane), which is a bioactive compound present in tumeric, was extensively studied and proved to be an inhibitor of several types of chemically induced neoplasia [35–37]. Dietary administration of curcumin reduces formation of focal areas of dysplasia and aberrant crypt foci in the colon, which are early preneoplastic lesions in rodents [37]. Continuous feeding of 0.2% curcumin during the initiation and post-initiation stages of AOM-induced colon carcinogenesis reduced adenocarcinoma incidence, multiplicity, and the total tumor burden in male F-344 rats [35]. Curcumin, given as a dietary supplement during the promotion/progression period, dramatically inhibited colon tumorigenesis in a dose-dependent manner [36].

Phenylethyl caffeate and its analogue, phenylethyl methylcaffeate, are major components of propolis in beehive honey that possess potent anti-inflammatory activities [38]. These compounds inhibit AOM-induced colonic aberrant crypt formation (ACF) and adenocarcinomas, skin carcinogenesis in rodent models, and also intestinal polyp formation in APC^{Min} mice [38–41]. Triterpenoids, such as oleanolic acid and its analogues, have been found to suppress COX-2 expression and activity in colon cancer cells, and to inhibit AOM-induced colonic ACF formation in a dose-dependent manner in rats [34]. Importantly, curcumin, phenylethyl methyl-caffeate, ursolic acid, oleanolic acid, and their analogues have no known side effects like those seen with synthetic and conventional NSAIDs. The inhibitory effect of curcumin and other anti-inflammatory phytochemicals is in part associated with increased apoptosis, suggesting that increased cell death may be one of the mechanisms by which these agents block carcinogenesis. This information suggests that phytochemicals that possess anti-inflammatory activity may retard growth and/or development of existing neoplastic lesions in the colon, and these agents may be effective chemopreventive agents for individuals at high risk for colon cancer development, such as patients with polyps.

With regard to their modes of action, curcumin and phenylethyl caffeate exhibit an array of metabolic, cellular, and molecular activities, including inhibition of arachidonic acid formation and its further metabolism to eicosanoids [6,37,42–44]. In our assays, dietary administration of these agents significantly inhibited phospholipase A2 (PLA_2) and PI-PLC in the colonic mucosa and tumor tissues, leading to the release of arachidonic acid from phospholipids; they also altered COX activity and modified prostaglandin (PGE_2) levels [6]. In contrast to NSAIDs, dietary curcumin and phenylethyl methylcaffeate inhibit lipoxygenase (LOX) activity, and block the production of the LOX metabolites, 5(S)-, 8(S)-, 12(S)- and 15(S)- hydroxyeicosatetraenoic acids (HETEs), in the colonic mucosa and in tumors [6, 42–44] and importantly, 12(S)-HETE formation in AOM-induced colonic tumors. Other studies indicate that curcumin and phenylethyl methylcaffeate also inhibit several mediators and enzymes involved in the mitogenic signal transduction pathways of the cell and in AP-1 and NFkB activation [43, 44]. Overall, naturally occurring anti-inflammatory agents predominantly block the expression of COX-2 activity by acting on upstream signaling pathways at the level of mRNA, suggesting that the mode of action of these agents is somewhat different from that of the NSAIDs, which modulate the COX-2 protein. This difference in mode of action between these anti-inflammatory phytochemicals and NSAIDs may, in part, explain the lack of toxicity of these agents in comparison with NSAIDs.

2.4. Combination of Low Doses of NSAIDs with other Chemopreventive Agents

An important strategy to improve the balance of benefits and risks associated with NSAID use is to identify combinations of agents with different modes of action that are effective at very low doses. This approach is extremely important when a promising chemopreventive agent demonstrates significant efficacy but may produce toxic side effects at effective higher doses. As an example, consider our study of the chemopreventive efficacy of combinations of piroxicam, an NSAID, and difluoromethylornithine (DFMO), a specific, irreversible enzyme-activated or suicide inhibitor of ornithine decarboxylase (ODC) in AOM-induced colon carcinogenesis in F-344 rats [45]. In the study, we tested effects of individual compounds at high dosages compared to low and high doses of piroxicam (100 and 200 ppm) combined with low and high doses of DFMO (1000 and 2000 ppm, respectively). As expected, higher dosages of the individual compounds (200 or 400 ppm of piroxicam, and 2000 or 4000 ppm of DFMO) in the diet reduced the incidence and multiplicity of AOM-induced colon adenocarcinomas. An important finding of the study was that the low dose levels of piroxicam (100 ppm) and DFMO (1000 ppm) administered together was more effective in inhibiting the incidence and multiplicity of colon adenocarcinomas than administration of these agents individually at high doses. Administration of these agents in combination at low doses suppressed colon adenocarcinomas more effectively than when these agents were given alone at high doses. These observations are of clinical significance because this can pave the way for use of combinations of these agents in small doses for the chemoprevention of colon neoplasms and other types of cancer.

Statins are a class of pharmaceutical agents that inhibit 3-hydroxy-3-methylglutaryl CoA reductase (HMG-CoA-reductase), a rate limiting enzyme in mevalonate synthesis, leading to inhibition of cholesterol biosynthesis. Statins have been shown to interfere with isoprenylation and subsequent membrane localization of G-proteins, including Ras and Ras-related proteins [46, 47]. Randomized controlled clinical trials designed to examine effects of statins in preventing cardiovascular disease provides evidence that statins may also prevent colorectal cancer [48]. Patients with coronary heart disease who took statins (provastatin or simvastatin) had a reduced incidence of colon cancer compared to those not taking the drugs during a 5-year follow-up period [48]. Nevertheless, chronic use of high doses of agents such as statins, COX-2-inhibitors, and NSAIDs may induce side effects in ostensibly normal individuals. In preclinical models, Agarwal et al. [49] observed that the combination of lovastatin and sulindac was more effective in inhibiting azoxymethane-induced colonic ACF in male F-344 rats than when these agents were given singularly, and we also found that treatment with combinations of low doses of celecoxib and lovastatin synergistically suppressed the growth of HT-29 human cancer cells and induced apoptosis [50].

In other studies we observed that a low-dose combinations of sulindac, an NSAID, and the cholesterol-lowering drug, lovastatin, were more effective in suppressing chemically-induced colon cancer in rodents and stimulating apoptosis in human tumor cells than when either drug was given alone at a high dose (51]. Our recent study provides convincing evidence that a very low dose of lovastatin in combination with a low dose of celecoxib suppressed invasive and noninvasive adenocarcinomas of the colon in the AOM-induced colon cancer model [51] (Figure 2). Furthermore, our recent study indicates that a very low dose of celecoxib administered in a high-fat diet containing omega-3 polyunsaturated fatty acids was more effective in inhibiting colon carcinogenesis than when it is administered in a high-fat diet containing mixed lipids (saturated and unsaturated fats) [52]. Thus, the use of a low dose of celecoxib in combination with a healthy diet and lifestyle may well be a promising approach for future human clinical trials. These animal data strongly support the view that combinations of chemopreventive agents that have diverse mechanisms of action can have beneficial applications in human cancer chemoprevention trials. This should be one of the approaches to future research and human intervention trials.

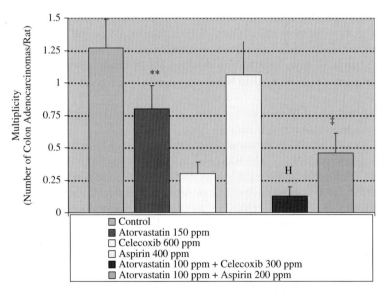

Figure 2. Effect of 150 ppm atorvastatin, 600 ppm celecoxib, and 400 ppm aspirin administered individually and 100 ppm atorvastatin + 300 ppm celecoxib and 100 ppm atorvastatin + 200 ppm aspirin on multiplicity of azoxymethane-induced colon adenocarcinomas (tmors/rat). Columns, means; bars, SE. *, $P < 0.05$, significantly different from the control group by Student's t test; ‡, $P < 0.01$, significantly different from the control diet group; **, $P < 0.001$, significantly different from the control diet group; H, $P < 0.0001$, significantly different from the control diet group

3. TRANSLATIONAL STUDIES

3.1. Randomized Clinical Trials

Randomized clinical trials have shown that sulindac suppresses adenomatous polyps and causes regression of existing polyps in patients with familial adenomatous polyposis (FAP) [53]. Labayle, et al. [54] reported that, in a randomized, placebo-controlled, double-blind crossover study of patients with FAP, administration of sulindac at a dosage of 300 mg/d for 6 to 12 months caused disappearance of all colonic polyps. In another study, the incidence and size of adenomas were reduced in FAP patients after long-term therapy with sulindac [53]. Although the dosage of sulindac administered in these studies varied from 150 to 400 mg/d, most of the patients treated with this drug exhibited full remission, whereas some patients showed a partial response. By contrast, some FAP patients developed rectal carcinoma, despite ongoing therapy with sulindac [55, 56], and adenomatous polyps resumed growth in FAP patients when NSAID treatment was stopped. With regard to sporadic adenomatous polyps, NSAID prophylaxis produced no statistically significant difference in polyp size (regression of small < 1 cm) among the 18 patients treated with sulindac (300 mg) for 4 months [57].

3.2. Curcuminoids

Lao, et al. [58] performed a dose escalation study to determine the maximum tolerated dose, safety profile and serum concentrations of a single dose of standardized powdered of turmeric. Healthy volunteers were administered escalating doses from 500–12,000 mg. Results indicate that the tolerance of curcumin in high single oral doses appears to be excellent [58].

3.3. Celecoxib

Clinical trials of celecoxib for the prevention of colonic polyps have produced mixed results. A randomized, double-blind trial of the COX-2 inhibitor, celecoxib, was conducted to evaluate its effects in the prevention of colorectal adenomas in 2035 patients who were randomized to receive placebo, 200 mg celecoxib or 400 mg celecoxib administered twice daily [59]. Follow-up colonoscopy was performed at 1 and 3 years after study randomization. Results indicate that celecoxib significantly suppressed formation of large intestinal adenomas at 1 and 3 years after polypectomy. However, an increased risk of cardiovascular events was observed among celecoxib users [59]. In another randomized, placebo-controlled, double-blind study, 400 mg of celecoxib taken once daily was evaluated for the prevention of colorectal adenomatous polyps among 1561 patients from 107 centers in 32 countries [60]. In this study, once daily use of 400 mg of celecoxib significantly reduced the occurrence of colorectal adenomas within 3 years after polypectomy. It is stated that "once daily dosing" offers not only a simpler chemopreventive regimen but may possibly provide an alternative to the benefit-risk profile of "twice daily dosing" [60]. Additional data will need to be collected and evaluated in order to determine the overall risk versus benefit profile of celecoxib in the prevention of colon cancer and other neoplasms.

4.   CONCLUSION

Large bowel cancer is not only the third most frequent cancer in the world but is one of the most common human malignancies in Western countries, including North America. In recent years, multidisciplinary research in epidemiology, molecular biology, and laboratory animal model studies have contributed much to our understanding of the etiology of this cancer; more importantly, it has enabled us to devise preventive strategies. Several epidemiological studies have detected a 40 to 50% decrease in risk of colorectal cancer in individuals who regularly use aspirin and other nonsteroidal anti-inflammatory drugs (NSAIDs). Clinical trials with NSAIDs in patients with familial adenomatous polyposis have demonstrated that treatment with NSAIDs caused regression of pre-existing adenomas. Preclinical efficacy studies using realistic laboratory animal models have provided scientifically sound evidence as to how NSAIDs act to retard, block, and reverse colonic carcinogenesis. Equally exciting are the opportunities for effective chemoprevention with selective COX-2 inhibitors in a variety of animal models of colon cancer. Selective COX-2 inhibitors such as celecoxib proven to be effective chemopreventive agents against colonic carcinogenesis with minimal gastrointestinal toxicity. Our exploration of the multistep process of carcinogenesis has provided substantial insights into the mechanisms by which anti-inflammatory agents modulate these events. There is growing optimism for the view that realization of preventive concepts in large bowel cancer will also serve as a model for preventing malignancies of the prostate, the breast, and many other types of cancer. There is increasing interest in the use of combinations of low doses of chemopreventive agents that differ in their modes of action in order to increase their efficacy and minimize toxicity. Preclinical studies conducted in our laboratory provide strong evidence that the administration of combinations of chemopreventive agents (NSAIDs, COX-2 inhibitors, DFMO, statins) at low dosages inhibits carcinogenesis more effectively and with less toxicity than when these agents are given alone.

ACKNOWLEDGEMENTS

Grant support: Current and past studies on chemoprevention of colon cancer are supported by USPHS Grants CA-17613, CA-8003, CA-37663, CP-33208, CN-85095, CN-45191, CN-2540, CP-05721, CN-55150, and CN-15122 from the National Cancer Institute. Thanks are due to Ms. Sandi Selby for preparation of the manuscript.

REFERENCES

1. Jamal A, Murray T, Ward E, Samuels A, et al: Cancer Statistics. *CA Cancer J Clin* 2005, 55:10–30.
2. World Cancer Research Fund and American Institute for Cancer Research, Panel on Food, Nutrition and Prevention. Washington DC: *American Institute for Cancer Research* 1997.
3. Potter JD, Steinmetz K. In: Principles of Chemoprevention. (Steward BW, McGregor D, Kleihues P. eds). IARC Scientific Publication No. 139. International Agency for Research on Cancer, Lyon, France. 1996:61–90.
4. Wattenberg L. Inhibition of tumorigenesis in animals. In: Principles of Chemoprevention (Stewart BW, McGregor D, Kleihues P. eds). IARC Scientific Publication No. 199, International Agency for Research on Cancer, Lyon, France. 1996:151–158.
5. Kelloff GJ. Perspectives on cancer prevention research and drug development. *Adv Cancer Res* 2000, 78:1999–2334.
6. Reddy BS, Rao CV. Chemoprophylaxis of Colon Cancer. *Current Gastroenterology Reports* 2005, 7(5):389–395.
7. Coussens LM, Werb Z. Inflammation and Cancer. *Nature* 2002, 420:56–867.
8. Balkwill F, Mantovani A. Inflammation and Cancer. *Lancet* 2001, 357:539–545.
9. Thun MJ, Namboodiri MM, Heath CJ Jr. Aspirin Use and Reduced Risk of Fatal Colon Cancer. *N. Engl. J. Med.* 1991, 325:1593–1596.
10. Thun MJ, Namboodiri MM, Calle EE, et al. Aspirin Use and Risk of Fatal Cancer. Cancer Res. 1993, 53:1322–1327.
11. Giovannucci E, Rimm EB, Stampfer M, et al. Aspirin Use and Risk for Colorectal Cancer and Adenoma in Male Health Professionals. *Ann. Intern. Med.* 1994, 121:241–246.
12. Kune G, Kune S, Watson LF. Colorectal Cancer Risk, Chronic Illnesses, Operations, and Medications: Case Control Results from the Melbourne Colorectal Cancer Study. *Cancer Res.* 1988, 48:4399–4404.
13. Reddy BS. Carcinogen-induced colon cancer models for chemoprevention and nutritional studies in: tumor models in Cancer Research. (ed., Teicher BA). *Human Press*, Totowa, NJ 2002, 183–191.
14. Narisawa T, Sato M, Tani M, et al. Inhibition of Development of Methylnitrosourea-Induced Rat Colon Tumors by Indomethacin Treatment. *Cancer Res.* 1981, 41:1954–1957.
15. Narisawa T, Sato M, Sano M, Takahashi T. Inhibition of Development of Methylnitrosourea-Induced Rat Colonic Tumors by Peroral Administration of Indomethacin. *Gann.* 1982, 73:377–381.
16. Pollard M, Luckert PH. Prolonged Anti-tumor Effect of Indomethacin on Autochthonous Intestinal Tumors in Rats. *J. Natl. Cancer Inst.* 1983, 70:1103–1105.
17. Reddy BS, Maruyama H, Kelloff G. Dose-Related Inhibition of colon Carcinogenesis by Dietary Piroxicam, A Nonsteroidal Anti-inflammatory Drug, During Different Stages of Rat Colon Tumor Development. *Cancer Res.* 1987, 47:5340–5346.
18. Reddy BS, Tokumo K, Kulkarni N, et al. Inhibition of Colon Carcinogenesis by Prostaglandin Synthesis Inhibitors and Related Compounds. *Carcinogenesis* 1992, 13:1019–1023.
19. Reddy BS, Rao CV, Rivenson A, Kelloff G. Inhibitory Effect of Aspirin on Azoxymethane-Induced Colon Carcinogenesis in F 344 Rats. *Carcinogenesis* 1993, 14:1493–1497.
20. Moorghen M, Ince P, Finney KJ, et al. The Effect of Sulindac on Colonic Tumor Formation in Dimethylhydrazine-Treated Mice. *Acta. Histochem. Suppl.* 1990, 39:195–199.
21. Skinner SA, Penney AG, O'Brien P. Sulindac Inhibits the Rate of Growth and Appearance of Colon Tumors in the Rat. *Arch. Surg.* 1991, 126:1094–1096.
22. Reddy BS, Kawamori T, Lubet RA, et al. Chemopreventive Efficacy of Sulindac sulfone Against Colon Cancer Depends on Time of Administration During Carcinogenic Process. *Cancer Res.* 1999, 59:3387–3391.
23. Wargovich MJ, Chen CD, Harris C, et al. Inhibition of Aberrant Crypt Growth by Non-Steroidal Anti-Inflammatory Agents and Differentiation Agents in the Rat Colon. *Int. J. Cancer.* 1995, 60:515–519.

24. Boolbol SK, Dannenberg AJ, Chadburn A, et al. Cyclooxygenase-2 Overexpression and Tumor Formation are Blocked by Sulindac in A Murine Model of Familial Adenomatous Polyposis. *Cancer Res.* 1996, 56:2556–2560.

25. Chiu CH, Mcentee MF, Whelan J. Sulindac Causes Rapid Regression of Preexisting Tumors in Min/+ Mice Independent of Prostaglandin Biosynthesis. *Cancer Res.* 1997, 57:4267–4273.

26. Mahmoud NN, Dannenberg AJ, Mestre J, et al. Aspirin Prevents Tumors in a Murine Model of Familial Adenomatous Polyposis. *Surgery* 1998, 124:225–231.

27. Dubois RN, Tsujii M, Bishop P, Awad JA, Makita K, Lanaham A. Cloning and characterization of growth factor-inducible cyclooxygenase gene from rat intestinal epithelial cells. *Am J Physiol.* 1994, 266(5 Pt 1):G822–G827.

28. Dannenberg AJ, Lippman SM, Mann JR, Subbaramaiah K, Dubois RN. Cyclooxygenase-2 and epidermal growth factor receptor: pharmacologic targets for chemoprevention. *J Clin Oncol* 2005, 23:254–266.

29. Oshima M, Murai N, Kargman S, et al. Chemoprevention of Intestinal Polyposis in the $APC^{\Delta 716}$ Mouse by Rofecoxib, A Specific Cyclooxygenase-2 Inhibitor. *Cancer Res.* 2001, 61: 1733–1740.

30. Reddy BS, Rao CV. Colon cancers: a role for cyclooxygenase-2 specific non-steroidal anti-inflammatory drugs. *Drugs & Aging* 2000, 16:329–334.

31. Jacoby RF, Seibert K, Cole CF, et al. The Cyclooxygenase-2 inhibitor celecoxib is a potent preventive and therapeutic agent in the Min mouse model of adenomatous polyposis. *Cancer Res.* 2000, 60:5040–5044.

32. Kawamori T, Rao CV, Seibert K, Reddy BS. Chemopreventive Activity of Celecoxib, A Specific Cyclooxygenase-2 Inhibitor, Against Colon Carcinogenesis. *Cancer Res.* 1998, 58:409–412.

33. Reddy BS, Hirose Y, Lubet R, et al. Chemoprevention of Colon Cancer by Specific Cyclooxygenase-2 Inhibitor, Celecoxib, Administered During Different Stages of Carcinogenesis. *Cancer Res.* 2000, 60:293–297.

34. Cooma I, Malisetty VS, Patlolla JM, et al. Chemoprevention of Colon Carcinogenesis by Oleanolic Acid and Its Analog in Male F 344 Rats and Modulation of Inos and COX-2, and Apoptosis in Human Colon Ht-29 Cancer Cells. *Am. Assoc. For Cancer Res.* 2002, 40:819.

35. Rao CV, Rivenson A, Simi B, Reddy BS. Chemoprevention of Colon Carcinogenesis by Dietary Curcumin, A Naturally Occurring Plant Phenolic Compound. *Cancer Res.* 1995, 55:259–266.

36. Kawamori T, Lubet R, Steele VE, et al. Chemopreventive Effect of Curcumin, A Naturally-Occurring Anti-inflammatory Agent, During the Promotion/Progression Stages of colon Cancer. *Cancer Res.* 1999, 59:597–601.

37. Rao CV, Simi B, Reddy BS. Inhibition by Dietary Curcumin of Azoxymethane-Induced Ornithine Decarboxylase, Tyrosine Protein Kinase, Arachidonic Acid Metabolism and Aberrant Crypt Foci in the Rat Colon. *Carcinogenesis* 1993, 14:2219–2225.

38. Rao CV, Desai D, Rivenson A, Simi B, et al. Chemoprevention of Colon Carcinogenesis by Phenlethyl-3-Methylcaffeate. *Cancer Res.* 1995, 55:2310–2315.

39. Rao CV, Desai D, Simi B, et al. Inhibitory Effects of Caffeic Acid Esters on Azoxymethane-Induced Biochemical Changes and Aberrant Crypt Foci Formation in Rat Colon. *Cancer Res.* 1993, 53:4182–4188.

40. Huang MT, Ma W, Yen P, et al. Inhibitory Effects of Caffeic Acid Phenethyl Ester (CAPE) on 12-O-Tetradecanoylphorbol-13-Acetate-Induced Tumor Promotion in Mouse Skin and the Synthesis of DNA, RNA and Protein in Hela Cells. *Carcinogenesis* 1996, 17:761–765.

41. Mahmoud NN, Carothers AM, Grunberger D, et al. Plant Phenolics Decrease Intestinal Tumors in an Animal Model of Familial Adenomatous Polyposis. *Carcinogenesis* 2000, 21:921–927.

42. Xu YX, Pindolia KR, Janakiraman N, et al. Curcumin Inhibits $1L$-1α and TNF-α Induction of AP-1 and NF-κB DNA-Binding Activity in Bone Marrow Stromal Cells. *Hematophathol. Mol. Hematol* 1998, 11:49–62.

43. Taylor JD. Lipoxygenase Regulation of Membrane Expression of Tumor Cell Glycoproteins and Subsequent Metastasis. *Adv. Prostaglandin Thromboxane Leukot. Res.* 1989, 19:439–443.

44. Natarajan K, Singh S, Burke TR Jr, et al. Caffeic Acid Phenethyl Ester is a Potent and Specific Inhibitor of Activation of Nuclear Transcription Factor Nf-Kappa B. 1996, 93:9090–9095.
45. Reddy BS, Nayani J, Tokumo K, et al. Chemoprevention of colon carcinogenesis by concurrent administration of piroxicam, a non-steroidal anti-inflammatory drug with D, L-α-difluoromethy-ornithine. An ornithine decarboxylase inhibitor, in diet. *Cancer Res.* 1990, 50:2562–2568.
46. Van der donk NWCI, Kamphuis MMJ, Lokhorst HM, Bloem AC. The choesterol lowering drug lovastatin induces cell death in myeloma plasma cells. *Leukemia* 2002, 16:1362–1371.
47. Cuthbert JA, Lipsky PE. Regulation of proliferation and Ras localization in transformed cells by products of mevalonate metabolism. *Cancer Res.* 1997, 57:3498–3505.
48. Demierre M-F, Higgins PDR, Gruber SB, Hawk E, Lippman SM. Statins and cancer prevention. *Nat Rev Cancer.* 2005, 5:930–942.
49. Agarwal B, Rao CV, Bhendwal S, et al. Lovastatin Augments Sulindac-Induced Apoptosis in Colon Cancer Cells and Potentiates Chemopreventive Effect of Sulindac. *Gastroenterology* 1999, 117:838–847.
50. Malisetty VS, Cooma I, Reddy BS, et al. Caspase-3-Activity, and Apoptosis Induction by a Combination of HMG-Coa Reductase Inhibitor and COX-2 Inhibitors: A Novel Approach in Developing Effective Chemopreventive Regimens. *Int. J. Oncol.* 2002, 20:753–759.
51. Reddy BS, Wang CX, KongA-N, et al. Prevention of Azoxymethane-Induced Colon Cancer by Combination of Low Doses of Atorvastatin, Aspirin, and Celecoxib in F 344 Rats. *Cancer Res.* 2006, 66(8):4542–4546.
52. Reddy BS, Patlolla JM, Simi B, et al. Prevention of Colon Cancer by Low Doses of Celecoxib, a Cyclooxygenase as Inhibitor, Administered in Diet Rich in ω-3 Polyunsaturated Fatty Acids. *Cancer Res.* 2005, 65(17):8022–8027.
53. Giardiello FM, Hamilton SR, Krush AJ, et al. Treatment of Colonic and Rectal Adenomas with Sulindac in Familial Adenomatous Polyposis. *N. Engl. J. Med.* 1993, 328:1313–1316.
54. Labayle D, Fischer D, Vielh P, et al. Sulindac Causes Regression of Rectal Polyps in Familial Adenomatous Polyposis. *Gastroenterology* 1991, 101:635–639.
55. Lynch HT, Thorson AG, Smyrk T. Rectal Cancer after Prolonged Sulindac Chemoprevention. A Case Report. *Cancer* 1995, 75:936–938.
56. Tonelli F, Valanzano R. Sulindac in Familial Adenomatous Polyposis. *Lancet* 1993, 342:1120.
57. Ladenheim J, Garcia G, Titzer D, et al. Effect of Sulindac on Sporadic Colonic Polyps. *Gastroenterology* 1995, 108:1083–1087.
58. Lao CD, Riffin MT, Normalle D, et al. Dose escalation of curcuminoid formulation. *BMC Complimentary and Alternative Medicine.* 2006, 6:10.
59. Bertagnolli MM, Eagle CJ, Hawk ET. Celecoxib reduces sporadic colorectal adenomas: results from adenoma prevention with celecoxib *(APC) trial. Proceedings of American Association for Cancer Research.* 2006; Abstract CP 3.
60. Arber N, Racz I, Spicak J, et al. Chemoprevention of colorectal adenomas with celecoxib in an international randomized, placebo-controlled, double-blind trials. *Proceedings of American Association for Cancer Research.* 2006; Abstract CP 4.

SECTION V

INFLAMMATION AND NEURODEGENERATIVE DISEASE

CHAPTER 11

NSAIDs FOR THE CHEMOPREVENTION
OF ALZHEIMER'S DISEASE

CHRISTINE A. SZEKELY[1], TERRENCE TOWN[2]
AND PETER P. ZANDI[1]

[1] Department of Mental Health, Johns Hopkins Bloomberg School of Public Health, Baltimore, MD
[2] Section of Immunobiology, Yale University School of Medicine, New Haven, CT

Abstract: Epidemiologic and laboratory studies suggest that non-steroidal anti-inflammatory drug (NSAID) use reduces the risk of Alzheimer's disease (AD). Initial reports in the early 1990's indicated that a history of arthritis, a presumed surrogate of NSAID use, was associated with a lower risk of AD. [1] These reports were followed by epidemiologic studies in which NSAID use was assessed directly and the majority of these reports confirmed the inverse association with risk for AD. [2, 3] Postmortem studies in humans [4], studies in animal models of AD [5, 6], and in vitro studies [7, 8] generally support the notion that NSAIDs can reduce the deleterious inflammation which surrounds amyloid beta (Aβ) plaques in the AD brain. In addition, some studies conducted in vitro and in rodents point to a subgroup of NSAIDs that may work by inhibiting amyloidogenic APP metabolism rather than through traditional anti-inflammatory mechanisms. [9–11] This novel property of NSAIDs is currently being explored in epidemiologic studies. Results from randomized clinical trials of NSAIDs and established AD and one trial on secondary prevention have not been promising and there have been no prevention trials completed. The feasibility of using NSAIDs as a chemopreventive agent in AD is discussed

R. E. Harris (ed.), Inflammation in the Pathogenesis of Chronic Diseases, 229–248.
© 2007 *Springer.*

1.   INTRODUCTION

AD is a neurodegenerative disease that causes progressive decline in cognitive function and behavior, culminating in dementia. Clinical disease onset is insidious and symptom progression is typically slow. It is estimated that between 2.5 and 4.5 million people in the United States are currently afflicted with AD. [12, 13] Age is the strongest risk factor and a meta-analysis of the annual incidence of AD indicates that rates approximately double for every five year age group over 60 starting at 0.06% in 60–65 year olds and increasing to 6.69% in those 95 years of age and older. [14] This, coupled with the fact that the age distribution of the population is shifting upward, may lead to a major public health problem in the future. Estimates in the United States alone indicate that the proportion of the population older than 65 years of age was 12% (35 million) in 2000 but is expected to increase to 20% (82 million) by 2050. [15, 16]

As noted by Alzheimer nearly a century ago, the brains of AD patients show three hallmark neuropathological and diagnostic features – neurofibrillary tangles, Aβ or "senile" plaques, and gliosis. These pathological features are present in more abundance in people with AD but are also present in brains of non-demented individuals. The neurofibrillary tangles are the main intracellular pathology of the disease and are primarily comprised of hyper-phosphorylated tau protein. [17] Neurofibrillary tangles gradually develop over decades and are used post-mortem to stage AD pathology. [18] In the AD brain, neurofibrillary tangles are thought to be the first stage preceding neuronal degeneration and loss, although their etiology still remains elusive. [19]

The extracellular "senile" plaques are primarily comprised of insoluble Aβ deposits and are often surrounded by activated astrocytes and microglia, and, in the case of mature plaques, contain dystrophic neurites. Aβ peptides are proteolytically derived from a much larger parent molecule, amyloid precursor protein (APP), a type I transmembrane protein. APP metabolism is a highly regulated process that is coordinated by a family of enzymes known as the secretases. There are two pathways for APP metabolism: non-amyloidogenic and amyloidogenic. In the former, APP is first acted upon by α-secretase and then γ-secretase cleavage, precluding the formation of Aβ. Amyloidogenic processing of APP occurs through sequential cleavage by extracellular β-secretase and intramembrane γ-secretase, and results in peptides from 38 to 43 amino acids in length. [20] $A\beta_{40}$ is a more abundant and more soluble variant of the peptide whereas $A\beta_{42}$ is not as readily cleaved (and therefore not as abundant), but is thought to be more toxic because it characteristically forms aggregates that may start the process of amyloid deposition in the AD brain. [21] Diffuse plaques, which are present early in the disease, are comprised mainly of $A\beta_{42}$ [22] and are also found in non-AD brains as early as the fourth or fifth decade. [18] It seems that, as the disease progresses, the diffuse plaques mature to form senile neuritic plaques that contain both $A\beta_{42}$ and $A\beta_{40}$. [21–23]

In addition to these two neuropathological features, Alzheimer originally identified a third type of pathology known as glial inflammation or simply "gliosis". [24] Although acute inflammatory responses are often beneficial in clearing foreign material from the brain, it is the chronic inflammation present in AD that may be pathogenic as it causes neurotoxicity, damage to neighboring cells, and is even thought to promote plaque pathology. [19, 25] The cellular and biochemical processes involved in brain inflammation in AD have been extensively studied (for detailed reviews see Akiyama et al. 2000 [26], McGeer et al. 2003 [27], and Eikelenboom et al. 2002 [28]). It is still not known whether this brain inflammation is an epiphenomenon (i.e., resulting from the disease process) or is pathoetiologically involved in disease initiation and/or progression. [19, 24] However, it is clear that the inflammatory response observed in the AD brain is typically localized around the Aβ plaques. For example, the numbers of proinflammatory cells such as microglia and astrocytes are elevated in AD brains compared to controls and these cells are co-localized with Aβ plaques. [29] Activated microglia, identified in vivo using positron emission tomography, have been found in patients with mild AD suggesting that the inflammatory process occurs at early stages of the disease. [30] Also, biochemical markers of inflammation, such as cyclooxygenase (COX), complement factors, chemokines, and cytokines, are in higher concentration in the AD brain. [31] Aβ-associated increases in activated microglia and related inflammatory markers have also been shown in studies using transgenic mouse models of AD. [32–35] Whether or not Aβ deposition precedes inflammation, once the deposition begins it is thought to activate proinflammatory glial cells which in turn produce a myriad of inflammatory molecules 26 which may lead to a feed-forward continuous cycle of deposition and inflammation.

A growing body of evidence suggests that non-steroidal anti-inflammatory drugs (NSAIDs), which are commonly used for pain relief and treatment of symptoms in inflammatory conditions such as arthritis, may protect against the neuropathogenesis of AD. [1–3] Epidemiologic data have accumulated over the last 15 years showing that the use of NSAIDs is associated with a reduced risk of AD. And, data from laboratory studies in cell culture and animal models are helping to clarify the mechanisms through which NSAIDs might exert their protective effects. These data are summarized below, and the potential for using NSAIDs as part of an intervention strategy in AD is discussed.

2. MECHANISMS OF ACTION

There are at least two possible mechanisms by which NSAIDs might protect against AD. One is by reducing inflammation via a COX-mediated pathway and the other is by altering APP metabolism to Aβ via a COX-independent pathway. Regarding the more traditional anti-inflammatory mechanism, NSAIDs competitively inhibit the active site of COX preventing it from binding arachidonic acid and converting it to prostaglandins, which are locally-acting hormones involved in inflammatory responses. [36, 37] At least two isoforms of the COX enzyme, referred to as COX-1 and COX-2, have been identified. [38] COX-1 is constitutively expressed in most tissues including the brain and gastric mucosa. By contrast, COX-2 is inducible and typically only detected in response to inflammation, except in the brain where it is constitutively present. [38] Commonly-used NSAIDs such as aspirin, ibuprofen, naproxen, and indomethacin, are non-selective in that they inhibit both COX-1 and COX-2 to varying degrees. The degree to which an NSAID blocks COX-1 relative to COX-2 is typically related to its toxicity. For example, NSAIDs that preferentially inhibit COX-1 generally have more gastrointestinal side effects. [38] Recently, COX-2 selective NSAIDs, such as celecoxib, rofecoxib, and valdecoxib, were approved for use in humans. These NSAIDs were widely touted at first because they have desirable anti-inflammatory properties presumably without the side effects of other traditional NSAIDs. However, they have since attracted considerable scrutiny due to emerging concerns over their potential cardiotoxicity. [39–41] Aspirin, unlike the other NSAIDs, inhibits COX by irreversibly acetylating the enzyme's active site. As a result, any new COX activity must be mediated by newly synthesized enzyme. [36] In platelets, the COX enzyme also plays an important role in converting arachidonic acid to thromboxanes, which are locally-acting hormones involved in the clotting activities of platelets. Because platelets cannot synthesize new COX enzyme, aspirin has potent anti-clotting effects even at low doses. It is this property which provides the rationale for using low-dose aspirin to prevent cardiovascular disease. Higher doses of aspirin may be required to see an anti-inflammatory effect.

Evidence from neuropathologic studies supports the notion that NSAIDs may protect against inflammation in the brain. MacKenzie and colleagues examined the brains of cognitively normal people who had osteoarthritis (OA) or rheumatoid arthritis (RA) and had been taking NSAIDs for one year or longer and compared them to age-matched controls. [42] They found, as expected, that some OA/RA brains and some control brains contained amyloid plaques. However, the number of activated microglia was lower in chronic NSAID users compared to non-users and this decrease was not dependent on the number of amyloid plaques. This decrease in inflammatory cells has been found in some studies [4, 42], but not all. [43]

The effect of NSAIDs on brain inflammation has also been investigated in cell culture and animal model studies. Aside from one contradictory finding [44], these studies have provided consistent evidence that NSAIDs have significant anti-inflammatory effects in the brain. [5–8, 45, 46] For example, in a mouse model of AD, Lim and colleagues found that chronic three or six-month treatment with the NSAID, ibuprofen, or the naturally-occurring NSAID, curcumin, reduced plaque-associated microglial activation, astrocytosis, and inflammatory products. [5, 6, 47] Similar anti-inflammatory properties have been found by others using ibuprofen [46] and indomethacin. [7, 8, 45]

Aside from their anti-inflammatory properties, recent evidence suggests that some NSAIDs may protect against AD independently of COX by directly reducing the metabolism of APP to Aβ. [9, 11] As described above, the metabolism of APP to Aβ is thought to play a central role in the pathogenesis of AD. APP is a type I transmembrane protein found in many cell types including neurons. Its normal physiological role is unknown, but it has been shown to inhibit certain enzymes, promote cell adhesion, and is associated with neuroprotection and neurodevelopment. [20, 48]

In AD, it undergoes sequential enzymatic cleavage first in the extracellular region by the enzyme β-secretase, which results in the release of a soluble protein denoted $sAPP_\beta$. The remaining piece of APP, embedded in the cell membrane, is then cleaved by the intramembrane enzyme, γ-secretase, after which the resulting Aβ fragment is secreted from the cell. [20] Gamma-secretase cleavage can occur at four sites resulting in Aβ fragments varying in length with 38, 40, 42, or 43 amino acids. Both the $A\beta_{40}$ and $A\beta_{42}$ peptides accumulate in the "senile" plaques that are pathognomic of AD, but it is the $A\beta_{42}$ species that is thought to be more damaging. Recent studies suggest that NSAIDs may modulate the activity of γ-secretase and shift the cleavage of APP towards the more benign $A\beta_{40}$ species. [9, 49]

Both in vivo [5, 6, 9, 11, 44–46, 50] and in vitro [9–11, 46, 50–55] studies have now documented that NSAID administration can modulate Aβ levels or Aβ plaques. Interestingly, some of these studies suggest that the effect on Aβ production may depend upon the type of NSAID. *In vivo* studies with ibuprofen [5, 6], indomethacin [45], and a derivative of flurbiprofen [44] all showed reduced Aβ levels in brain regions classically associated with Alzheimer-like pathology. However, one study could not replicate the ibuprofen finding and failed to show any evidence that celecoxib treatment mitigated Aβ pathology. [44] In a more detailed series of studies, Weggen and colleagues fed ibuprofen or naproxen to Alzheimer's mice and measured both soluble $A\beta_{42}$ and $A\beta_{40}$ levels. [11] They found that although ibuprofen selectively lowered $A\beta_{42}$ compared to $A\beta_{40}$, naproxen did not. In a follow-up study, they fed numerous NSAIDs to mice for three days and, as before, found that only some NSAIDs (e.g., diclofenac, diflunisal, fenoprofen, flurbiprofen, ibuprofen, indomethacin, meclofen, piroxicam, R-flurbiprofen, S-flurbiprofen, and sulindac) selectively lowered $A\beta_{42}$ compared to $A\beta_{40}$ whereas other NSAIDs (e.g., aspirin, ketoprofen, nabumetone, and naproxen) did not. [9] Yan and colleagues [46] found a similar reduction in $A\beta_{42}$ after mice were fed ibuprofen for four months, but a recent study by Lanz et al. [50] failed to show consistent reductions in brain $A\beta_{42}$ after three-day administration of flurbiprofen, ibuprofen, or sulindac. Cell culture studies appear to support the notion that some, but not all, NSAIDs selectively decrease $A\beta_{42}$ levels. However, the results are more difficult to interpret because many different cell types (i.e., derived from humans vs. other animals, and from peripheral vs. glial cells or neuronal cells) and varying doses of NSAIDs have been used. For example, in hamster ovary, human neuroglioma, human kidney, or mouse fibroblasts, a selective reduction in $A\beta_{42}$ was found with diclofenac, fenoprofen, flurbiprofen, ibuprofen, indomethacin, meclofen, R-ibuprofen, R-flurbiprofen, S-flurbiprofen, and sulindac, but not with aspirin, celecoxib, diflunisal, etodolac, fenbufen, ketorolac, ketoprofen, mefanamic acid, meloxicam, nabumetone, naproxen, phenylbutazone, piroxicam, sulindac sulphone, and suprofen. [9, 11, 46, 52] In contrast, Gasparini and colleagues tested a neuroblastoma cell line and found that flurbiprofen, sulindac sulfide, and aspirin produced a reduction in both $A\beta_{42}$ and $A\beta_{40}$, while in primary neurons, sulindac sulfide reduced both $A\beta_{42}$ and $A\beta_{40}$ and celecoxib reduced $A\beta_{40}$ and increased levels of $A\beta_{42}$. [54] Although the results from the cell culture studies are not entirely consistent with the animal model studies, there appears to be some consensus that NSAIDs such as ibuprofen, flurbiprofen, indomethacin and sulindac tend to lower $A\beta_{42}$ whereas others such as naproxen and celecoxib do not.

The mechanisms underlying the apparent differences between NSAIDs need clarification, but in any case $A\beta_{42}$ reduction is probably not mediated through COX as compounds that lack COX activity (e.g., R-flurbiprofen, R-ibuprofen) still showed the capacity to decrease $A\beta_{42}$. [9–11, 51, 52, 55] To demonstrate that the effect on $A\beta_{42}$ reduction is independent of COX, Weggen and colleagues treated COX-deficient cells with sulindac sulphide and then monitored $A\beta_{42}$ levels. [11] Interestingly, the COX-deficient cells did not demonstrate any alteration in basal $A\beta_{42}$ vs. wild-type cells, but treatment with sulindac did reduce $A\beta_{42}$. In another study, Sagi et al. showed that other known targets of NSAIDs besides COX, including lipoxygenases, peroxisome proliferator-activated receptor, or nuclear factor kappa B, are also not required for $A\beta_{42}$-reduction. [10] Studies with a broken cell γ-secretase assay have suggested that the $A\beta_{42}$ lowering NSAIDs may in fact directly target the γ-secretase complex. [9, 49] In order to elucidate how such NSAIDs might interact with γ-secretase, Lleo and colleagues utilized a fluorescence resonance energy transfer technique. [56] They found that these NSAIDs influence the proximity between APP and presenilin-1 (PS1), which is thought to activate or be part of the γ-secretase complex, and as a result alter PS1 conformation. They proposed a model in which the allosteric change in PS1 conformation shifts the cleavage of APP toward shorter $A\beta$ species. [56]

However these compounds work to reduce amyloidogenic APP processing, a key question is whether such drugs will be effective in the prevention or treatment of clinical AD. One study with a transgenic mouse model of AD showed that treatment with ibuprofen was associated not only with a reduction in amyloid burden but also with mitigation of behavioral deficits as assayed by an open field task. These results are encouraging because they suggest that AD-like clinical features can be ameliorated by NSAID treatment. [6] However, another study with a transgenic mouse model suggested that the neuroprotective effects of such NSAIDs may depend upon when they are used. Jankowsky and colleagues made an inducible APP transgenic mouse (where the mutant APP transgene is controlled by the antibiotic tetracycline and its analogues, designed to mimic γ-secretase inhibition) and turned the transgene "off" once AD-like pathology was established. Strikingly, these authors were unable to reverse $A\beta$ plaque, astroglial, or neuritic pathology in these mice, even after six months of transgene inactivation. [57] These results suggest that inhibition of γ-secretase would need to be started early in the course of the disease in order to have any efficacy.

3.   EVIDENCE FROM EPIDEMIOLOGIC STUDIES

3.1.   Observational Studies

At least 25 epidemiologic studies have reported on the relationship between NSAIDs and the risk of AD in humans. [58-83] Many of the early studies from the 1990's examined inflammatory conditions such as arthritis, with some [59, 60, 62, 63, 66, 67] but not all [58, 61, 64] finding an inverse association with AD. In a meta-analysis of these earlier studies, McGeer and colleagues reported that a history of arthritis was associated with a 44% reduction in risk of AD. [1]

It was suggested that a history of arthritis was a surrogate for NSAID exposure [63], and that the chronic use of NSAIDs among those with arthritis was responsible for the observed reduction in risk of AD. Thus, later studies began to focus specifically on the use of NSAIDs. Of twelve such studies that examined the use of non-aspirin NSAIDs using a non-prospective study design (i.e., case-control or cross-sectional) [68–71, 73–76, 79, 81, 84, 85], ten concluded that AD cases were less likely to have been using these agents whereas two concluded there was no association. [73, 79] The odds ratios (ORs) reported in these studies ranged from 0.19 (95% CI = 0.06 to 0.64) in a sibling study conducted by Breitner and colleagues [70] to 0.79 (95% CI = 0.45 to 1.38) in a retrospective case-control study conducted as part of the Rochester Epidemiology Project. [73] Eight of the twelve non-prospective studies are summarized in a meta-analysis in Figure 1a. To be included in the meta-analysis the studies had to have an outcome of AD that was diagnosed by formal criteria (e.g., the Diagnostic and Statistical Manual of Mental Disorders [87] or the National Institute of Neurological and Communicative Disorders and Stroke and the Alzheimer's Disease and Related Disorders Association [88]), the original data must have been reported for both the cases and the controls, and the criteria for exposure to non-aspirin NSAIDs must have been well-documented. The combined OR from these studies, which is based on a total of 1,833 AD cases and 13,780 controls, indicates a 53% risk reduction of AD in those participants who reported using a non-aspirin NSAID (combined OR = 0.47, 95% CI = 0.36 to 0.62).

In two studies conducted by Breitner and colleagues, an effort was made to tease apart the separate effects of NSAID use and arthritis on AD risk. [70, 85] When this was done, the OR for individuals who had a history of arthritis but did not use NSAIDs was 0.60 (95% CI = 0.10 to 3.50) in a study of twins and 0.68 (95% CI = 0.38 to 1.22) in a study of siblings. For individuals who used NSAIDs but did not have a history of arthritis the OR was 0.08 (95% CI = 0.01 to 0.69) in the twin study and indeterminate in the other study due to limited sample size. Although not definitive, these results provided evidence that the previously observed reduction in AD risk was due to the use of NSAIDs and not arthritis.

Seven of the non-prospective studies also had data available on aspirin use. [70, 73, 75, 76, 81, 83, 85] As seen in Figure 1b, which is based on data from 1,509 AD cases and 7,923 controls, aspirin use was also associated with a reduced risk of AD (combined OR = 0.55, 95% CI = 0.44 to 0.70), but in nearly half of the studies the confidence interval included the null. As discussed above, aspirin is like other NSAIDs in that it inhibits the COX enzyme, but it does so in a different manner by irreversibly blocking the active site. Another consideration with aspirin is that it is typically taken by the elderly for cardioprophylaxis at lower doses that will not have a potent anti-inflammatory effect.

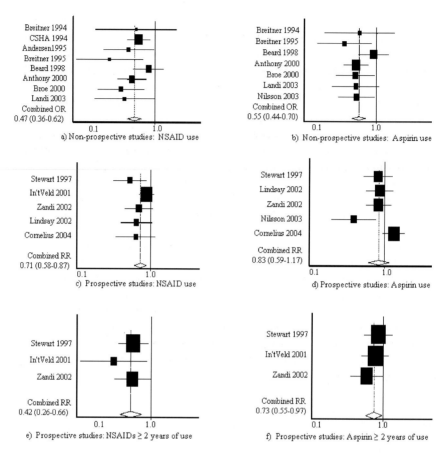

Figure 1. Meta-analyses showing the relationship between 1a) non-aspirin NSAID use and AD in non-prospective studies, 1b) aspirin use and AD in non-prospective studies, 1c) non-aspirin NSAID use and AD in prospective studies, 1d) aspirin use and AD in prospective studies, 1e) two or more years of non-aspirin NSAID use and AD in prospective studies, and 1f) two or more years of aspirin use and AD in prospective studies. (OR = odds ratio; RR = risk ratio). Figures 1a, c, and e modified from Szekely et al: Neuroepidemiology 2004;23:159–169 with permission from S. Karger AG, Basel; Statistical analysis performed using Stata 8.0 [86]

A major limitation of non-prospective observational studies like the ones discussed above is that they are unable to establish the temporality between NSAID use and AD, making it difficult to draw firm conclusions about the causal relationship between the two. Furthermore, such studies can be biased by differential recall of NSAID exposure in patient and control groups. This recall may be especially problematic in studies of diseases affecting memory such as AD. As a result, prospective studies in which information on exposure to NSAIDs is collected prior to diagnosis of AD can provide more conclusive evidence about their putative association.

Five prospective studies including a total of 836 AD cases and 16,294 controls have been published on the relation between NSAID use and incidence of AD. The findings from these studies are summarized in Figure 1c. [72, 77, 78, 80, 82] The combined risk ratio (RR) for lifetime use of non-aspirin NSAIDs and AD was 0.71 (95% CI 0.58 to 0.87). All five studies showed a trend for an inverse association between NSAIDs and AD, but it should be noted that all but one risk estimate included the null. In three of the studies in which data on duration was available, [72, 77, 80] the combined RR for two or more years of NSAID use was 0.42 (95% CI 0.26 to 0.66) (Figure 1e), suggesting a greater reduction in risk of AD with longer user. Interestingly, these three studies were also able to examine lag effects between NSAID use and onset of AD. In particular, two of these studies [77, 80] reported evidence suggesting that NSAID use was effective in reducing the risk of AD only if taken several years before the clinical onset of disease. By contrast, NSAID use within several years of the onset of disease did not appear to have any protective effect. These latter findings appear to be consistent with those from the study by Jankowsky and colleagues described above in which they showed using a transgene mouse model that it was not possible to reverse the AD pathology by simulating γ-secretase inhibition once the pathology was established. [57]

Five prospective studies also reported data on aspirin use. Figure 1d. shows a marginal reduction in risk of AD with lifetime use (RR = 0.83, 95% CI 0.59 to 1.17). However, as shown in Figure 1f, the reduction in risk became more apparent for use of aspirin greater than two years (RR = 0.73, 95% CI 0.55 to 0.97), again suggesting a duration effect similar to what is found with the other non-aspirin NSAIDs.

Other than aspirin, the effects of individual NSAIDs on AD risk have not been systematically examined in the published observational studies. The problem is that the sample sizes in these studies have typically been too small to allow for such investigations. Aspirin is an exception because it is used much more widely among the elderly for cardioprophylaxis. Consequently, it remains an open question whether those NSAIDs that have been shown to lower $A\beta_{42}$ in cell cultures and in animal models are associated with lower risk of AD in observational studies compared to NSAIDs that do not possess this property. An abstract from the Rotterdam Study [89], one of the five prospective studies that found a reduced risk of AD with NSAIDs, attempted to address this question and was reported at a research conference. The authors suggested that the observed reduction in AD risk was attributable to the use of $A\beta_{42}$-lowering NSAIDs such as ibuprofen and flurbiprofen, but the findings were inconclusive because of very small sample sizes. To overcome this limitation, we have pooled data from prospective studies of AD with the goal of assembling a sample that has sufficient power to adequately assess the neuroprotective effects of the different types of NSAIDs. Preliminary findings from this individual-patient-data meta-analysis, based on three published studies, suggested that NSAID exposure was associated with decreased risk of AD, but the reduction was not dependent on the $A\beta_{42}$-lowering capability of the NSAID. [90] We are currently nearing completion of this project and hope that the results from the larger pooled sample will provide more definitive conclusions regarding the role of type of NSAID on AD risk.

It should be noted that even though data from observational studies provide invaluable information about the relationship between NSAID use and AD, there are confounders and biases inherent in the design of these studies that must be considered when interpreting their results. One type of confounding that is a particular problem in studies of pharmacologic treatments is confounding by indication, in which a drug under investigation is used as a treatment for a disease which is, in itself, associated with the outcome of interest. [91, 92] For example, the apparent risk reduction with NSAID use and AD could be due to the presence of arthritic disease, for which NSAIDs are routinely taken. However, the studies that attempted to address this issue provided some evidence that NSAID use, in the absence of arthritis, still reduced risk for AD. Results from studies of medication can also be influenced by the healthy drug user bias in which individuals who use medications may be more health conscious or may have greater access to health care compared to non-users. [93] This is probably not a substantive bias for studies on NSAID use, as compared to hormone replacement therapy or vitamin use, as NSAIDs are often taken for chronic pain relief and not as preventive therapies. Also, many of the observational studies found null results when looking at a control medication, acetaminophen (also used for pain management), suggesting that this is not an important source of bias. Another potential source of bias in prospective studies could result from differences in mortality between exposed groups, or mortality bias. If participants exposed to NSAIDs have a higher rate of mortality due to NSAID-related complications compared to those unexposed to NSAIDs, the relationship between NSAID use and mortality could then result in an apparent inverse relationship between NSAID use and AD because the NSAID users are removed from the risk set (they die) before they have a chance to develop dementia. This issue was addressed in both the Rotterdam [94] and Cache County (unpublished data) cohorts where it was found that NSAID use was associated with a reduced risk of AD but not with all-cause mortality. Despite these (and other) limitations of observational studies, the consistency of findings across many studies does support the notion that NSAIDs might, in theory, be efficacious in reducing the risk of AD.

3.2.   Randomized Trials

The encouraging findings from the observational studies have provided a rationale for carrying out randomized controlled trials (RCT) to formally test the effects of NSAIDs on AD. To date, seven RCTs have been carried out to test whether NSAIDs can slow the progression of clinically established AD (see Table 1). Such trials are often referred to as tertiary prevention or treatment trials. The NSAIDs tested thus far include indomethacin [95], diclofenac [96], nimesulide [97], naproxen [98] and the more recently developed selective COX-2 inhibitors celecoxib and rofecoxib. [98–100] Sample sizes of these RCTs ranged from 40 to 692 subjects, and the

Table 1. Randomized placebo-controlled trials using NSAIDs (or related compounds) for treatment, secondary prevention, and primary prevention

PI and year	Drug and dose per day	Sample size	Duration (months)	Main outcome measures	Main findings or trial status
Treatment trials					
Rogers 1993 [95]	Indomethacin (100 to 150 mg)	44	6	Cognitive measures	Indomethacin group improved, placebo group declined; significant difference between groups on composite cognitive score
Scharf 1999 [96]	Diclofenac (50 mg)	41	6	Cognitive measures, clinical rating, ADL	No significant differences
Sainati 2000 [100]	Celecoxib (400 mg)	425	6	Cognitive measures, clinical rating, ADL, psychiatric symptoms	No significant differences
Aisen 2002 [97]	Nimesulide (200 mg)	40	6	Cognitive measures, clinical rating, ADL, psychiatric symptoms	No significant differences
Aisen 2003 [98]	Rofecoxib (25 mg) Naproxen (440 mg)	351	12	Cognitive measures, clinical rating, psychiatric symptoms, quality of life	No significant differences; trend for rofecoxib group to deteriorate more on cognitive measure and ADL vs placebo
Reines 2004 [99]	Rofecoxib (25 mg)	692	12	Cognitive measures, clinical rating	No significant differences
Black 2005 [101]	R-flurbiprofen (800 mg) R-flurbiprofen (1600 mg)	207	12	Cognitive measures, clinical rating, ADL	In mild AD with 1600 mg/day there was a trend for benefit on all three measures

(*Continued*)

Table 1. (Continued)

PI and year	Drug and dose per day	Sample size	Duration (months)	Main outcome measures	Main findings or trial status
Treatment trials					
Ringman [102]	Curcumin (2 doses)	33 exp	12	Cognitive and behavioral measures, Aβ and tau levels	Recruiting
Laughlin [103]	R-flurbiprofen (800 mg)	1600 exp	18	Cognitive measures, ADL	Recruiting
Baum [104]	Curcumin (1 g) Curcumin (4 g)	30 exp	6	Cognitive measures, Aβ and isoprostane levels	Recruiting
Secondary prevention trials					
Thal 2005 [105]	Rofecoxib (25 mg)	1457	48	Time to clinically diagnosed AD, cognitive measures, clinical rating	Risk to convert to AD higher in rofecoxib vs. placebo group; No significant differences on other measures
Small [106]	Celecoxib (400 mg)	135 exp	18	Further cognitive decline, neuroimaging changes	Recently completed
Primary prevention trial					
Breitner [107]	Celecoxib (400 mg) Naproxen (440 mg)	2528	20	Time to clinically diagnosed AD, cognitive measures, clinical rating	Recently completed/ treatment suspended

PI=principal investigator/author; mg=milligrams; g=grams; exp=expected; ADL=activities of daily living; AD=Alzheimer's disease; Aβ =amyloid-beta duration of follow-up was typically 6 to 12 months. Only one of these trials showed a mild benefit in slowing cognitive decline [95], while the others did not offer any evidence of a therapeutic effect. More recently, preliminary results were reported from a RCT of 207 subjects testing an enantiomer of flurbiprofen which was selected specifically because it modulates γ-secretase but has little activity against COX. This trial showed slightly less decline in cognitive ability in patients with mild AD over a 12 month period among subjects taking 1600 mg of R-flurbiprofen compared to placebo. [101] While the results do not show a striking improvement, they are promising and are currently being followed-up by a RCT with a larger sample and longer period of follow-up. [103, 108] Two other RCTs for the treatment of AD are also currently recruiting subjects to test curcumin. [102, 104] This compound, derived from the spice turmeric, may be of interest as it has strong anti-inflammatory and anti-oxidant properties and has been shown in animal models of AD to decrease levels of plaque burden, circulating amyloid, and proinflammatory cytokines. [47, 109]

Only one RCT has been carried out to test whether NSAIDs can delay the progression of prodromal mild cognitive impairment (MCI) to AD. [105] Such trials are often referred to as secondary prevention trials. In this secondary prevention trial, a total of 1,457 subjects were randomized to receive either 25 mg of rofecoxib or placebo and followed for up to four years. Surprisingly, subjects on rofecoxib converted to AD at a faster rate than those on placebo, but there were no significant differences in other functional measures. Another secondary prevention trial using 400 mg of celecoxib with 135 subjects followed for 18 months was recently completed, but the results have not yet been reported. [106]

Only one RCT has been initiated to test whether an NSAID can delay the progression to AD among cognitively normal elderly individuals. Such trials are often referred to as primary prevention trials. The Alzheimer's Disease Anti-inflammatory Prevention Trial [110], known as ADAPT, began recruiting participants in 2001 with an expected follow-up of up to seven years. The trial was designed to test two NSAIDs, naproxen and celecoxib, for the prevention of AD in approximately 2,625 elderly individuals who were cognitively normal with no evidence of MCI but who were at higher risk of AD than the general population because they had at least one first-degree relative with a history of dementia. Other exclusion criteria were based on a number of safety measures related to potential toxic side effects of NSAIDs. Participants were asked to travel to the clinics for routine biannual safety monitoring and annual cognitive assessments as well as additional safety-related visits. As ADAPT progressed, evidence from other studies emerged raising concerns about the cardiovascular safety of COX-2 inhibitors. [111, 112] More definitive evidence that these drugs, particularly rofecoxib, increased the risk of cardiovascular events was later reported. [113, 114] This led to withdrawal of rofecoxib from the market and to suspension of two cancer trials using celecoxib. In December of 2004, ADAPT investigators decided to suspend treatment in ADAPT due to the findings from outside trials and also because preliminary data suggested an increased risk of cardiovascular events in the naproxen group. [107, 115] ADAPT participants were asked to stop taking study drug, but were asked to continue followup visits for safety and outcome monitoring. The results pertaining to cardiovascular events, AD, or cognitive decline are not available at the time of this writing.

4.   SUMMARY AND CONCLUSIONS

The evidence is growing that NSAIDs may be useful in combating AD. Laboratory studies indicate there are compelling, biologically plausible reasons to believe that NSAIDs have a potent neuroprotective effect. By inhibiting COX, NSAIDs may reduce inflammatory responses in the brain thought to be associated with AD pathogenesis. Furthermore, certain NSAIDs may also modulate the activity of γ-secretase to reduce amyloid plaque production by shifting APP metabolism away from the more toxic $A\beta_{42}$ species. In line with this, epidemiologic studies carried out since the early 1990's have consistently shown that NSAIDs are associated with a lower risk of AD. A meta-analysis of the most rigorously conducted observational studies suggested that the use of non-aspirin NSAIDs for more than two years is associated with a 60% reduction in risk of AD, while the use of aspirin for more than two years is associated with a 30% reduction. The less apparent effect with aspirin may be due to the fact that it is typically taken by the elderly at low doses for cardioprophylaxis. Although observational studies have not had sufficient sample size to examine whether the reduction in risk is different for specific NSAIDs shown to selectively reduce $A\beta_{42}$, preliminary findings from a pooled analysis that we are carrying out suggest this may not be the case. Results from randomized trials have not been as encouraging. Seven trials with NSAIDs have been reported in the literature. With the possible exception of the most recent trial with R-flurbiprofen, the results from these trials suggest that NSAIDs (or related agents) may not be effective for the tertiary or secondary prevention of AD. These results are not surprising, and in fact appear to be consistent with observational studies that have shown that NSAIDs need to be taken several years prior to the clinical onset of disease in order to have any effect on lowering AD risk. Thus, it is reasonable to conclude that NSAIDs may be particularly effective for the primary prevention of AD before the course of disease has progressed to a point beyond remediation.

The best way to formally demonstrate the efficacy of NSAIDs on primary prevention is through randomized trials. Unfortunately, the one existing trial that was appropriately designed to address this important question, ADAPT, suspended treatment early due to safety concerns. Primary prevention trials of AD, like ADAPT, present significant challenges. These challenges include attaining an adequate sample size, allowing for a sufficient follow-up time, maintaining compliance, and implementing a cost-effective data collection schedule. [116] Participants willing to enroll in trials may have lower disease rates and mortality compared to others, and therefore either the sample size must be increased or the follow-up lengthened to ensure accrual of sufficient disease endpoints. [117]

Additionally, a longer trial may be needed to accommodate agents that require a certain amount of time to fully exert a protective effect. However, as trials become bigger and longer, the threat of non-compliance increases [116] and the costs quickly become prohibitive. Finally, there are considerable ethical concerns in giving drugs like NSAIDs, which can have significant toxic side effects, to elderly subjects who do not have the disease.

Despite these challenges, it is important that efforts continue to further clarify the neuroprotective role of NSAIDs. Because many elderly take NSAIDs regularly for a variety of indications such as arthritis, it is crucial to establish the risks of taking NSAIDs in regards to potential gastrointestinal and cardiovascular adverse effects relative to the benefits including any concomitant salutary effects on cognition. Furthermore, by elucidating the mechanisms by which NSAIDs may protect against AD, more rational interventions can be adapted that maximize the benefits while minimizing the risks, and certain groups of participants who might tolerate the new treatments better than others can be more successfully identified. Thus, future studies should continue to investigate the relative contribution of COX and γ-secretase mediated effects of NSAIDs and how these different effects translate into a reduced risk of AD in human populations. Additionally, it will be important for investigators to focus on the issue of how the timing of NSAID exposure and the duration of use influences the underlying progression of AD. With 2.5 to 4.5 million prevalent cases in the United States alone and projections that these numbers will likely quadruple in the United States over the coming 50 years [12], AD is a major public health problem that threatens to worsen. Thus, there is considerable motivation to develop effective strategies for delaying or even preventing the disease.

REFERENCES

1. McGeer PL, Schulzer M, McGeer EG. Arthritis and anti-inflammatory agents as possible protective factors for Alzheimer's disease: a review of 17 epidemiologic studies. Neurology. 1996;47(2):425–432.
2. Etminan M, Gill S, Samii A. Effect of non-steroidal anti-inflammatory drugs on risk of Alzheimer's disease: systematic review and meta-analysis of observational studies. BMJ. 2003;327:128–132.
3. Szekely CA, Thorne JE, Zandi PP et al. Nonsteroidal anti-inflammatory drugs for the prevention of Alzheimer's disease: a systematic review. Neuroepidemiology. 2004;23:159–169.
4. Mackenzie IR, Munoz DG. Effect of anti-inflammatory medications on neuropathological findings in Alzheimer disease. Arch Neurol. 2001;58(3):517–9.
5. Lim GP, Yang F, Chu T et al. Ibuprofen suppresses plaque pathology and inflammation in a mouse model for Alzheimer's disease. J Neurosci. 2000;20(15):5709–5714.
6. Lim GP, Yang F, Chu T et al. Ibuprofen effects on Alzheimer pathology and open field activity in APPsw transgenic mice. Neurobiol Aging. 2001;22(6):983–991.
7. Dzenko KA, Weltzien RB, Pachter JS. Suppression of A beta-induced monocyte neurotoxicity by antiinflammatory compounds. J Neuroimmunol. 1997;80(1-2):6–12.
8. Netland EE, Newton JL, Majocha RE, Tate BA. Indomethacin reverses the microglial response to amyloid beta-protein. Neurobiol Aging. 1998;19(3):201–204.

9. Eriksen JL, Sagi SA, Smith TE et al. NSAIDs and enantiomers of flurbiprofen target gamma-secretase and lower Abeta 42 in vivo. J Clin Invest. 2003;112(3):440–449.

10. Sagi SA, Weggen S, Eriksen J, Golde TE, Koo EH. The non-cyclooxygenase targets of non-steroidal anti-inflammatory drugs, lipoxygenases, peroxisome proliferator-activated receptor, inhibitor of kappa B kinase, and NF kappa B, do not reduce amyloid beta 42 production. J Biol Chem. 2003;278(34):31825–31830.

11. Weggen S, Eriksen JL, Das P et al. A subset of NSAIDs lower amyloidogenic Abeta42 independently of cyclooxygenase activity. Nature. 2001;414(6860):212–216.

12. Brookmeyer R, Gray S. Methods for projecting the incidence and prevalence of chronic diseases in aging populations: application to Alzheimer's disease. Stat Med. 2000;19(11-12):1481–1493.

13. Hebert LE, Scherr PA, Bienias JL, Bennett DA, Evans DA. Alzheimer disease in the US population: prevalence estimates using the 2000 census. Arch Neurol. 2003;60(8):1119–1122.

14. Gao S, Hendrie HC, Hall KS, Hui S. The relationships between age, sex, and the incidence of dementia and Alzheimer disease: a meta-analysis. Arch Gen Psychiatry. 1998;55(9):809–815.

15. U.S. Census Bureau. Annual projections of the resident population by age, sex, race, and hispanic origin: lowest, middle, highest series and zero international migration series, 1999 to 2100. [http://www.census.gov/publication/www/projections/natdet-D1A.html] Accessed 07 April 2004.

16. Centers for Disease Control. Public health and aging: Trends in aging – United States and worldwide. Morbidity and Mortality Weekly Report. 2003;52(6):101–106.

17. Goedert M, Wischik CM, Crowther RA, Walker JE, Klug A. Cloning and sequencing of the cDNA encoding a core protein of the paired helical filament of Alzheimer disease: identification as the microtubule-associated protein tau. Proc Natl Acad Sci U S A. 1988;85(11):4051–4055.

18. Braak H, Braak E. Frequency of stages of Alzheimer-related lesions in different age categories. Neurobiol Aging. 1997;18(4):351–357.

19. Selkoe DJ. Alzheimer's disease: genes, proteins, and therapy. Physiol Rev. 2001;81(2):741–766.

20. Selkoe DJ. Alzheimer disease: mechanistic understanding predicts novel therapies. Ann Intern Med. 2004;140(8):627–638.

21. Jarrett JT, Berger EP, Lansbury PT Jr. The C-terminus of the beta protein is critical in amyloidogenesis. Ann N Y Acad Sci. 1993;695:144–148.

22. Iwatsubo T, Odaka A, Suzuki N, Mizusawa H, Nukina N, Ihara Y. Visualization of A beta 42(43) and A beta 40 in senile plaques with end-specific A beta monoclonals: evidence that an initially deposited species is A beta 42(43). Neuron. 1994;13(1):45–53.

23. Lemere CA, Blusztajn JK, Yamaguchi H, Wisniewski T, Saido TC, Selkoe DJ. Sequence of deposition of heterogeneous amyloid beta-peptides and APO E in Down syndrome: implications for initial events in amyloid plaque formation. Neurobiol Dis. 1996;3(1):16–32.

24. Selkoe DJ. Toward a comprehensive theory for Alzheimer's disease. Hypothesis: Alzheimer's disease is caused by the cerebral accumulation and cytotoxicity of amyloid beta-protein. Ann N Y Acad Sci. 2000;924:17–25.

25. McGeer PL, McGeer EG. Mechanisms of cell death in Alzheimer disease–immunopathology. J Neural Transm Suppl. 1998;54:159–166.

26. Akiyama H, Barger S, Barnum S et al. Inflammation and Alzheimer's disease. Neurobiol Aging. 2000;21(3):383–421.

27. McGeer EG, McGeer PL. Inflammatory processes in Alzheimer's disease. Prog Neuropsychopharmacol Biol Psychiatry. 2003;27(5):741–749.

28. Eikelenboom P, Bate C, Van Gool WA et al. Neuroinflammation in Alzheimer's disease and prion disease. Glia. 2002;40(2):232–239.

29. Vehmas AK, Kawas CH, Stewart WF, Troncoso JC. Immune reactive cells in senile plaques and cognitive decline in Alzheimer's disease. Neurobiol Aging. 2003;24(2):321–331.

30. Cagnin A, Brooks DJ, Kennedy AM et al. In-vivo measurement of activated microglia in dementia. Lancet. 2001;358(9280):461–467.

31. Yasojima K, Schwab C, McGeer EG, McGeer PL. Human neurons generate C-reactive protein and amyloid P: upregulation in Alzheimer's disease. Brain Res. 2000;887(1):80–89.

32. Rogers J, Cooper NR, Webster S et al. Complement activation by beta-amyloid in Alzheimer disease. Proc Natl Acad Sci U S A. 1992;89(21):10016–10020.

33. Bradt BM, Kolb WP, Cooper NR. Complement-dependent proinflammatory properties of the Alzheimer's disease beta-peptide. J Exp Med. 1998;188(3):431–438.

34. Mehlhorn G, Hollborn M, Schliebs R. Induction of cytokines in glial cells surrounding cortical beta-amyloid plaques in transgenic Tg2576 mice with Alzheimer pathology. Int J Dev Neurosci. 2000;18(4-5):423–431.

35. Benzing WC, Wujek JR, Ward EK et al. Evidence for glial-mediated inflammation in aged APP(SW) transgenic mice. Neurobiol Aging. 1999;20(6):581–589.

36. Vane JR. Inhibition of prostaglandin synthesis as a mechanism of action for aspirin-like drugs. Nat New Biol. 1971;231(25):232–235.

37. Meade EA, Smith WL, Dewitt DL. Differential inhibition of prostaglandin endoperoxide synthase (cyclooxygenase) isozymes by aspirin and other non-steroidal anti-inflammatory drugs. J Biol Chem. 1993;268(9):6610–6614.

38. DuBois RN, Abramson SB, Crofford L et al. Cyclooxygenase in biology and disease. FASEB J. 1998;12(12):1063–1073.

39. Couzin J. Drug safety. Withdrawal of Vioxx casts a shadow over COX-2 inhibitors. Science. 2004;306(5695):384–385.

40. Drazen JM. COX-2 inhibitors–a lesson in unexpected problems. N Engl J Med. 2005;352(11):1131–1132.

41. Psaty BM, Furberg CD. COX-2 inhibitors–lessons in drug safety. N Engl J Med. 2005;352(11):1133–1135.

42. Mackenzie IR, Munoz DG. Nonsteroidal anti-inflammatory drug use and Alzheimer-type pathology in aging. Neurology. 1998;50(4):986–90.

43. Halliday GM, Shepherd CE, McCann H et al. Effect of anti-inflammatory medications on neuropathological findings in Alzheimer disease. Arch Neurol. 2000;57(6):831–6.

44. Jantzen PT, Connor KE, DiCarlo G et al. Microglial activation and beta -amyloid deposit reduction caused by a nitric oxide-releasing nonsteroidal anti-inflammatory drug in amyloid precursor protein plus presenilin-1 transgenic mice. J Neurosci. 2002;22(6):2246–2254.

45. Quinn J, Montine T, Morrow J, Woodward WR, Kulhanek D, Eckenstein F. Inflammation and cerebral amyloidosis are disconnected in an animal model of Alzheimer's disease. J Neuroimmunol. 2003;137(1-2):32–41.

46. Yan Q, Zhang J, Liu H et al. Anti-inflammatory drug therapy alters beta-amyloid processing and deposition in an animal model of Alzheimer's disease. J Neurosci. 2003;23(20):7504–7509.

47. Lim GP, Chu T, Yang F, Beech W, Frautschy SA, Cole GM. The curry spice curcumin reduces oxidative damage and amyloid pathology in an Alzheimer transgenic mouse. J Neurosci. 2001;21(21):8370–8377.

48. Kerr ML, Small DH. Cytoplasmic domain of the beta-amyloid protein precursor of Alzheimer's disease: function, regulation of proteolysis, and implications for drug development. J Neurosci Res. 2005;80(2):151–159.

49. Weggen S, Eriksen JL, Sagi SA et al. Evidence that nonsteroidal anti-inflammatory drugs decrease amyloid beta 42 production by direct modulation of gamma-secretase activity. J Biol Chem. 2003;278(34):31831–31837.

50. Lanz TA, Fici GJ, Merchant KM. Lack of specific amyloid-beta(1-42) suppression by nonsteroidal anti-inflammatory drugs in young, plaque-free Tg2576 mice and in guinea pig neuronal cultures. J Pharmacol Exp Ther. 2005;312(1):399–406.

51. Beher D, Clarke EE, Wrigley JD et al. Selected non-steroidal anti-inflammatory drugs and their derivatives target gamma-secretase at a novel site. Evidence for an allosteric mechanism. J Biol Chem. 2004;279(42):43419–43426.

52. Morihara T, Chu T, Ubeda O, Beech W, Cole GM. Selective inhibition of Abeta42 production by NSAID R-enantiomers. J Neurochem. 2002;83(4):1009–1012.

53. Takahashi Y, Hayashi I, Tominari Y et al. Sulindac sulfide is a noncompetitive gamma-secretase inhibitor that preferentially reduces Abeta 42 generation. J Biol Chem. 2003;278(20):18664–18670.

54. Gasparini L, Rusconi L, Xu H, del SP, Ongini E. Modulation of beta-amyloid metabolism by non-steroidal anti-inflammatory drugs in neuronal cell cultures. J Neurochem. 2004;88(2):337–348.

55. Peretto I, Radaelli S, Parini C et al. Synthesis and biological activity of flurbiprofen analogues as selective inhibitors of beta-amyloid(1)(-)(42) secretion. J Med Chem. 2005;48(18):5705–5720.

56. Lleo A, Berezovska O, Herl L et al. Nonsteroidal anti-inflammatory drugs lower Abeta42 and change presenilin 1 conformation. Nat Med. 2004;10(10):1065–1066.

57. Jankowsky JL, Slunt HH, Gonzales V et al. Persistent amyloidosis following suppression of Abeta production in a transgenic model of Alzheimer disease. PLoS Med. 2005;2(12):e355.

58. Heyman A, Wilkinson WE, Stafford JA, Helms MJ, Sigmon AH, Weinberg T. Alzheimer's disease: a study of epidemiological aspects. Ann Neurol. 1984;15(4):335–41.

59. French LR, Schuman LM, Mortimer JA, Hutton JT, Boatman RA, Christians B. A case-control study of dementia of the Alzheimer type. Am J Epidemiol. 1985;121(3):414–21.

60. Jenkinson ML, Bliss MR, Brain AT, Scott DL. Rheumatoid arthritis and senile dementia of the Alzheimer's type. Br J Rheumatol. 1989;28(1):86–8.

61. Graves AB, White E, Koepsell TD et al. A case-control study of Alzheimer's disease. Ann Neurol. 1990;28(6):766–74.

62. Broe GA, Henderson AS, Creasey H et al. A case-control study of Alzheimer's disease in Australia. Neurology. 1990;40(11):1698–707.

63. McGeer PL, McGeer E, Rogers J, Sibley J. Anti-inflammatory drugs and Alzheimer disease. Lancet. 1990;335(8696):1037.

64. Beard CM, Kokman E, Kurland LT. Rheumatoid arthritis and susceptibility to Alzheimer's disease. Lancet. 1991;337(8754):1426.

65. McGeer, P. L., Harada, N., Kimura, H., and McGeer, E. G. Prevalence of dementia amongst elderly Japanese with leprosy: Apparent effect of chronic drug therapy. Dementia. 1992;3(3):146–149.

66. Li G, Shen YC, Li YT, Chen CH, Zhau YW, Silverman JM. A case-control study of Alzheimer's disease in China. Neurology. 1992;42(8):1481–8.

67. Myllykangas-Luosujarvi R, Isomaki H. Alzheimer's disease and rheumatoid arthritis. Br J Rheumatol. 1994;33(5):501–2.

68. Lucca U, Tettamanti M, Forloni G, Spagnoli A. Nonsteroidal antiinflammatory drug use in Alzheimer's disease. Biol Psychiatry. 1994;36(12):854–6.

69. Andersen K, Launer LJ, Ott A, Hoes AW, Breteler MM, Hofman A. Do nonsteroidal anti-inflammatory drugs decrease the risk for Alzheimer's disease? The Rotterdam Study. Neurology. 1995;45(8):1441–5.

70. Breitner JC, Welsh KA, Helms MJ et al. Delayed onset of Alzheimer's disease with nonsteroidal anti-inflammatory and histamine H2 blocking drugs. Neurobiol Aging. 1995;16(4):523–30.

71. Rich JB, Rasmusson DX, Folstein MF, Carson KA, Kawas C, Brandt J. Nonsteroidal anti-inflammatory drugs in Alzheimer's disease. Neurology. 1995;45(1):51–5.

72. Stewart WF, Kawas C, Corrada M, Metter EJ. Risk of Alzheimer's disease and duration of NSAID use. Neurology. 1997;48(3):626–32.

73. Beard CM, Waring SC, O'Brien PC, Kurland LT, Kokmen E. Nonsteroidal anti-inflammatory drug use and Alzheimer's disease: a case-control study in Rochester, Minnesota, 1980 through 1984. Mayo Clin Proc. 1998;73(10):951–5.

74. in 't Veld BA, Launer LJ, Hoes AW et al. NSAIDs and incident Alzheimer's disease. The Rotterdam Study. Neurobiol Aging. 1998;19(6):607–11.

75. Anthony JC, Breitner JC, Zandi PP et al. Reduced prevalence of AD in users of NSAIDs and H2 receptor antagonists: the Cache County study. Neurology. 2000;54(11):2066–71.

76. Broe GA, Grayson DA, Creasey HM et al. Anti-inflammatory drugs protect against Alzheimer disease at low doses. Arch Neurol. 2000;57(11):1586–91.

77. in 't Veld BA, Ruitenberg A, Hofman A et al. Nonsteroidal antiinflammatory drugs and the risk of Alzheimer's disease. N Engl J Med. 2001;345(21):1515–21.

78. Lindsay J, Laurin D, Verreault R et al. Risk factors for Alzheimer's disease: a prospective analysis from the Canadian Study of Health and Aging. Am J Epidemiol. 2002;156(5):445–453.

79. Wolfson C, Perrault A, Moride Y, Esdaile JM, Abenhaim L, Momoli F. A case-control analysis of nonsteroidal anti-inflammatory drugs and Alzheimer's disease: are they protective? Neuroepidemiology. 2002;21(2):81–86.

80. Zandi PP, Anthony JC, Hayden KM, Mehta K, Mayer L, Breitner JC. Reduced incidence of AD with NSAID but not H2 receptor antagonists: the Cache County Study. Neurology. 2002;59(6):880–886.

81. Landi F, Cesari M, Onder G, Russo A, Torre S, Bernabei R. Non-steroidal anti-inflammatory drug (NSAID) use and Alzheimer disease in community-dwelling elderly patients. Am J Geriatr Psychiatry. 2003;11(2):179–185.

82. Cornelius C, Fastbom J, Winblad B, Viitanen M. Aspirin, NSAIDs, risk of dementia, and influence of the apolipoprotein E epsilon 4 allele in an elderly population. Neuroepidemiology. 2004;23(3):135–143.

83. Nilsson SE, Johansson B, Takkinen S et al. Does aspirin protect against Alzheimer's dementia? A study in a Swedish population-based sample aged > or = 80 years. Eur J Clin Pharmacol. 2003;59(4):313–319.

84. The Canadian Study of Health and Aging: risk factors for Alzheimer's disease in Canada. Neurology. 1994;44(11):2073–80.

85. Breitner JC, Gau BA, Welsh KA et al. Inverse association of anti-inflammatory treatments and Alzheimer's disease: initial results of a co-twin control study. Neurology. 1994;44(2):227–32.

86. Stata Statistical Software: Release 8.0. College Station, Texas: Stata Corporation; 2003.

87. American Psychiatric Association. Diagnostic and statistical manual of mental disorders: DSM-III-R. 3rd, revised ed. Washington, DC: American Psychiatric Association; 1987.

88. McKhann G, Drachman D, Folstein M, Katzman R, Price D, Stadlan EM. Clinical diagnosis of Alzheimer's disease: report of the NINCDS-ADRDA Work Group under the auspices of Department of Health and Human Services Task Force on Alzheimer's Disease. Neurology. 1984;34(7):939–944.

89. Breteler MB, in 't Veld BA, Hofman A, and Stricker BH. AB-42 peptide lowering NSAIDs and Alzheimer's disease. Neurobiol Aging. 2002;23(S1):S286

90. Zandi PP, Szekely CA, Green RC, Breitner JC, Welsh-Bohmer KA. Pooled analysis of the association between different NSAIDs and AD: Preliminary findings. Neurobiol Aging. 2004;25(S2):S5.

91. Salas M, Hofman A, Stricker BH. Confounding by indication: an example of variation in the use of epidemiologic terminology. Am J Epidemiol. 1999;149(11):981–983.

92. Psaty BM, Koepsell TD, Lin D et al. Assessment and control for confounding by indication in observational studies. J Am Geriatr Soc. 1999;47(6):749–754.

93. Barrett-Connor E, Grady D. Hormone replacement therapy, heart disease, and other considerations. Annu Rev Public Health. 1998;19:55–72.

94. Stricker BH, Hofman A, Breteler MB. Letter to the Editor: Nonsteroidal drugs and Alzheimer's disease. N Engl J Med. 2002;346(15):1171–1173.

95. Rogers J, Kirby LC, Hempelman SR et al. Clinical trial of indomethacin in Alzheimer's disease. Neurology. 1993;43(8):1609–1611.

96. Scharf S, Mander A, Ugoni A, Vajda F, Christophidis N. A double-blind, placebo-controlled trial of diclofenac/misoprostol in Alzheimer's disease. Neurology. 1999;53(1):197–201.

97. Aisen PS, Schmeidler J, Pasinetti GM. Randomized pilot study of nimesulide treatment in Alzheimer's disease. Neurology. 2002;58(7):1050–1054.

98. Aisen PS, Schafer KA, Grundman M et al. Effects of rofecoxib or naproxen vs placebo on Alzheimer disease progression: a randomized controlled trial. JAMA. 2003;289(21):2819–2826.

99. Reines SA, Block GA, Morris JC et al. Rofecoxib: no effect on Alzheimer's disease in a 1-year, randomized, blinded, controlled study. Neurology. 2004;62(1):66–71.

100. Sainati S, Ingram D, Talwalker S, Geis G. Results of a double-blind, randomized, placebo-controlled study of celecoxib in the treatment of progression of Alzheimer's Disease. 6th International Stockholm-Springfield Symposium of Advances in Alzheimer's Therapy; 2000; Stockholm, Sweden.

101. Black SE, Wilcock G, Haworth J, et al. A placebo-controlled, double-blind trial of the selective Abeta42-lowering agent Flurizan in patients with mild to moderate Alzheimer's disease:

Efficacy, safety, and follow-on results. 2005. Program No. 585.6. Washington, DC: Society for Neuroscience.

102. www.clinicaltrials.gov. Curcumin in patients with mild to moderate Alzheimer's disease; Ringman J, Study Director; sponsored by John Douglas French Foundation and ISOA. [www.clinicaltrials.gov]. Accessed 22 March 2006.

103. www.clinicaltrials.gov. Efficacy study of MPC-7869 to treat patients with Alzheimer's; Laughlin M, Study Director; sponsored by Myriad Pharmaceuticals. [www.clinicaltrials.gov]. Accessed 22 March 2006.

104. www.clinicaltrials.gov. A pilot study of curcumin and ginkgo for treating Alzheimer's disease; Baum L, Principal Investigator; sponsored by BUPA Foundation and Institute of Chinese Medicine of the Chinese University of Hong Kong. [www.clinicaltrials.gov]. Accessed 22 March 2006.

105. Thal LJ, Ferris SH, Kirby L et al. A randomized, double-blind, study of rofecoxib in patients with mild cognitive impairment. Neuropsychopharmacology. 2005;30(6):1204–1215.

106. www.clinicaltrials.gov. Anti-inflammatory treatment for age-associated memory impairment: a double-blind placebo-controlled trial; Small GW, Principal Investigator; sponsored by NIMH. [www.clinicaltrials.gov]. Accessed 22 March 2006.

107. ADAPT Steering Committee. Statement from the Steering Committee of the Alzheimer's Disease Anti-inflammatory Prevention Trial (ADAPT) to FDA. [www.jhucct.com/adapt/documents.htm]. Accessed 07 April 2006.

108. Myriad Genetics Incorporated. Flurizan™ Alzheimer's disease phase 3 clinical trial. [http://www.myriad.com/research/trial_ad.php]. Accessed 22 March 2006.

109. Yang F, Lim GP, Begum AN et al. Curcumin inhibits formation of amyloid beta oligomers and fibrils, binds plaques, and reduces amyloid in vivo. J Biol Chem. 2005;280(7):5892–5901.

110. Martin BK, Meinert CL, Breitner JC. Double placebo design in a prevention trial for Alzheimer's disease. Control Clin Trials. 2002;23(1):93–99.

111. Mukherjee D, Nissen SE, Topol EJ. Cox-2 inhibitors and cardiovascular risk: we defend our data and suggest caution. Cleve Clin J Med. 2001;68(11):963–964.

112. Mukherjee D, Nissen SE, Topol EJ. Risk of cardiovascular events associated with selective COX-2 inhibitors. JAMA. 2001;286(8):954–959.

113. Solomon SD, McMurray JJ, Pfeffer MA et al. Cardiovascular risk associated with celecoxib in a clinical trial for colorectal adenoma prevention. N Engl J Med. 2005;352(11):1071–1080.

114. Bresalier RS, Sandler RS, Quan H et al. Cardiovascular events associated with rofecoxib in a colorectal adenoma chemoprevention trial. N Engl J Med. 2005;352(11):1092–1102.

115. Federal Drug Administration. FDA statement on naproxen. December 20 2004. [http://www.fda.gov/bbs/topics/news/2004/NEW01148.html]. Accessed 18 June 2005.

116. Buring JE. Special issues related to randomized trials of primary prevention. Epidemiol Rev. 2002;24(1):67–71.

117. Sesso HD, Gaziano JM, VanDenburgh M, Hennekens CH, Glynn RJ, Buring JE. Comparison of baseline characteristics and mortality experience of participants and nonparticipants in a randomized clinical trial: the Physicians' Health Study. Control Clin Trials. 2002;23(6):686–702.

CHAPTER 12

INFLAMMATION IN PARKINSON'S DISEASE
Causative or epiphenomenal?

ANDREAS HALD[1], JOHAN VAN BEEK[2] AND JULIE LOTHARIUS[2,*]

[1] *Department of Pharmacology and Pharmacotherapeutics, The Danish University of Pharmaceutical Sciences, Universitetsparken 2, 2100 Copenhagen, Denmark*
[2] *Department of Disease Biology, H. Lundbeck A/S, Ottiliavej 9, 2500 Valby, Denmark*

---

* Disease Biology, Department 807, H. Lundbeck A/S, Ottiliavej 9, 2500 Valby, Denmark.
  E-mail: MJL@Lundbeck.com

R. E. Harris (ed.), Inflammation in the Pathogenesis of Chronic Diseases, 249–279.
© 2007 *Springer.*

Abstract: Parkinson's disease (PD) is a neurodegenerative disorder characterized by a dramatic loss of dopaminergic neurons in the substantia nigra (SN). Several pathogenic mechanisms have been implicated in the demise of these cells, including dopamine-dependent oxidative stress, mitochondrial dysfunction, excitotoxicity, and proteasomal impairment. In recent years, the involvement of neuroinflammatory processes in nigral degeneration has gained increasing attention. Not only have activated microglia and increased levels of inflammatory mediators been detected in the striatum of PD patients, but a large body of animal studies points to a contributory role of inflammation in dopaminergic cell loss. For example, post-mortem examination of human subjects exposed to the parkinsonism-inducing toxin, 1-methyl-4-phenyl-1,2,3,6-tetrahydropyridine, revealed the presence of activated microglia decades after drug exposure, suggesting that even a brief pathogenic insult can induce an ongoing inflammatory response. Perhaps not surprisingly, non-steroidal anti-inflammatory drugs have been shown to reduce the risk of developing PD. In the past few years, various pathways have come to light that could link neurodegeneration and microglial activation, finally ascribing a pathogenic trigger to the chronic inflammatory response characteristic of PD

1.   PATHOGENESIS OF PARKINSON'S DISEASE

1.1.   Clinical Characteristics

Parkinson's disease is one of the leading causes of neurologic disability in elderly people, with an estimated one million North Americans currently affected by the disease. The clinical features of PD involve tremor, rigidity, bradykinesia and postural instability. The mean age of onset is 55 years of age, with the risk for developing PD increasing 5-fold by the age of 70. Two forms of the disease have been identified: a sporadic form, which affects 95% of all cases and whose etiology is unknown, and a familial form accounting for about 5–10% of affected persons, which is linked to mutations in a restricted number of genes (see reviews by (Dauer and Przedborski, 2003; Zimprich et al., 2004; Cookson et al., 2005). The symptoms observed in PD are caused by a > 50% loss of dopaminergic neurons in the substantia nigra (SN) pars compacta corresponding to a > 80% reduction in dopamine levels in the striatum (Figure 1), with a more severe depletion seen in the putamen (thought to be involved in the regulation of movement) than in the caudate nucleus (involved in higher cognitive functions) (Kish et al., 1988; Hirsch et al., 1988; Fearnley and Lees, 1991; Pakkenberg et al., 1991; Hornykiewicz, 1998). A reduction in dopamine is also seen in other dopaminergic projection areas such as the neocortex and hippocampus (Scatton et al., 1982). In addition, cell loss is also found in other brain areas such as the noradrenergic locus coeruleus, dorsal vagal nucleus and medullary nuclei, serotonergic dorsal raphe, nucleus basalis of Meynert and other cholinergic brainstem nuclei (Jellinger, 1999).

1.2.   Molecular Pathways Leading to Neurodegeneration in PD

Several hypotheses exist which attempt to explain the selective loss of dopaminergic neurons in PD (Figure 2). One theory proposes that nigral neurons are selectively vulnerable to environmental contaminants triggering mitochondrial

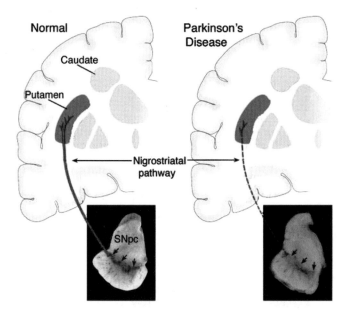

Figure 1. Schematic showing regions in the human brain affected in PD

dysfunction, produce an endogenous mitochondrial toxin, or harbor endogenous defects in mitochondrial enzymes such as Complex I (NADH dehydrogenase) of the electron transport chain that lead to impaired energy metabolism (see review by Orth and Schapira, 2002). This theory arose from the fortuitous finding that the meperidine analog, 1-methyl-4-phenyl-1,2,3,6- tetrahydropyridine (MPTP), and other mitochondrial poisons such as rotenone can induce a parkinsonian condition in humans, non-human primates, and rodents. In support of the mitochondrial dysfunction hypothesis are neuropathological studies reporting a $\approx 30\%$ defect in Complex I function in the SN and platelets from deceased PD patients (see reviews by Schapira, 1994; Sherer et al., 2002). Furthermore, mutations in mitochondrial DNA genes such as *12SrRNA*, have been linked in recent years to rare maternally-inherited forms of parkinsonism with additional clinical features not found in idiopathic PD. Mutations in a nuclear-encoded mitochondrial gene, DNA polymerase g or *POLG*, have also been linked to familial parkinsonism but again the clinical characteristics of this disorder differ from classical PD and caution should be used when extrapolating disease mechanisms active in these diseases to PD (Abou-Sleiman et al., 2006).

The proteolytic stress hypothesis ascribes the loss of nigral neurons in PD to the toxic accumulation of misfolded and aggregated proteins. This theory is supported by studies showing a significant defect in the 20S proteasome, the primary cellular machinery responsible for degrading non-ubiquinated proteins, in post-mortem nigral tissue from sporadic PD patients, and by linkage of two genes encoding

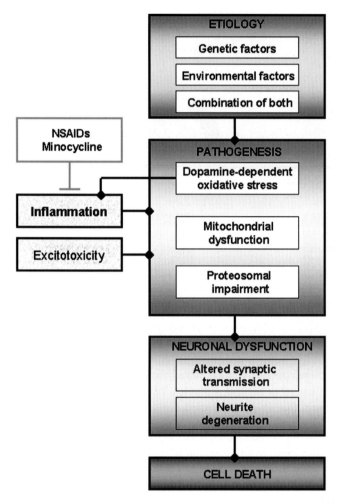

Figure 2. Potential etiological triggers and pathogenic mechanims contributing to the loss of dopaminergic cells in PD. White boxes indicate key events occuring during the etiology and pathogenesis stages of the disease that could play a causative role in dopaminergic cell dysfunction and ultimately cell death. Gray boxes boxes outside the mainstream cascade represent events thought to contribute to the pathogenesis of the disease

enzymes essential for the proper function of the ubiquitin-proteasome system (UPS), namely ubiquitin carboxyl-terminal hydrolase 1 (UCHL1) and parkin, a ubiquitin E3 ligase, to early-onset, familial forms of PD (see reviews by McNaught and Olanow, 2003; Greenamyre and Hastings, 2004). Interestingly, Complex I inhibitors such as rotenone have been shown to reduce proteasomal activity through ATP depletion, leading to increased toxicity in neurons with a compromised proteasome. This may constitute a link between mitochondrial activity, proteasomal insufficiency and cell death in PD (Hoglinger et al., 2003).

In an alternative hypothesis, the preferential loss of nigral neurons in PD has been attributed to the highly-oxidative intracellular environment within dopaminergic neurons arising mainly from the highly labile nature of their endogenous neurotransmitter dopamine (Lotharius and Brundin, 2002a; Lotharius and Brundin, 2002b). Indeed, post-mortem studies of PD patients show a significant and selective increase in various oxidative stress markers in the SN compared to control subjects (Table 1). These indices of oxidation are not found in other brain regions unaffected in the disease. PD-linked mutations in genes encoding proteins such as DJ-1, a putative oxidative sensor (Bonifati et al., 2004), further support a causative role of oxidative stress in this disorder.

1.3. Dopamine-dependent Oxidative Stress: Evidence and Implications

Intracellularly, dopamine is either degraded by monoamine oxidase A (MAO-A) (Gotz et al., 1994) or by autooxidation. Dopamine metabolism by MAO-A leads to the production of dihydroxyphenylacetic acid (DOPAC) and H_2O_2 under the consumption of O_2 and H_2O (Maker et al., 1981; Gesi et al., 2001) (Figure 3). Intracellular autooxidation of dopamine generates H_2O_2 and dopamine-quinone (Graham, 1978; Sulzer and Zecca, 2000). The latter of which participates in nucleophilic addition reactions with protein sulfhydryl groups (Tse et al., 1976; Graham, 1978; Stokes et al., 1999), leading to structural modifications in proteins and reduced levels of the tripeptide thiol glutathione (GSH), the major redox buffer used by cells to counteract oxidative stress. In this context, dopamine-quinones were shown to inhibit glutamate and dopamine transporter function in synaptosomes (Berman et al., 1996; Berman and Hastings, 1997), inhibit tyrosine hydroxylase (TH) in cell free systems (Kuhn et al., 1999), and promote H^+ leakage from mitochondria resulting in uncoupling of respiration to ATP synthesis (Berman and Hastings, 1999; Khan et al., 2001).

H_2O_2, produced during the metabolism of dopamine (Graham, 1978; Maker et al., 1981), can be converted through the Fenton reaction in the presence of ferrous iron (Fe^{2+}) to hydroxyl radicals ($OH^•$). Hydroxyl radicals are highly reactive species capable of covalently modified cellular macromolecules including proteins. Iron-mediated catalysis of hydroxyl radicals could be a key pathogenic mechanism contributing to oxidative stress in PD, given that the iron levels in the SN are not only higher than in other areas of the brain (Gerlach et al., 1994), but are increased by approximately 35% in PD patients compared to age-matched controls (Sofic et al., 1988; Dexter et al., 1989). A similar increase in iron levels has not been found in progressive supranuclear palsy, a neurodegenerative disease of the brainstem, suggesting that increased iron levels are not a mere consequence of neurodegeneration (Hirsch et al., 1991). Thus, it appears that dopamine oxidation may underlie the selective vulnerability of dopaminergic neurons to cell death in PD.

Table 1. Evidence of oxidative stress in PD

Evidence	References
I. Experimental data	
• MPTP-treated mice show upregulation of iNOS and increased levels of nitrotyrosine	Liberatore et al., 1999
• iNOS knockout mice show decreased sensitivity to MPTP	Liberatore et al., 1999
• Mice overexpressing either Cu/Zn (cytoplasmic) or Mn (mitochondrial) superoxide dismutase are more resistant to MPTP, a combination of paraquat and maneb, and 6-OHDA	Przedborski et al., 1992; Callio et al., 2005; Thiruchelvam et al., 2005
• Cu/Zn knockout mice are more susceptible to MPTP	Zhang et al., 2000
• Glutathione peroxidase knockout mice are more susceptible to MPTP	Klivenyi et al., 2000; Zhang et a., 2000
• Both autooxidation and MAO-A dependent oxidation of dopamine leads to the production of H_2O_2, $O_2^{\bullet-}$, $OH^\bullet$, and dopamine quinones	Maker et al., 1981; Graham, 1978
• Dopamine metabolism by MAO-A increases GSSG levels in synaptosomes	Spina and Cohen, 1988
• MPP$^+$-induced Complex I inhibition leads to the formation of H_2O_2 and $O_2^{\bullet-}$	Kalivendi et al., 2003
• *Drosophila* overexpressing glutathione S-transferase are protected from dopaminergic neuronal loss	Whithworth et al., 2005
• Synthetic superoxide dismutase/catalase mimetics protects against dopaminergic cell death both *in vitro* and *in vivo*	Peng et al., 2005
II. Human data	
• Decreased levels of GSH in the SN of PD patients	Sofic et al., 1992; Pearce et al., 1997
• Increased levels superoxide dismutase activity in the SN of PD patients	Radunovic et al., 1997; Saggu et al., 1989
• Increased iron levels in the SN of healthy individuals and PD patients	Gerlach et al., 1994; Sofic et al., 1988; Dexter et al., 1989
• Increased levels of 8-hydroxyguanosine, protein carbonyls, and HNE in PD brains	Yoritaka et al., 1996; Alam et al, 1997; Zhang et al., 1999
• Increased levels of toxic dopamine derivatives (e.g. NM(R) salsollinol, DMDHIQ+) in the nigrostriatal system of PD patients	Maruyama et al., 1997
• Increased levels of cysteinyl-dopamine conjugates in the SN and putamen of deceased PD patients compared to controls	Spencer et al., 1998
• Uric acid protects against PD	de Lau et al., 2005

1.4.   Evidence of Oxidative Stress in PD

In addition to a wide body of experimental evidence suggesting that oxidative stress plays an active role in the pathogenesis of PD (*in vitro* and *in vivo* studies summarized in Table 1), post-mortem investigations have consistently shown that oxidative stress is a hallmark not only of healthy but diseased human nigral tissue

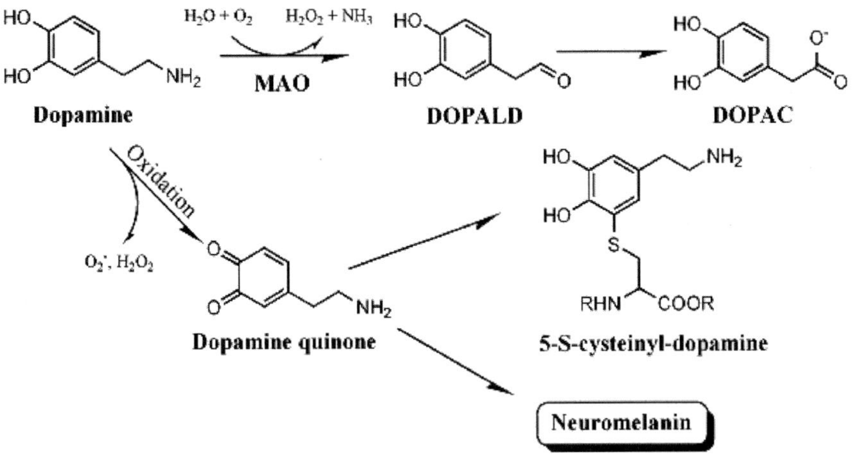

Figure 3. Oxidation of dopamine. Oxidation of dopamine by MAO or by autooxidation leads to the production of H_2O_2, which when converted to $OH^\bullet$ radicals, can lead to the oxidization of proteins, lipids and nucleosides. Autooxidation of dopamine also leads to the generation of dopamine-quinone, which may covalently bind to proteins or further be converted to neuromelanin. The modification of biomolecules by $OH^\bullet$ or dopamine quinone may exert toxic effects on dopaminergic neurons

(Table 1). Carbonyl modifications, which are indicative of protein oxidation, are increased 2-fold in the SN compared to the basal ganglia and prefrontal cortex of normal subjects (Floor and Wetzel, 1998). Levels of 4-hydroxy-2,3-nonenal (HNE), an aldehyde generated during lipid peroxidation and 8-hydroxyguanosine, a nucleoside oxidation product, are increased approximately 6- and 16-fold, respectively, in the SN of PD brains compared to controls (Yoritaka et al., 1996; Zhang et al., 1999). Decreased levels of GSH localized to surviving neurons in the SN in parkinsonian patients have also been reported (Sofic et al., 1992; Pearce et al., 1997). These reactive oxygen species (ROS) appear to arise from increased oxidation and metabolism of dopamine, since salsolinol, an endogenous dopamine-derived neurotoxin, appears to be elevated in the cerebrospinal fluid of newly diagnosed PD patients (Maruyama et al., 2000). In fact, cysteinyl-dopamine conjugates are found to be increased in the SN and putamen of PD patients compared to controls (Spencer et al., 1998).

2. INFLAMMATORY PROCESS IN PARKINSON'S DISEASE

2.1. Brain Inflammation in PD

The brain is an immunologically isolated site, largely sheltered from circulating cells and proteins of the immune system. A number of diseases that lead to injury of the central nervous system (CNS) are mediated by classic autoimmunity or inflammatory reactions in the brain. Multiple sclerosis is a typical autoimmune disease characterized by the breakdown of the blood-brain barrier

(BBB), recruitment of leukocytes and secretion of antibodies by plasma cells (Matyszak, 1998; van der Goes A. et al., 1999) Although dysfunction of midbrain efflux pumps for small molecules has recently been identified in the BBB of PD patients as assessed by positron emission tomography (PET) (Kortekaas et al., 2005), there is little evidence that either the BBB or the blood-cerebrospinal fluid barrier (CSF) are compromised in PD (Haussermann et al., 2001). Recently, Orr and colleagues observed IgG deposition at the surface of SN dopamine neurons in post-mortem PD brain samples without evidence of BBB compromise (Orr et al., 2005). However, classical inflammatory mediators such as acute-phase proteins, complement factors and cytokines can be rapidly induced in the brain (Allan and Rothwell, 2001). The role of inflammation in neurodegenerative conditions such as PD is not well understood, primarily because the events triggering the inflammatory response observed in PD are still obscure (see reviews by McGeer and McGeer, 2004; Hald and Lotharius, 2005).

2.2.   The Role of Astrocytes in Inflammation and in PD

In higher species, including humans, astrocytes are the most abundant cell type in the CNS, outnumbering neurons 10 to 1 (Magistretti and Ransom, 2002) Under physiological conditions, they are responsible for household tasks such as providing energy in the form of carbohydrates to neurons (Pellerin, 2005; Hertz, 2004), regulating cerebral blood flow as well as controlling water and ion homeostasis (Simard and Nedergaard, 2004). In addition to these functions, astrocytes are known to play an important role in modulating neuronal activity through the uptake and release of neurotransmitters such as glutamate and adenosine triphosphate (ATP) (Hertz et al., 1999; Volterra and Meldolesi, 2005).

In a wide range of neurological disorders, astrocytes undergo a remarkable transition from quiet nursing cells to a state, referred to as "reactive", in which, they bear some resemblance to cells of the immune system. They are distinguished from resting astrocytes by hypertrophy, proliferation (astrogliosis) and a changed gene expression (Sofroniew, 2005). In the reactive state, astrocytes secrete a wide variety of neurotrophic factors that may promote neuronal survival (Liberto et al., 2004) but also pro-inflammatory factors and putative neurotoxic factors such as ROS and reactive nitrogen species (RNS) (Hald and Lotharius, 2005; McNaught and Jenner, 2000; Cacquevel et al., 2004; Falsig et al., 2004; Chung and Benveniste, 1990). They also express MHC class II, making astrocytes antigen-presenting cells capable of driving inflammatory processes within the CNS (Benveniste et al., 1989).

Experimental and human data supporting the presence of reactive astrogliosis in PD is not as substantial as for activated microglia. Though several groups have reported astrogliosis, astrocytic hypertrophy and upregulation of the astrocyte marker glial fibrillary acidic protein (GFAP) in the 6-OHDA and MPTP animal models of PD (Miklossy et al., 2006; Reinhard et al., 1988; Chen et al., 2002; Stromberg et al., 1986; O'Callaghan and Seidler, 1992; Schneider and Denaro, 1988; Sheng et al., 1993), the same observations in PD patients are more sparse and have been disputed (Damier et al., 1993; Mirza et al., 2000; Schipper et al., 1998; Miklossy et al., 2006).

Theoretically there is good reason to believe that some degree of reactive astrogliosis could take place in PD, as cytokines such as tumor necrosis factor alpha (TNF-α), interleukin 1beta (IL-1β), IL-6, the levels of which are upregulated in PD patients as well as in animal models of PD, are capable of inducing astrocytes into their reactive state (Giulian et al., 1988; Selmaj et al., 1990) and stimulate astrocyte-mediated production of TNF-α, IL-1β, IL-6, ROS and nitric oxide (NO) (McNaught and Jenner, 2000; Chung and Benveniste, 1990; Benveniste et al., 1990; Lee et al., 1993; Cacquevel et al., 2004).

In CNS pathologies such as Alzheimer's disease (AD) (Yermakova and O'Banion, 2001), amyotrophic lateral sclerosis (Barbeito et al., 2004) and ischemia (Maslinska et al., 1999) as well as in *in vitro* (Xu et al., 2003; Falsig et al., 2004) and *in vivo* models of reactive astrogliosis (Minghetti, 2004), upregulation of cyclooxygenase-2 (COX-2) in astrocytes precedes an increase in prostaglandin synthesis (Xu et al., 2003; Falsig et al., 2004). This suggests that COX inhibitors could provide tools for treating CNS diseases involving reactive astrogliosis. Epidemiological data have shown that COX inhibitors have a beneficial effect on disease progression in AD patients whose brains are marked by widespread astrogliosis (In t' Veld et al., 2001). However, a one-year, controlled clinical trial using the non-specific COX inhibitor Naproxen and the selective COX-2 inhibitor Rofecoxib did not support these findings (Aisen et al., 2003).

The possibility that reactive astrocytes produce a combination of putative neurotrophic and neurotoxic factors could result in mixed beneficial and detrimental effects of utilizing COX inhibitors in regards to damaged or stressed neurons. Modulating or partly blocking the production of toxic substances from reactive astrocytes or enhancing the neuroprotective processes like increased GSH release, solely produced in the brain by astrocytes (Dringen and Hirrlinger, 2003), could turn out to be valuable as a PD therapy. Indeed, ONO-2506 (arundic acid) a specific modulator of reactive astrogliosis, blocks astrocytic expression of neuritic extension factor, S100B, nerve growth factor beta (NGF-β), COX-2 and inducible nitric oxide synthase (iNOS) while increasing the expression of GSH *in vitro* (Asano et al., 2005). In animal models of ischemia-induced brain damage and in the MPTP model of PD ONO-2506 was found to partially block neurodegeneration (Asano et al., 2005; Kato et al., 2003; Kato et al., 2004).

2.3. The Role of Microglia in Inflammation and in PD

Under normal conditions, microglia display a ramified morphology and are called "resting" microglia, but upon subtle changes in their micro-environment, or as a consequence of pathological changes, they rapidly transform into an activated state displaying a plastic amoeboid morphology (Kreutzberg, 1996). Microglial activation can be triggered by pathogenically-modified CNS proteins, antigens from infectious agents, such as the gram-negative bacterial cell wall component lipopolysaccharide

(LPS), prion proteins, or by a complex combination of biomolecules including ATP, cyclic adenosine monophosphate (cAMP), IL-1β, IL-6 and IL-10 (Hanisch, 2002; Nakamura, 2002). Activated microglia release pro-inflammatory molecules such as IL-1β, TNF-α, and NO, the overproduction of which can be neurotoxic. NO readily reacts with superoxide ($O_2^{\bullet-}$), also produced by activated microglia, to produce highly reactive peroxynitrite anions ($ONOO^-$). $ONOO^-$ can lead to DNA base modifications and strand breaks (Kennedy et al., 1997), as well as covalently modify tyrosine residues leading to a disruption of enzyme function and structural protein integrity, events that can trigger cellular apoptosis or necrosis (Beckman and Koppenol, 1996; Estevez and Jordan, 2002).

The proinflammatory cytokines TNF-α and IL-1 can also trigger direct toxicity in neurons (Allan and Rothwell, 2001; Clarke and Branton, 2002) and can potentiate an ongoing inflammatory response by enhancing microglial NO production (Possel et al., 2000; Hunot et al., 1999). Microglia activated with LPS upregulate levels of COX-2, a key enzyme responsible for the synthesis of inflammation-related prostaglandins (Hoozemans et al., 2002). The prostaglandins can be directly toxic to neurons through activation of caspase 3 or indirectly through astrocyte-mediated release of glutamate, increased levels of which have been linked to excitotoxicity (Consilvio et al., 2004). Whether microglial activation protects or exacerbates neuronal loss is presently debated (Hirsch et al., 2003), though a majority of evidence gained from both *in vitro* and *in vivo* studies suggests that activated microglia exert a toxic effect on neurons. However, moderately activated microglia appear to play a homeostatic role in the CNS by scavenging excess neurotoxins, removing dying cells and cellular debris (for review see Nakamura, 2002), and by promoting collateral sprouting in normal or injury states via the release of trophic factors like brain-derived neurotrophic factor (BDNF) (see review by Aloisi, 1999; Batchelor et al., 1999).

In PD, the degeneration of dopaminergic neurons is associated with robust microglial activation (McGeer et al., 1988; Fearnley and Lees, 1991; Imamura et al., 2003; Ouchi et al., 2005; Orr et al., 2005) which could be seen as an epiphenomenon rather than having a direct involvement in the pathogenesis of the disease. However, recent PET studies conducted in early-stage, untreated PD patients using a radiotracer for activated microglia, [^{11}C](R)-PK11195 and the dopamine transporter tracer [^{11}C]CFT demonstrated parallel changes in microglial activation and corresponding dopaminergic terminal loss in the nigrostriatal pathway in early PD (Ouchi et al., 2005). Furthermore, activation of microglia as visualised by PET scanning or immunohistochemistry is not a regionally-unspecific phenomenom in PD but is highly localized to the midbrain (Ouchi et al., 2005; Orr et al., 2005). These data support the view that neuroinflammatory responses mediated by microglia contribute significantly to the progressive degeneration process in the disease.

Animals treated with MPTP, rotenone and 6-OHDA exhibit levels of microglial activation similar to those found in PD (Cicchetti et al., 2002; Czlonkowska et al., 1996; Sherer et al., 2003). In the rotenone model, microglial activation was detected before the appearance of a dopaminergic lesion (Sherer et al., 2003). In post-mortem investigations of humans exposed to MPTP, activated microglia have been detected up to 16 years after the last drug exposure (McGeer et al., 2003). Activated microglia and dopaminergic cell loss are also found in the SN of primates years after they were treated with MPTP (Langston et al., 1999). These findings suggest that microglia play an active role in the pathology of PD and may indeed perpetuate the degeneration of dopaminergic neurons once activated. Both human and preclinical data supporting an active role of inflammation in PD are shown in Table 2.

Direct evidence that microglial activation can trigger cell loss comes from *in vivo* studies using LPS. Intranigral injection of LPS in rats results in activation

Table 2. Evidence of inflammation in PD

Evidence	References
I. Human data	
• Elevated level of antibodies to proteins modified by dopamine oxidation products in PD patients	Rowe et al., 1998
• Increased levels of cytokines in the CSF and striatum in PD brains	Blum-Degen et al., 1995; Mogi et al., 1994b Mogi et al., 1994a; Muller et al., 1998
• Increased number of activated microglia in PD brains	McGeer et al., 1988
• Sustained microglial activity in humans exposed to MPTP years after drug exposure	Langston et al., 1999
• Decreased risk of developing PD in regular NSAID users	Chen et al., 2003
II. Experimental data	
• Several animal models of PD (MPTP, rotenone and 6-OHDA) show microglial activation	Clcchetti et al., 2002; Czlonkowska et al., 1996 Sherer et al., 2003
• LPS-induced microglial activation leads to dopaminergic degeneration *in vitro* and *in vivo*	Gao et al., 2002; Wang et al., 2002; Liu et al., 2003; Gayle et al., 2002; Hemmer et al., 2001 Le et al., 2001; Castano et al., 1998; Herrera et al., 2000; Iravani et al., 2002; Li et al., 2004 Arimoto and Bing, 2003
• Conditioned medium from LPS-stimulated microglial cultures is toxic to neurons	Taylor et al., 2003
• COX-2 knockout mice show decreased responsiveness to MPTP	Feng et al., 2002
• Anti-Inflammatory drugs (VIP, Silymarin, Dextromethorphan, Minocycline and PPAR-*v*) are neuroprotective in several animal models of PD	Delgado and Ganea, 2003; Wang et al., 2002 Liu et al., 2003; Wu et al., 2002; Breider et al., 2002
• INOS is upregulated in experimental PD models	Iravani et al., 2002; Liberatore et al., 1999; Wu et al., 2002
• INOS inhibitors confer neuroprotection in PD models	Hemmer et al., 2001; Le et al., 2001; Iravani et al., 2002
• TNF-α, IL-1, IL-6 and NO are toxic to neurons	Sriram et al., 2002; Ma et al., 2002; Gayle et al., 2002; Liu et al., 2002; Allan and Rothwell, 2001 Fisher et al., 2001; Ladenheim et al., 2000 Campbell et al., 1993

of microglia and degeneration of the dopaminergic system (Castano et al., 1998; Herrera et al., 2000) These results are supported by *in vitro* experiments showing that mixed neuron-glia cultures treated with LPS rapidly display microglial activation and subsequently neuronal death (Gao et al., 2002). Experiments using microglial conditioned medium also demonstrate that the toxic effect of LPS on neurons is at least partly mediated by stable substances secreted from activated microglia and not by LPS acting directly on these cells (this is shown by the lack of neurotoxicity of LPS given to pure neuronal cultures) (Taylor et al., 2003).

2.4.   The Role of Cytokines in PD

In support of a role of inflammation in PD, the concentration of several inflammatory cytokines including TNF-α, IL-1β and IL-6, are found to be elevated in the CSF and basal ganglia of PD patients (Blum-Degen et al., 1995; Mogi et al., 1994a and 1994b; Muller et al., 1998). For instance, TNF-α levels in patients with PD were increased by 366% in the striatum and by 432% in the CSF (Mogi et al., 1994b). Furthermore, post-mortem histopathological studies have reported increased immunoreactivity for TNF-α and IL-1β in activated glial cells in the SN of PD patients (Boka et al., 1994; Hunot et al., 1999).

In humans, TNF-α receptor (TNF-R)-1, but not TNF-R2, is expressed in dopaminergic neurons of the SN (Hirsch et al., 2003). While the exact role of TNF-α and its two receptors is not completely understood, the observation that mice lacking both TNF-α receptors are resistant to MPTP may underline the importance of TNF-α in PD. However, the effect of MPTP in mice lacking TNF-R1 or TNF-R2 or both TNF receptors is disputed (Rousselet et al., 2002). Aditionnally, both *in vivo* and *in vitro* studies using TNF-R1 and TNF-R2 knockout mice suggest that activation of TNF-R1 is toxic to neurons while activation of TNF-R2 is neuroprotective (Fontaine et al., 2002; Kassiotis and Kollias, 2001). This could explain the conflicting reports describing neurotoxic or neuroprotective properties of TNF-α depending on experimental set-up and cell types examined (Barger et al., 1995; Hemmer et al., 2001; Zassler et al., 2003). Exposing mesencephalic cultures to TNF-α triggers dopaminergic cell death by apoptosis, while non-dopaminergic cells remain unaffected (Clarke and Branton, 2002). Gayle et al. (2002) reported that the toxic effect of LPS on rat primary dopaminergic neurons co-cultured with microglia is reduced to approximately 50% by the addition of neutralizing antibodies to TNF-α, while Le et al (2001) observed no effect of such neutralizing antibodies in a similar system using a rat dopaminergic cell line (MES 23.5) cultured with primary microglia, which could be explained by differences in receptor expression or signaling between the dopaminergic cell line and primary dopaminergic cells. Nevertheless, the toxic effects of TNF-α on dopaminergic neurons is still under question.

The signal transduction pathway downstream of the IL-1 receptor interconnects with that of TNF-R1 in terms of activation/translocation of the transcription factors nuclear factor kappa beta (NF-κB) and c-Jun. However, work is still needed to elucidate the various effects of IL-1 receptor activation on the regulation of cell survival and death (Martin and Wesche, 2002). Results from *in vivo* experiments suggest that IL-1β is toxic to neurons, while *in vitro* experiments using low- to moderate concentrations of IL-1β often report a neuroprotective effect (Allan and Rothwell, 2001). IL-1β-neutralizing antibodies have been shown to significantly abrogate neuronal toxicity induced by microglia in cortical neuron-microglial co-cultures treated with LPS and INF-γ (Ma et al., 2002). A similar result has been reported for primary dopaminergic neuron-microglial co-cultures activated with LPS (Gayle et al., 2002). This suggests that IL-1β can work in concert with other mediators to induce toxicity in neurons but is not toxic when administered alone. In contrast to these findings, another group did not find a protective effect of IL-1β-neutralizing antibodies on LPS-activated microglia-mediated toxicity on a murine dopaminergic cell line (MES 23.5) (Le et al., 2001). The discrepancy between these results could again reflect different endpoints for measuring toxicity or lower susceptibility to IL-1β in the dopaminergic cell line compared to primary neurons.

Binding of IL-6 to its receptor leads to the activation of signal transducers and activators of transcription (STAT) and members of the mitogen activated protein kinase (MAPK) pathway that have been shown to protect human tumor cells from apoptosis induced by staurosporine (Leu et al., 2003). Nevertheless, IL-6 knockout mice show reduced neurodegeneration in response to experimental autoimmune encephalitis, a model of multiple sclerosis, and glutamate toxicity (Fisher et al., 2001), suggesting that IL-6 has neurotoxic properties. These findings are supported by the decreased dopaminergic toxicity found in IL-6 knockout mice exposed to methamphetamine, which induces nigrostriatal degeneration, (Ladenheim et al., 2000) as well as from examinations of mice overexpressing IL-6, which exhibit spontaneous neuronal degeneration (Campbell et al., 1993). In contrast to this, IL-6, which is upregulated at the mRNA level in the striatum of mice injected with MPTP (Ciesielska et al., 2003), has been shown to rescue cultured dopaminergic neurons exposed to the active, neurotoxic metabolite of MPTP, 1-methyl-4-phenylpyridium ion (MPP^+), in a dose-dependent manner (Akaneya et al., 1995). Thus, IL-6 may have both neuroprotective and neurotoxic effects on dopaminergic neurons.

2.5. The Role of NO in PD

Reports on rodent models of PD have implicated NO in cell death. For example, nigral injection of LPS in rats resulted in upregulation of iNOS and NO production and led to the loss of dopaminergic neurons, which could be effectively blocked by iNOS inhibitors (Iravani et al., 2002; Arimoto and Bing, 2003). *In vitro*, direct inhibition of iNOS reduced the toxicity of LPS or LPS and INF-γ activated microglia on dopaminergic neurons by 75% (Hemmer et al., 2001; Le et al., 2001). Mice treated with the parkinsonian pro-toxin, MPTP, also showed increased levels of iNOS in the SN (Liberatore et al., 1999). Consistent with a contributory role of this enzyme in MPTP toxicity, iNOS deficient mice were more resistant to MPTP-induced dopaminergic cell loss than their wild-type littermates (Liberatore et al.,

1999). However, studies with NO donors have shown that NO is sufficient to kill various neuronal subtypes, but that the concentration of NO has to be higher (high μM to low mM) than what is produced by microglial cultures exposed to LPS (Liu et al., 2002). Moreover, human microglial cells, unlike rodent, are found to produce very little NO (McGeer and McGeer, 2004). Therefore, it is still uncertain whether NO plays an important role in PD.

2.6.   The Role of Complement in Neurodegeneration in PD

The complement system is a key component of the innate immune system (for review see Frank and Fries, 1991). Functions of the complement system include (i) defence against invading pathogens by triggering the generation of the membranolytic C5b-9 complex, known as the membrane attack complex (MAC), and complement fragments (named opsonins, i.e., C1q, C3b and iC3b) mediating phagocytosis. Soluble complement anaphylatoxins (C4a, C3a and C5a) control the local pro-inflammatory response through the chemotaxis and activation of leukocytes; (ii) safe disposal of immune complexes and the products of the inflammatory injury (e.g., toxic cell debris and apoptotic corpses) to ensure the protection and healing of the host. The regulatory mechanisms of complement are finely balanced so that, on the one hand, invading micro-organisms are recognized and killed and, on the other hand, deposition of complement on normal "self" cells is limited by several key complement regulators. However, if inadequately controlled, the complement cascade may cause bystander lysis and stimulate inflammation.

Complement activation has been demonstrated in numerous inflammatory and degenerative diseases of the brain including multiple sclerosis, AD, ischemic stroke and trauma (see reviews by Barnum, 2002; van Beek et al., 2003). Immunostaining for complement activation products of the classical pathway and the MAC is seen in the SN in PD (Yamada et al., 1992). C1q and C9 mRNA levels are increased in the SN and caudate nucleus (McGeer and McGeer, 2004) suggesting that complement proteins found in PD brains may originate from local synthesis. Indeed, in the CNS, astrocytes, microglia, and nerve cells are, together, capable of providing a functional intraparenchymal complement system (Morgan and Gasque, 1996). Recently, postmortem analysis of idiopathic and genetic PD cases showed pigmented dopamine neurons coated with IgG and associated with activated microglia (Orr et al., 2005). Moreover, there was a strong association between neuronal IgG labelling in PD and progression of neurodegeneration (Orr et al., 2005).

Opsonisation of dopamine neurones may contribute to the pathogenesis of dopamine neuronal cell death by triggering activation of the classical complement cascade (Frank and Fries, 1991). The presence of antibodies recognizing specific epitopes of dopaminergic neurons in serum from PD patients as well as their capability to induce neuronal damage has been previously suggested (Defazio et al., 1994). Indeed, exposure of mesencephalic neuronal cultures to serum from PD patients induced cell death only in the presence of complement (Defazio et al.,

1994). Although the mediator responsible for complement activation in serum was not identified, work by (Orr et al., 2005) suggests it could be IgG. Alternatively, C1q can bind specifically to the membrane of neurons, leading to spontaneous activation of the classical pathway in an antibody-independent manner and to cell death (Singhrao et al., 2000; van Beek et al., 2005). Studies are warranted to clarify the role of complement activation in the neurodegeneration process observed in PD.

2.7. Linking Pathogenic Mechanisms in Nigral Dopaminergic Neurons to Activation of Surrounding Microglia

Though it is clear that degeneration of dopaminergic neurons leads to the activation of microglia, the exact mechanism whereby this occurs remains unknown. Direct interaction between neurons and microglia was found to be important for microglial activation in neuron-microglial co-cultures (Sudo et al., 1998). Immunohisto-chemical examination of SN from PD patients, showed major histocompatibility complex II (HLA) and IgG receptor expression on microglial cells and IgG bound to dopaminergic neurons (Orr et al., 2005). A subset of PD patients were found to produce antibodies against proteins that were modified by dopamine oxidation products (Rowe et al., 1998), and microglia exposed to a combination of antibodies from PD patients and to dopamine-quinone or H_2O_2-modified dopaminergic cell membranes showed signs of activation such as ROS and cytokine production (Le et al., 2001).

HNE is capable of inducing COX-2 in macrophages, the peripheral counterpart to microglia (Kumagai et al., 2004), suggesting yet another mechanism of microglial activation in PD. Furthermore, neuromelanin, which is released by dying dopamin-ergic neurons, was shown to activate microglia *in vitro* (Wilms et al., 2003) and complement proteins have been found to be associated with filamentous inclusions known as Lewy bodies (Yamada et al., 1992), which may result from accumulating mutant, abnormal or oxidized proteins (Betarbet et al., 2005). These findings suggest a possible link between oxidative stress from dopamine metabolism to the inflam-matory reactions reported in PD. Furthermore, in pathophysiological conditions not related to PD, such as systemic lupus erythematosus and rheumatoid arthritis, ROS-modified DNA has been suggested to play an important role in the development of autoimmunity (Ahsan et al., 2003), and in atherogenesis, oxidized low-density lipoproteins may potentiate the inflammatory reaction through scavenger receptors, leading to increased cytokine production from macrophages (Osterud and Bjorklid, 2003). This suggests that ROS may lead to or potentiate an inflammatory reaction through modifications of biomolecules.

Stressed dopaminergic neurons may be more susceptible to toxic mediators secreted by activated microglia (Figure 4). For instance, MPP^+ or rotenone enhance LPS-induced, microglia-mediated superoxide release in mixed neuron-glia mesen-cephalic cultures resulting in greater toxicity of primary dopaminergic neurons

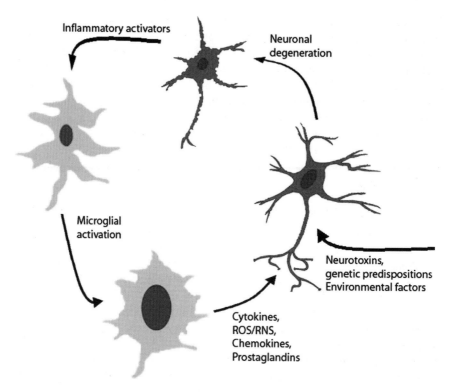

Figure 4. Neuron-microglia interactions in PD. Neurons whose viability has been compromised by an intracellular insult such as dopamine-derived metabolites may release factors that activate resting microglia. In experimental conditions, microglia activated directly by pro-inflammatory agents such as LPS or indirectly by dying neurons in human disease may induce or exacerbate neuronal toxicity. This could result in a self-amplifying cycle of inflammatory-mediated neurodegeneration

(Gao et al., 2003a and 2003b). If activated microglia indeed exacerbate neurode-generative processes in PD and in animal models of the disease, blocking their activation with anti-inflammatory drugs should lead to increased neuronal survival. Indeed, vasoactive intestinal peptide (VIP), a neuropeptide with anti-inflammatory effects, blocked microglial activation in mesencephalic cultures induced by MPP$^+$. This was shown by a decrease in microglial TNF-α production and accompanying increase in dopaminergic cell survival. A similar effect of VIP was found in mice treated with MPTP (Delgado and Ganea, 2003).

In vitro, silymarin and dextromethorphan both prevented microglial activation by LPS and the ensuing dopaminergic degeneration in mesencephalic neuron-glia cultures (Wang et al., 2002; Liu et al., 2003). Furthermore, dextromethorphan did not have a rescuing effect on pure dopaminergic cultures treated with MPP$^+$, suggesting that its effect was mediated by a blockade of microglial activation and not through general neuroprotection (Liu et al., 2003). Lastly, the tetracycline derivative, minocycline, currently in clinical trials for PD, has been shown to block microglial activation and protect against nigrostriatal dopaminergic neurodegeneration in animals treated with parkinsonian neurotoxins such as 6-OHDA and MPTP (see review by Thomas and Le, 2004). However, recent reports claim that although minocycline is able to decrease microglial activation it fails to afford neuroprotection in response to MPTP (Sriram et al., 2006) and has even been shown to worsen motor dysfunction in monkeys treated with this toxin (Diguet et al., 2004). Nevertheless, the neuroprotective efficacy of a majority of anti-inflammatory compounds in various animal models of PD suggests not only that inflammation contributes to dopaminergic cell loss but that anti-inflammatory therapies might be useful for treating PD.

2.8. Cyclooxygenases Revisited

NSAIDs induce their pharmacological effect through inhibition of the cyclooxygenase enzymes (Vane, 1971), which are key enzymes in the metabolism of arachidonic acid into prostanoids (Smith et al., 1996). After arachidonic acid is released from the plasma membrane by phospholipase A_2, the COX enzymes catalyze, at first, the rate limiting cyclooxygenase reaction in which arachidonic acid is converted to PGG_2 and next a peroxidation of PGG_2 to PGH_2, which is further metabolized to different prostanoids (PGD_2, PGE_2, $PGF_{2\alpha}$, TxA2, PGI_2) (Figure 5). (Patrignani et al., 2005; Smith et al., 1996). In humans, two different COX enzymes exist, denoted COX-1 and COX-2. COX-1 is constitutively expressed in various tissues and its products serve a variety of functions, such as controlling platelet aggregation, renal blood flow regulation and cytoprotection of the stomach. However, the inducible COX-2 is mainly expressed in the cells of the immune system and its degree of expression seems to depend on regulation of mRNA stability and rate of transcription, which is, in turn, regulated through a complicated network of signalling cascades involving NF-κB, p38 MAPK, C-jun N terminal kinase (JNK), and extracellular signal regulated kinases (ERK1/2) (Chun and Surh, 2004).

Among the intercellular signalling molecules capable of inducing transcription of the COX-2 genes and a concomitant release of prostaglandins are the classical proinflammatory compounds TNF-α (Yamamoto et al., 1995), IL-1β (Guan et al., 1998) and IFN-γ (Falsig et al., 2004), which may also produce synergistic effects (Falsig et al., 2004). Furthermore, the inflammatory initiator LPS triggers extensive upregulation of COX-2 and prostaglandin synthesis in immune cells such as macrophages and microglia (Lee et al., 1992; Ikeda-Matsuo et al., 2005).

The mechanism whereby NSAIDs inhibit the COX enzymes depends on the specific type of drug and ranges from reversible inhibition by ibuprofen to irreversible acetylation in the active site by aspirin (Walker et al., 2001; Roth et al., 1975). The human COX-1 and COX-2 share approximately 60% amino acid homology (Hla and Neilson, 1992) but a single amino acid difference in the active site between the two isoenzymes has made the synthesis of selective COX-2 inhibitors (coxibs) possible in recent years (Gierse et al., 1996; Warner and Mitchell,

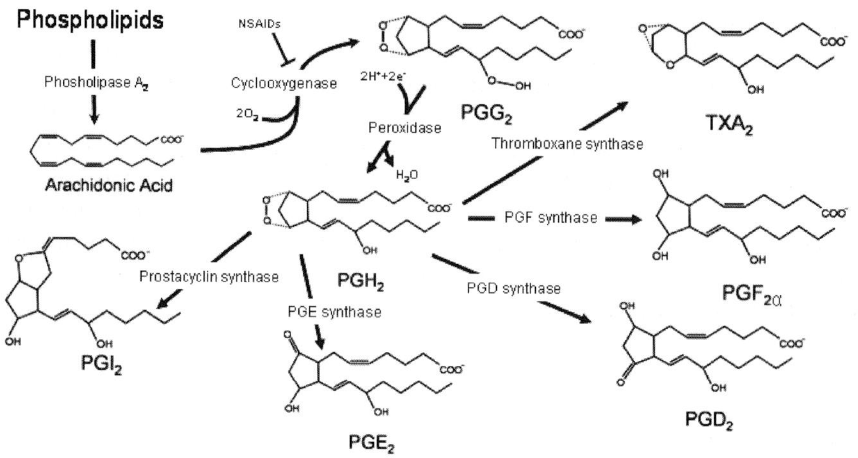

Figure 5. Metabolism of arachidonic acid into prostanoids

2004). The main pharmaceutical argument for developing coxibs is to produce drugs with the beneficial effects of regular NSAIDs on pain and inflammation but without the adverse effects of COX-1 inhibition, especially the ones related to the gastrointestinal tract (Graham and Chan, 2004). Clinical trials have now shown that coxibs induce fewer gastrointestinal complications compared to non-selective COX inhibitors (Silverstein et al., 2000; Schnitzer et al., 2004; Mamdani et al., 2002; Norgard et al., 2004), while disturbing data has emerged suggesting an increased rate of cardiovascular complications following coxib treatment.

2.9.   The Effect of COX Inhibition on Neurotoxicity

Surmounting evidence suggests a neuroprotective role of COX inhibition in various models of neuropathology. For instance, ibuprofen has proven beneficial in a mouse model of AD (Lim et al., 2000) and rofecoxib (a selective COX-2 inhibitor) has been shown to block both astrocytic and microglial activation in response to quisqualic acid injection into the nucleus basalis in rats and ensuing neuronal death (Scali et al., 2003). SC58125 (a selective COX-2 inhibitor) protects against ischemia-induced neurotoxicity (Nakayama et al., 1998). In the same way, microglial activation and ensuing neurotoxic effect of LPS infusion into the CNS are both blocked by administration of CI987 (a selective COX-2 inhibitor) (Willard et al., 2000).

In relation to PD, MPTP administration in mice has been shown to induce an upregulation of COX-2 mRNA and protein followed by prostaglandin synthesis while COX-1 expression remains unaltered (Przybylkowski et al., 2004; Hunot et al., 2004). Blocking the activity of the COX enzymes by ibuprofen (a non-selective COX inhibitor) leads to neuroprotection in pure mesencephalic neurons against both MPP^+- and 6-OHDA-induced toxicity (Carrasco et al., 2005) and selective COX-2 inhibitors are found to reduce dopaminergic cell death in response to MPP^+ in mixed dopaminergic neuron-glia cultures (Wang et al., 2005) as well in co-cultures containing microglia actived by a combination of IFN-γ and CD40 agonists (Okuno et al., 2005).

In support of a beneficial effect of COX inhibition in PD, both acetylsalicylic acid and meloxicam (a selective COX-2 inhibitor) were found to protect mice from MPTP intoxication (Teismann and Ferger, 2001; Mohanakumar et al., 2000) and celecoxib (a selective COX-2 inhibitor) was found to protect mice from 6-OHDA-induced toxicity (Sanchez-Pernaute et al., 2004). In contrast, rofecoxib did not rescue dopaminergic neurons in mice treated with MPTP (Przybylkowski et al., 2004), though the different outcome of these two experiments could result from different experimental techniques and treatment protocols. In agreement with findings suggesting a fundamental role of COX-2 in PD pathology, COX-2 knockout mice have marked resistance against MPTP-induced toxicity (Feng et al., 2002; Feng et al., 2003; Hunot et al., 2004).

2.10. The Effect of Anti-inflammatory Drugs in Parkinson's Disease

Whether inflammatory reactions play a beneficial or detrimental role in the pathogenesis of PD, by blocking microglial activation or the effect of specific inflammatory mediators on dopaminergic neurons, remains to be determined. Therefore, it is difficult to predict whether an anti-inflammatory drug would alter disease progression. One caveat to using anti-inflammatory therapy for neurodegenerative disorders is that the type of anti-inflammatory drugs shown to arrest progression of dopaminergic cell loss in animal models of PD are likely not suitable for long-term use in humans, as in the case of steroids. Thus, assuming that their use is beneficial in halting ongoing cell loss, addressing what types of anti-inflammatory drugs are adequate for the treatment of PD is of utmost importance.

In deceased PD patients and normal subjects, dopaminergic neurons express COX-2, while COX-2 expression in microglia and astrocytes is found only in PD (Knott et al., 2000). Comparing the intake of NSAIDs by a large cohort of Americans (n = 50, 000) showed that the risk for developing PD in persons regularly taking NSAIDs was decreased by 45% (Chen et al., 2003). This finding was later confirmed by analysing epidemiological data from another large American cohort where ibuprofen but not aspirin was found to decrease the risk of developing PD (Chen et al., 2005). Thus, the use of NSAIDs may result in neuroprotection in PD, though mechanisms other than the modulation of inflammatory state cannot be ruled out.

For instance, the ability of NSAIDs to scavenge $OH^\bullet$ and NO could result in protection of dopaminergic neurons exposed to oxidative stress (Chen et al., 2003). Deletion of COX-2 in mice resulted in protection against MPTP-induced dopaminergic cell loss (Feng et al., 2002), suggesting that NSAIDs do in fact exert their neuroprotective effects via inhibition of COX-2. However, a recent report claimed that the neuroprotective effect of COX-2 inhibition against MPTP *in vivo* was not due to decreased microglial activation but was more likely related to the blockade of COX-2-mediated dopamine oxidation by COX-2 inhibitors (Teismann et al., 2003). Indeed, COX-2 has been shown to catalyse the oxidation of dopamine to dopamine-quinone in the presence of H_2O_2 *in vitro* (Hastings, 1995). Thus, blocking COX-2 may lead to a decrease in neurotoxic cysteinyl-dopamine-mediated protein modifications *in vivo*. In conclusion, the exact mechanism that lies behind COX inhibition mediated-neuroprotection in PD models is still largely unknown; it may depend on blockade of an inflammatory response, decreased oxidation of dopamine by the COX-enzymes or a combination of the two.

Agonists of the peroxisome proliferator-activated receptor-γ (PPAR-γ), which has anti-inflammatory qualities, have been found to attenuate glial activation and rescue nigral dopaminergic cells in MPTP-treated mice. Again, PPAR-γ agonists may induce direct dopaminergic protection against MPP$^+$ toxicity by increasing neuronal glucose uptake, which would, turn, decrease glial activation (Breidert et al., 2002). A derivative of a naturally occurring rocaglamid, referred to as compound A, exhibits anti-inflammatory characteristics such as decreasing cytokine and NO production in glial cells. Compound A rescues dopaminergic neurons from MPP$^+$-induced toxicity *in vitro* and MPTP *in vivo* (Fahrig et al., 2005). Lastly, as mentioned earlier, minocycline, a putative blocker of microglial activation which has shown mixed benefits in animal models of PD, is currently in clinical trials for this condition.

2.11.   A Vicious Cycle

The agent responsible for triggering dopaminergic toxicity in the SN of PD patients is yet unknown. However, the neurotransmitter dopamine itself may induce dopaminergic toxicity through mitochondrial inhibition, and dopamine breakdown products such as ROS and dopamine-quinones may trigger toxicity through deleterious modifications important cellular macromolecules. Such modified biomolecules as well as neuromelanin released from dying dopaminergic neurons could activate microglia, which in turn may lead to increased dopaminergic toxicity through the production of cytokines, ROS, and/or RNS. This may lead to the generation of a vicious cycle that further increases dopaminergic toxicity in the SN (Figure 4). A better understanding of how inflammatory reactions are initiated in PD and what the specific effects of various inflammatory mediators are on dopaminergic neurons of the SN may lead to a new generation of disease-modifying treatments for PD.

ACKNOWLEDGEMENTS

Part of this work was supported by a grant from The Danish University of Pharmaceutical Sciences. We would like to thank Dr. Arne Schousboe for critically reading this manuscript.

ABBREVIATIONS

ATP	adenosine triphosphate
cAMP	cclic adenosine monophosphate
BBB	blood brain barrier
BDNF	brain derived neurotrophic factor
CNS	central nervous system
CSF	cerebral spinal fluid
COX-1	cyclooxygenase-1
COX-2	cyclooxygenase-2
DOPAC	dihydroxyphenylacetic acid
DOPALD	dihydroxyphenylacetaldehyde
eNOS	endothelial nitric oxide synthase
ERK1/2	extracellular signal-regulated kinases 1/2
GFAP	glial fibrillary acidic protein
GSH	reduced glutathione
GSSG	oxidized glutathione
H_2O	water
H_2O_2	hydrogen peroxide
HLA	major histocompatibility complex II
HNE	4-hydroxy-2,3-nonenal
6-OHDA	6-hydroxydopamine
IFN-γ	interferon-gamma
IL	interleukin
iNOS	inducible NOS
JNK	c-Jun N-terminal kinase
LPS	lipopolysaccharide
MAC	membrane attack complex
MAO	monoamine oxidase
MAPK	mitogen-activated protein kinase
MPP^+	1-methyl-4-phenylpyridium ion
MPTP	1-methyl-4-phenyl-1,2,3,6-tetrahydropyridine
NGF	nerve growth factor
nNOS	neuronal NOS
NO	nitric oxide
NOS	nitric oxide synthase
NSAIDs	non-steroidal anti-inflammatory drugs
NF-κB	nuclear factor-kappaB
$O_2{}^{\bullet-}$	superoxide anion
$OH^\bullet$	hydroxyl radical
PD	Parkinson's disease
PET	positron emission tomography
PHOX	phagocyte oxidase
POLG	DNA polymerase g

RNS reactive nitrogen species
ROS reactive oxygen species
S100B neurite extension factor
SN substantia nigra
STAT signal transducer and activator of transcription
TH tyrosine hydroxylase
TNF tumor necrosis factor
TNF-R tumor necrosis factor receptor
TxA2 collagen-induced thromboxane-A2
UCHL1 ubiquitin carboxyl-terminal hydrolase 1
UPS ubiquitin-proteasome system
VIP vasoactive intestinal peptide

REFERENCES

Abou-Sleiman PM, Muqit MM, Wood NW (2006) Expanding insights of mitochondrial dysfunction in Parkinson's disease. Nat Rev Neurosci 7:207–219.

Ahsan H, Ali A, Ali R (2003) Oxygen free radicals and systemic autoimmunity. Clin Exp Immunol 131:398–404.

Aisen PS, Schafer KA, Grundman M, Pfeiffer E, Sano M, Davis KL, Farlow MR, Jin S, Thomas RG, Thal LJ (2003) Effects of rofecoxib or naproxen vs placebo on Alzheimer disease progression: a randomized controlled trial. JAMA 289:2819–2826.

Akaneya Y, Takahashi M, Hatanaka H (1995) Interleukin-1 beta enhances survival and interleukin-6 protects against MPP+ neurotoxicity in cultures of fetal rat dopaminergic neurons. Exp Neurol 136:44–52.

Allan SM, Rothwell NJ (2001) Cytokines and acute neurodegeneration. Nat Rev Neurosci 2:734–744.

Aloisi F (1999) The role of microglia and astrocytes in CNS immune surveillance and immunopathology. Adv Exp Med Biol 468:123–133.

Arimoto T, Bing G (2003) Up-regulation of inducible nitric oxide synthase in the substantia nigra by lipopolysaccharide causes microglial activation and neurodegeneration. Neurobiol Dis 12:35–45.

Asano T, Mori T, Shimoda T, Shinagawa R, Satoh S, Yada N, Katsumata S, Matsuda S, Kagamiishi Y, Tateishi N (2005) Arundic acid (ONO-2506) ameliorates delayed ischemic brain damage by preventing astrocytic overproduction of S100B. Curr Drug Targets CNS Neurol Disord 4:127–142.

Barbeito LH, Pehar M, Cassina P, Vargas MR, Peluffo H, Viera L, Estevez AG, Beckman JS (2004) A role for astrocytes in motor neuron loss in amyotrophic lateral sclerosis. Brain Res Brain Res Rev 47:263–274.

Barger SW, Horster D, Furukawa K, Goodman Y, Krieglstein J, Mattson MP (1995) Tumor necrosis factors alpha and beta protect neurons against amyloid beta-peptide toxicity: evidence for involvement of a kappa B-binding factor and attenuation of peroxide and Ca2+ accumulation. Proc Natl Acad Sci U S A 92:9328–9332.

Barnum SR (2002) Complement in central nervous system inflammation. Immunol Res 26:7–13.

Batchelor PE, Liberatore GT, Wong JY, Porritt MJ, Frerichs F, Donnan GA, Howells DW (1999) Activated macrophages and microglia induce dopaminergic sprouting in the injured striatum and express brain-derived neurotrophic factor and glial cell line-derived neurotrophic factor. J Neurosci 19:1708–1716.

Beckman JS, Koppenol WH (1996) Nitric oxide, superoxide, and peroxynitrite: the good, the bad, and ugly. Am J Physiol 271:C1424–C1437.

Benveniste EN, Sparacio SM, Bethea JR (1989) Tumor necrosis factor-alpha enhances interferon-gamma-mediated class II antigen expression on astrocytes. J Neuroimmunol 25:209–219.

Benveniste EN, Sparacio SM, Norris JG, Grenett HE, Fuller GM (1990) Induction and regulation of interleukin-6 gene expression in rat astrocytes. J Neuroimmunol 30:201–212.

Berman SB, Hastings TG (1999) Dopamine oxidation alters mitochondrial respiration and induces permeability transition in brain mitochondria: implications for Parkinson's disease. J Neurochem 73:1127–1137.

Berman SB, Hastings TG (1997) Inhibition of glutamate transport in synaptosomes by dopamine oxidation and reactive oxygen species. J Neurochem 69:1185–1195.

Berman SB, Zigmond MJ, Hastings TG (1996) Modification of dopamine transporter function: effect of reactive oxygen species and dopamine. J Neurochem 67:593–600.

Betarbet R, Sherer TB, Greenamyre JT (2005) Ubiquitin-proteasome system and Parkinson's diseases. Exp Neurol 191(1):S17–S27.

Blum-Degen D, Muller T, Kuhn W, Gerlach M, Przuntek H, Riederer P (1995) Interleukin-1 beta and interleukin-6 are elevated in the cerebrospinal fluid of Alzheimer's and de novo Parkinson's disease patients. Neurosci Lett 202:17–20.

Boka G, Anglade P, Wallach D, Javoy-Agid F, Agid Y, Hirsch EC (1994) Immunocytochemical analysis of tumor necrosis factor and its receptors in Parkinson's disease. Neurosci Lett 172:151–154.

Bonifati V, Oostra BA, Heutink P (2004) Linking DJ-1 to neurodegeneration offers novel insights for understanding the pathogenesis of Parkinson's disease. J Mol Med 82:163–174.

Breidert T, Callebert J, Heneka MT, Landreth G, Launay JM, Hirsch EC (2002) Protective action of the peroxisome proliferator-activated receptor-gamma agonist pioglitazone in a mouse model of Parkinson's disease. J Neurochem 82:615–624.

Cacquevel M, Lebeurrier N, Cheenne S, Vivien D (2004) Cytokines in neuroinflammation and Alzheimer's disease. Curr Drug Targets 5:529–534.

Campbell IL, Abraham CR, Masliah E, Kemper P, Inglis JD, Oldstone MB, Mucke L (1993) Neurologic disease induced in transgenic mice by cerebral overexpression of interleukin 6. Proc Natl Acad Sci U S A 90:10061–10065.

Carrasco E, Casper D, Werner P (2005) Dopaminergic neurotoxicity by 6-OHDA and MPP+: differential requirement for neuronal cyclooxygenase activity. J Neurosci Res 81:121–131.

Castano A, Herrera AJ, Cano J, Machado A (1998) Lipopolysaccharide intranigral injection induces inflammatory reaction and damage in nigrostriatal dopaminergic system. J Neurochem 70:1584–1592.

Chen H, Jacobs E, Schwarzschild MA, McCullough ML, Calle EE, Thun MJ, Ascherio A (2005) Nonsteroidal antiinflammatory drug use and the risk for Parkinson's disease. Ann Neurol 58:963–967.

Chen H, Zhang SM, Hernan MA, Schwarzschild MA, Willett WC, Colditz GA, Speizer FE, Ascherio A (2003) Nonsteroidal anti-inflammatory drugs and the risk of Parkinson disease. Arch Neurol 60:1059–1064.

Chen LW, Wei LC, Qiu Y, Liu HL, Rao ZR, Ju G, Chan YS (2002) Significant up-regulation of nestin protein in the neostriatum of MPTP-treated mice. Are the striatal astrocytes regionally activated after systemic MPTP administration? Brain Res 925:9–17.

Chun KS, Surh YJ (2004) Signal transduction pathways regulating cyclooxygenase-2 expression: potential molecular targets for chemoprevention. Biochem Pharmacol 68:1089–1100.

Chung IY, Benveniste EN (1990) Tumor necrosis factor-alpha production by astrocytes. Induction by lipopolysaccharide, IFN-gamma, and IL-1 beta. J Immunol 144:2999–3007.

Cicchetti F, Brownell AL, Williams K, Chen YI, Livni E, Isacson O (2002) Neuroinflammation of the nigrostriatal pathway during progressive 6-OHDA dopamine degeneration in rats monitored by immunohistochemistry and PET imaging. Eur J Neurosci 15:991–998.

Ciesielska A, Joniec I, Przybylkowski A, Gromadzka G, Kurkowska-Jastrzebska I, Czlonkowska A, Czlonkowski A (2003) Dynamics of expression of the mRNA for cytokines and inducible nitric synthase in a murine model of the Parkinson's disease. Acta Neurobiol Exp (Wars) 63:117–126.

Clarke DJ, Branton RL (2002) A role for tumor necrosis factor alpha in death of dopaminergic neurons following neural transplantation. Exp Neurol 176:154–162.

Consilvio C, Vincent AM, Feldman EL (2004) Neuroinflammation, COX-2, and ALS–a dual role? Exp Neurol 187:1–10.

Cookson MR, Xiromerisiou G, Singleton A (2005) How genetics research in Parkinson's disease is enhancing understanding of the common idiopathic forms of the disease. Curr Opin Neurol 18:706–711.

Czlonkowska A, Kohutnicka M, Kurkowska-Jastrzebska I, Czlonkowski A (1996) Microglial reaction in MPTP (1-methyl-4-phenyl-1,2,3,6-tetrahydropyridine) induced Parkinson's disease mice model. Neurodegeneration 5:137–143.

Damier P, Hirsch EC, Zhang P, Agid Y, Javoy-Agid F (1993) Glutathione peroxidase, glial cells and Parkinson's disease. Neuroscience 52:1–6.

Dauer W, Przedborski S (2003) Parkinson's disease: mechanisms and models. Neuron 39:889–909.

Defazio G, Dal TR, Benvegnu D, Minozzi MC, Cananzi AR, Leon A (1994) Parkinsonian serum carries complement-dependent toxicity for rat mesencephalic dopaminergic neurons in culture. Brain Res 633:206–212.

Delgado M, Ganea D (2003) Neuroprotective effect of vasoactive intestinal peptide (VIP) in a mouse model of Parkinson's disease by blocking microglial activation. FASEB J 17:944–946.

Dexter DT, Wells FR, Lees AJ, Agid F, Agid Y, Jenner P, Marsden CD (1989) Increased nigral iron content and alterations in other metal ions occurring in brain in Parkinson's disease. J Neurochem 52:1830–1836.

Diguet E, Fernagut PO, Wei X, Du Y, Rouland R, Gross C, Bezard E, Tison F (2004) Deleterious effects of minocycline in animal models of Parkinson's disease and Huntington's disease. Eur J Neurosci 19:3266–3276.

Dringen R, Hirrlinger J (2003) Glutathione pathways in the brain. Biol Chem 384:505–516.

Estevez AG, Jordan J (2002) Nitric oxide and superoxide, a deadly cocktail. Ann N Y Acad Sci 962:207–211.

Fahrig T, Gerlach I, Horvath E (2005) A synthetic derivative of the natural product rocaglaol is a potent inhibitor of cytokine-mediated signaling and shows neuroprotective activity in vitro and in animal models of Parkinson's disease and traumatic brain injury. Mol Pharmacol 67:1544–1555.

Falsig J, Latta M, Leist M (2004) Defined inflammatory states in astrocyte cultures: correlation with susceptibility towards CD95-driven apoptosis. J Neurochem 88:181–193.

Fearnley JM, Lees AJ (1991) Ageing and Parkinson's disease: substantia nigra regional selectivity. Brain 114 (Pt 5):2283–2301.

Feng Z, Li D, Fung PC, Pei Z, Ramsden DB, Ho SL (2003) COX-2-deficient mice are less prone to MPTP-neurotoxicity than wild-type mice. Neuroreport 14:1927–1929.

Feng ZH, Wang TG, Li DD, Fung P, Wilson BC, Liu B, Ali SF, Langenbach R, Hong JS (2002) Cyclooxygenase-2-deficient mice are resistant to 1-methyl-4-phenyl1, 2, 3, 6-tetrahydropyridine-induced damage of dopaminergic neurons in the substantia nigra. Neurosci Lett 329:354–358.

Fisher J, Mizrahi T, Schori H, Yoles E, Levkovitch-Verbin H, Haggiag S, Revel M, Schwartz M (2001) Increased post-traumatic survival of neurons in IL-6-knockout mice on a background of EAE susceptibility. J Neuroimmunol 119:1–9.

Floor E, Wetzel MG (1998) Increased protein oxidation in human substantia nigra pars compacta in comparison with basal ganglia and prefrontal cortex measured with an improved dinitrophenylhydrazine assay. J Neurochem 70:268–275.

Fontaine V, Mohand-Said S, Hanoteau N, Fuchs C, Pfizenmaier K, Eisel U (2002) Neurodegenerative and neuroprotective effects of tumor Necrosis factor (TNF) in retinal ischemia: opposite roles of TNF receptor 1 and TNF receptor 2. J Neurosci 22:RC216.

Frank MM, Fries LF (1991) The role of complement in inflammation and phagocytosis. Immunol Today 12:322–326.

Gao HM, Hong JS, Zhang W, Liu B (2003a) Synergistic dopaminergic neurotoxicity of the pesticide rotenone and inflammogen lipopolysaccharide: relevance to the etiology of Parkinson's disease. J Neurosci 23:1228–1236.

Gao HM, Jiang J, Wilson B, Zhang W, Hong JS, Liu B (2002) Microglial activation-mediated delayed and progressive degeneration of rat nigral dopaminergic neurons: relevance to Parkinson's disease. J Neurochem 81:1285–1297.

Gao HM, Liu B, Zhang W, Hong JS (2003b) Critical role of microglial NADPH oxidase-derived free radicals in the in vitro MPTP model of Parkinson's disease. FASEB J 17:1954–1956.

Gayle DA, Ling Z, Tong C, Landers T, Lipton JW, Carvey PM (2002) Lipopolysaccharide (LPS)-induced dopamine cell loss in culture: roles of tumor necrosis factor-alpha, interleukin-1beta, and nitric oxide. Brain Res Dev Brain Res 133:27–35.

Gerlach M, Ben-Shachar D, Riederer P, Youdim MB (1994) Altered brain metabolism of iron as a cause of neurodegenerative diseases? J Neurochem 63:793–807.

Gesi M, Santinami A, Ruffoli R, Conti G, Fornai F (2001) Novel aspects of dopamine oxidative metabolism (confounding outcomes take place of certainties). Pharmacol Toxicol 89:217–224.

Gierse JK, McDonald JJ, Hauser SD, Rangwala SH, Koboldt CM, Seibert K (1996) A single amino acid difference between cyclooxygenase-1 (COX-1) and -2 (COX-2) reverses the selectivity of COX-2 specific inhibitors. J Biol Chem 271:15810–15814.

Giulian D, Woodward J, Young DG, Krebs JF, Lachman LB (1988) Interleukin-1 injected into mammalian brain stimulates astrogliosis and neovascularization. J Neurosci 8:2485–2490.

Gotz ME, Kunig G, Riederer P, Youdim MB (1994) Oxidative stress: free radical production in neural degeneration. Pharmacol Ther 63:37–122.

Graham DG (1978) Oxidative pathways for catecholamines in the genesis of neuromelanin and cytotoxic quinones. Mol Pharmacol 14:633–643.

Graham DY, Chan FK (2004) Is the use of COX-2 inhibitors in gastroenterology cost-effective? Nat Clin Pract Gastroenterol Hepatol 1:60–61.

Greenamyre JT, Hastings TG (2004) Biomedicine. Parkinson's–divergent causes, convergent mechanisms. Science 304:1120–1122.

Guan Z, Buckman SY, Miller BW, Springer LD, Morrison AR (1998) Interleukin-1beta-induced cyclooxygenase-2 expression requires activation of both c-Jun NH2-terminal kinase and p38 MAPK signal pathways in rat renal mesangial cells. J Biol Chem 273:28670–28676.

Hald A, Lotharius J (2005) Oxidative stress and inflammation in Parkinson's disease: is there a causal link? Exp Neurol 193:279–290.

Hanisch UK (2002) Microglia as a source and target of cytokines. Glia 40:140–155.

Hastings TG (1995) Enzymatic oxidation of dopamine: the role of prostaglandin H synthase. J Neurochem 64:919–924.

Haussermann P, Kuhn W, Przuntek H, Muller T (2001) Integrity of the blood-cerebrospinal fluid barrier in early Parkinson's disease. Neurosci Lett 300:182–184.

Hemmer K, Fransen L, Vanderstichele H, Vanmechelen E, Heuschling P (2001) An in vitro model for the study of microglia-induced neurodegeneration: involvement of nitric oxide and tumor necrosis factor-alpha. Neurochem Int 38:557–565.

Herrera AJ, Castano A, Venero JL, Cano J, Machado A (2000) The single intranigral injection of LPS as a new model for studying the selective effects of inflammatory reactions on dopaminergic system. Neurobiol Dis 7:429–447.

Hertz L (2004) The astrocyte-neuron lactate shuttle: a challenge of a challenge. J Cereb Blood Flow Metab 24:1241–1248.

Hertz L, Dringen R, Schousboe A, Robinson SR (1999) Astrocytes: glutamate producers for neurons. J Neurosci Res 57:417–428.

Hirsch E, Graybiel AM, Agid YA (1988) Melanized dopaminergic neurons are differentially susceptible to degeneration in Parkinson's disease. Nature 334:345–348.

Hirsch EC, Brandel JP, Galle P, Javoy-Agid F, Agid Y (1991) Iron and aluminum increase in the substantia nigra of patients with Parkinson's disease: an X-ray microanalysis. J Neurochem 56:446–451.

Hirsch EC, Breidert T, Rousselet E, Hunot S, Hartmann A, Michel PP (2003) The role of glial reaction and inflammation in Parkinson's disease. Ann N Y Acad Sci 991:214–228.

Hla T, Neilson K (1992) Human cyclooxygenase-2 cDNA. Proc Natl Acad Sci U S A 89:7384–7388.

Hoglinger GU, Carrard G, Michel PP, Medja F, Lombes A, Ruberg M, Friguet B, Hirsch EC (2003) Dysfunction of mitochondrial complex I and the proteasome: interactions between two biochemical deficits in a cellular model of Parkinson's disease. J Neurochem 86:1297–1307.

Hoozemans JJ, Veerhuis R, Janssen I, van Elk EJ, Rozemuller AJ, Eikelenboom P (2002) The role of cyclo-oxygenase 1 and 2 activity in prostaglandin E(2) secretion by cultured human adult microglia: implications for Alzheimer's disease. Brain Res 951:218–226.

Hornykiewicz O (1998) Biochemical aspects of Parkinson's disease. Neurology 51:S2–S9.

Hunot S, Dugas N, Faucheux B, Hartmann A, Tardieu M, Debre P, Agid Y, Dugas B, Hirsch EC (1999) FcepsilonRII/CD23 is expressed in Parkinson's disease and induces, in vitro, production of nitric oxide and tumor necrosis factor-alpha in glial cells. J Neurosci 19:3440–3447.

Hunot S, Vila M, Teismann P, Davis RJ, Hirsch EC, Przedborski S, Rakic P, Flavell RA (2004) JNK-mediated induction of cyclooxygenase 2 is required for neurodegeneration in a mouse model of Parkinson's disease. Proc Natl Acad Sci U S A 101:665–670.

Ikeda-Matsuo Y, Ikegaya Y, Matsuki N, Uematsu S, Akira S, Sasaki Y (2005) Microglia-specific expression of microsomal prostaglandin E2 synthase-1 contributes to lipopolysaccharide-induced prostaglandin E2 production. J Neurochem 94:1546–1558.

Imamura K, Hishikawa N, Sawada M, Nagatsu T, Yoshida M, Hashizume Y (2003) Distribution of major histocompatibility complex class II-positive microglia and cytokine profile of Parkinson's disease brains. Acta Neuropathol (Berl) 106:518–526.

In t' Veld, Ruitenberg A, Hofman A, Launer LJ, van Duijn CM, Stijnen T, Breteler MM, Stricker BH (2001) Nonsteroidal antiinflammatory drugs and the risk of Alzheimer's disease. N Engl J Med 345:1515–1521.

Iravani MM, Kashefi K, Mander P, Rose S, Jenner P (2002) Involvement of inducible nitric oxide synthase in inflammation-induced dopaminergic neurodegeneration. Neuroscience 110:49–58.

Jellinger KA (1999) Post mortem studies in Parkinson's disease–is it possible to detect brain areas for specific symptoms? J Neural Transm Suppl 56:1–29.

Kassiotis G, Kollias G (2001) Uncoupling the proinflammatory from the immunosuppressive properties of tumor necrosis factor (TNF) at the p55 TNF receptor level: implications for pathogenesis and therapy of autoimmune demyelination. J Exp Med 193:427–434.

Kato H, Araki T, Imai Y, Takahashi A, Itoyama Y (2003) Protection of dopaminergic neurons with a novel astrocyte modulating agent (R)-(−)-2-propyloctanoic acid (ONO-2506) in an MPTP-mouse model of Parkinson's disease. J Neurol Sci 208:9–15.

Kato H, Kurosaki R, Oki C, Araki T (2004) Arundic acid, an astrocyte-modulating agent, protects dopaminergic neurons against MPTP neurotoxicity in mice. Brain Res 1030:66–73.

Kennedy LJ, Moore K Jr, Caulfield JL, Tannenbaum SR, Dedon PC (1997) Quantitation of 8-oxoguanine and strand breaks produced by four oxidizing agents. Chem Res Toxicol 10:386–392.

Khan FH, Saha M, Chakrabarti S (2001) Dopamine induced protein damage in mitochondrial-synaptosomal fraction of rat brain. Brain Res 895:245–249.

Kish SJ, Shannak K, Hornykiewicz O (1988) Uneven pattern of dopamine loss in the striatum of patients with idiopathic Parkinson's disease. Pathophysiologic and clinical implications. N Engl J Med 318:876–880.

Knott C, Stern G, Wilkin GP (2000) Inflammatory regulators in Parkinson's disease: iNOS, lipocortin-1, and cyclooxygenases-1 and -2. Mol Cell Neurosci 16:724–739.

Kortekaas R, Leenders KL, van Oostrom JC, Vaalburg W, Bart J, Willemsen AT, Hendrikse NH (2005) Blood-brain barrier dysfunction in parkinsonian midbrain in vivo. Ann Neurol 57:176–179.

Kreutzberg GW (1996) Microglia: a sensor for pathological events in the CNS. Trends Neurosci 19:312–318.

Kuhn DM, Arthur RE Jr, Thomas DM, Elferink LA (1999) Tyrosine hydroxylase is inactivated by catechol-quinones and converted to a redox-cycling quinoprotein: possible relevance to Parkinson's disease. J Neurochem 73:1309–1317.

Kumagai T, Matsukawa N, Kaneko Y, Kusumi Y, Mitsumata M, Uchida K (2004) A lipid peroxidation-derived inflammatory mediator: identification of 4-hydroxy-2-nonenal as a potential inducer of cyclooxygenase-2 in macrophages. J Biol Chem 279:48389–48396.

Ladenheim B, Krasnova IN, Deng X, Oyler JM, Polettini A, Moran TH, Huestis MA, Cadet JL (2000) Methamphetamine-induced neurotoxicity is attenuated in transgenic mice with a null mutation for interleukin-6. Mol Pharmacol 58:1247–1256.

Langston JW, Forno LS, Tetrud J, Reeves AG, Kaplan JA, Karluk D (1999) Evidence of active nerve cell degeneration in the substantia nigra of humans years after 1-methyl-4-phenyl-1,2,3,6-tetrahydropyridine exposure. Ann Neurol 46:598–605.

Le W, Rowe D, Xie W, Ortiz I, He Y, Appel SH (2001) Microglial activation and dopaminergic cell injury: an in vitro model relevant to Parkinson's disease. J Neurosci 21:8447–8455.

Lee SC, Dickson DW, Liu W, Brosnan CF (1993) Induction of nitric oxide synthase activity in human astrocytes by interleukin-1 beta and interferon-gamma. J Neuroimmunol 46:19–24.

Lee SH, Soyoola E, Chanmugam P, Hart S, Sun W, Zhong H, Liou S, Simmons D, Hwang D (1992) Selective expression of mitogen-inducible cyclooxygenase in macrophages stimulated with lipopolysaccharide. J Biol Chem 267:25934–25938.

Leu CM, Wong FH, Chang C, Huang SF, Hu CP (2003) Interleukin-6 acts as an antiapoptotic factor in human esophageal carcinoma cells through the activation of both STAT3 and mitogen-activated protein kinase pathways. Oncogene 22:7809–7818.

Liberatore GT, Jackson-Lewis V, Vukosavic S, Mandir AS, Vila M, McAuliffe WG, Dawson VL, Dawson TM, Przedborski S (1999) Inducible nitric oxide synthase stimulates dopaminergic neurodegeneration in the MPTP model of Parkinson disease. Nat Med 5:1403–1409.

Liberto CM, Albrecht PJ, Herx LM, Yong VW, Levison SW (2004) Pro-regenerative properties of cytokine-activated astrocytes. J Neurochem 89:1092–1100.

Lim GP, Yang F, Chu T, Chen P, Beech W, Teter B, Tran T, Ubeda O, Ashe KH, Frautschy SA, Cole GM (2000) Ibuprofen suppresses plaque pathology and inflammation in a mouse model for Alzheimer's disease. J Neurosci 20:5709–5714.

Liu B, Gao HM, Wang JY, Jeohn GH, Cooper CL, Hong JS (2002) Role of nitric oxide in inflammation-mediated neurodegeneration. Ann N Y Acad Sci 962:318–331.

Liu Y, Qin L, Li G, Zhang W, An L, Liu B, Hong JS (2003) Dextromethorphan protects dopaminergic neurons against inflammation-mediated degeneration through inhibition of microglial activation. J Pharmacol Exp Ther 305:212–218.

Lotharius J, Brundin P (2002a) Pathogenesis of Parkinson's disease: dopamine, vesicles and alpha-synuclein. Nat Rev Neurosci 3:932–942.

Lotharius J, Brundin P (2002b) Impaired dopamine storage resulting from alpha-synuclein mutations may contribute to the pathogenesis of Parkinson's disease. Hum Mol Genet 11:2395–2407.

Ma XC, Gottschall PE, Chen LT, Wiranowska M, Phelps CP (2002) Role and mechanisms of interleukin-1 in the modulation of neurotoxicity. Neuroimmunomodulation 10:199–207.

Magistretti PJ, Ransom BR (2002) Astrocytes. In: Neuropsychopharmacology: The Fifth Generation of Progress (Charney DMD, Coyle JT, Nemeroff C, eds), Lippincott Williams & Wilkins (LWW) 133–145.

Maker HS, Weiss C, Silides DJ, Cohen G (1981) Coupling of dopamine oxidation (monoamine oxidase activity) to glutathione oxidation via the generation of hydrogen peroxide in rat brain homogenates. J Neurochem 36:589–593.

Mamdani M, Rochon PA, Juurlink DN, Kopp A, Anderson GM, Naglie G, Austin PC, Laupacis A (2002) Observational study of upper gastrointestinal haemorrhage in elderly patients given selective cyclo-oxygenase-2 inhibitors or conventional non-steroidal anti-inflammatory drugs. BMJ 325:624.

Martin MU, Wesche H (2002) Summary and comparison of the signaling mechanisms of the Toll/interleukin-1 receptor family. Biochim Biophys Acta 1592:265–280.

Maruyama W, Strolin-Benedetti M, Naoi M (2000) N-methyl(R)salsolinol and a neutral N-methyltransferase as pathogenic factors in Parkinson's disease. Neurobiology (Bp) 8:55–68.

Maslinska D, Wozniak R, Kaliszek A, Modelska I (1999) Expression of cyclooxygenase-2 in astrocytes of human brain after global ischemia. Folia Neuropathol 37:75–79.

Matyszak MK (1998) Inflammation in the CNS: balance between immunological privilege and immune responses. Prog Neurobiol 56:19–35.

McGeer PL, Itagaki S, Boyes BE, McGeer EG (1988) Reactive microglia are positive for HLA-DR in the substantia nigra of Parkinson's and Alzheimer's disease brains. Neurology 38:1285–1291.

McGeer PL, McGeer EG (2004) Inflammation and neurodegeneration in Parkinson's disease. Parkinsonism Relat Disord 10 (1):S3–S7.

McGeer PL, Schwab C, Parent A, Doudet D (2003) Presence of reactive microglia in monkey substantia nigra years after 1-methyl-4-phenyl-1,2,3,6-tetrahydropyridine administration. Ann Neurol 54:599–604.

McNaught KS, Jenner P (2000) Extracellular accumulation of nitric oxide, hydrogen peroxide, and glutamate in astrocytic cultures following glutathione depletion, complex I inhibition, and/or lipopolysaccharide-induced activation. Biochem Pharmacol 60:979–988.

McNaught KS, Olanow CW (2003) Proteolytic stress: a unifying concept for the etiopathogenesis of Parkinson's disease. Ann Neurol 53 Suppl 3:S73–S84.

Miklossy J, Doudet DD, Schwab C, Yu S, McGeer EG, McGeer PL (2006) Role of ICAM-1 in persisting inflammation in Parkinson disease and MPTP monkeys. Exp Neurol 197:275–283.

Minghetti L (2004) Cyclooxygenase-2 (COX-2) in inflammatory and degenerative brain diseases. J Neuropathol Exp Neurol 63:901–910.

Mirza B, Hadberg H, Thomsen P, Moos T (2000) The absence of reactive astrocytosis is indicative of a unique inflammatory process in Parkinson's disease. Neuroscience 95:425–432.

Mogi M, Harada M, Kondo T, Riederer P, Inagaki H, Minami M, Nagatsu T (1994a) Interleukin-1 beta, interleukin-6, epidermal growth factor and transforming growth factor-alpha are elevated in the brain from parkinsonian patients. Neurosci Lett 180:147–150.

Mogi M, Harada M, Riederer P, Narabayashi H, Fujita K, Nagatsu T (1994b) Tumor necrosis factor-alpha (TNF-alpha) increases both in the brain and in the cerebrospinal fluid from parkinsonian patients. Neurosci Lett 165:208–210.

Mohanakumar KP, Muralikrishnan D, Thomas B (2000) Neuroprotection by sodium salicylate against 1-methyl-4-phenyl-1,2,3, 6-tetrahydropyridine-induced neurotoxicity. Brain Res 864:281–290.

Morgan BP, Gasque P (1996) Expression of complement in the brain: role in health and disease. Immunol Today 17:461–466.

Muller T, Blum-Degen D, Przuntek H, Kuhn W (1998) Interleukin-6 levels in cerebrospinal fluid inversely correlate to severity of Parkinson's disease. Acta Neurol Scand 98:142–144.

Nakamura Y (2002) Regulating factors for microglial activation. Biol Pharm Bull 25:945–953.

Nakayama M, Uchimura K, Zhu RL, Nagayama T, Rose ME, Stetler RA, Isakson PC, Chen J, Graham SH (1998) Cyclooxygenase-2 inhibition prevents delayed death of CA1 hippocampal neurons following global ischemia. Proc Natl Acad Sci U S A 95:10954–10959.

Norgard B, Pedersen L, Johnsen SP, Tarone RE, McLaughlin JK, Friis S, Sorensen HT (2004) COX-2-selective inhibitors and the risk of upper gastrointestinal bleeding in high-risk patients with previous gastrointestinal diseases: a population-based case-control study. Aliment Pharmacol Ther 19: 817–825.

O'Callaghan JP, Seidler FJ (1992) 1-Methyl-4-phenyl-1,2,3,6-tetrahydropyridine (MPTP)-induced astrogliosis does not require activation of ornithine decarboxylase. Neurosci Lett 148:105–108.

Okuno T, Nakatsuji Y, Kumanogoh A, Moriya M, Ichinose H, Sumi H, Fujimura H, Kikutani H, Sakoda S (2005) Loss of dopaminergic neurons by the induction of inducible nitric oxide synthase and cyclooxygenase-2 via CD 40: relevance to Parkinson's disease. J Neurosci Res 81: 874–882.

Orr CF, Rowe DB, Mizuno Y, Mori H, Halliday GM (2005) A possible role for humoral immunity in the pathogenesis of Parkinson's disease. Brain 128:2665–2674.

Orth M, Schapira AH (2002) Mitochondrial involvement in Parkinson's disease. Neurochem Int 40:533–541.

Osterud B, Bjorklid E (2003) Role of monocytes in atherogenesis. Physiol Rev 83:1069–1112.

Ouchi Y, Yoshikawa E, Sekine Y, Futatsubashi M, Kanno T, Ogusu T, Torizuka T (2005) Microglial activation and dopamine terminal loss in early Parkinson's disease. Ann Neurol 57:168–175.

Pakkenberg B, Moller A, Gundersen HJ, Mouritzen DA, Pakkenberg H (1991) The absolute number of nerve cells in substantia nigra in normal subjects and in patients with Parkinson's disease estimated with an unbiased stereological method. J Neurol Neurosurg Psychiatry 54:30–33.

Patrignani P, Tacconelli S, Sciulli MG, Capone ML (2005) New insights into COX-2 biology and inhibition. Brain Res Brain Res Rev 48:352–359.

Pearce RK, Owen A, Daniel S, Jenner P, Marsden CD (1997) Alterations in the distribution of glutathione in the substantia nigra in Parkinson's disease. J Neural Transm 104:661–677.

Pellerin L (2005) How astrocytes feed hungry neurons. Mol Neurobiol 32:59–72.

Possel H, Noack H, Putzke J, Wolf G, Sies H (2000) Selective upregulation of inducible nitric oxide synthase (iNOS) by lipopolysaccharide (LPS) and cytokines in microglia: in vitro and in vivo studies. Glia 32:51–59.

Przybylkowski A, Kurkowska-Jastrzebska I, Joniec I, Ciesielska A, Czlonkowska A, Czlonkowski A (2004) Cyclooxygenases mRNA and protein expression in striata in the experimental mouse model of Parkinson's disease induced by 1-methyl-4-phenyl-1,2,3,6-tetrahydropyridine administration to mouse. Brain Res 1019:144–151.

Reinhard JF Jr, Miller DB, O'Callaghan JP (1988) The neurotoxicant MPTP (1-methyl-4-phenyl-1,2,3,6-tetrahydropyridine) increases glial fibrillary acidic protein and decreases dopamine levels of the mouse striatum: evidence for glial response to injury. Neurosci Lett 95:246–251.

Roth GJ, Stanford N, Majerus PW (1975) Acetylation of prostaglandin synthase by aspirin. Proc Natl Acad Sci U S A 72:3073–3076.

Rousselet E, Callebert J, Parain K, Joubert C, Hunot S, Hartmann A, Jacque C, Perez-Diaz F, Cohen-Salmon C, Launay JM, Hirsch EC (2002) Role of TNF-alpha receptors in mice intoxicated with the parkinsonian toxin MPTP. Exp Neurol 177:183–192.

Rowe DB, Le W, Smith RG, Appel SH (1998) Antibodies from patients with Parkinson's disease react with protein modified by dopamine oxidation. J Neurosci Res 53:551–558.

Sanchez-Pernaute R, Ferree A, Cooper O, Yu M, Brownell AL, Isacson O (2004) Selective COX-2 inhibition prevents progressive dopamine neuron degeneration in a rat model of Parkinson's disease. J Neuroinflammation 1:6.

Scali C, Giovannini MG, Prosperi C, Bellucci A, Pepeu G, Casamenti F (2003) The selective cyclooxygenase-2 inhibitor rofecoxib suppresses brain inflammation and protects cholinergic neurons from excitotoxic degeneration in vivo. Neuroscience 117:909–919.

Scatton B, Rouquier L, Javoy-Agid F, Agid Y (1982) Dopamine deficiency in the cerebral cortex in Parkinson disease. Neurology 32:1039–1040.

Schapira AH (1994) Evidence for mitochondrial dysfunction in Parkinson's disease–a critical appraisal. Mov Disord 9:125–138.

Schipper HM, Liberman A, Stopa EG (1998) Neural heme oxygenase-1 expression in idiopathic Parkinson's disease. Exp Neurol 150:60–68.

Schneider JS, Denaro FJ (1988) Astrocytic responses to the dopaminergic neurotoxin 1-methyl-4-phenyl-1,2,3,6-tetrahydropyridine (MPTP) in cat and mouse brain. J Neuropathol Exp Neurol 47:452–458.

Schnitzer TJ, Burmester GR, Mysler E, Hochberg MC, Doherty M, Ehrsam E, Gitton X, Krammer G, Mellein B, Matchaba P, Gimona A, Hawkey CJ (2004) Comparison of lumiracoxib with naproxen and ibuprofen in the Therapeutic Arthritis Research and Gastrointestinal Event Trial (TARGET), reduction in ulcer complications: randomised controlled trial. Lancet 364:665–674.

Selmaj KW, Farooq M, Norton WT, Raine CS, Brosnan CF (1990) Proliferation of astrocytes in vitro in response to cytokines. A primary role for tumor necrosis factor. J Immunol 144:129–135.

Sheng JG, Shirabe S, Nishiyama N, Schwartz JP (1993) Alterations in striatal glial fibrillary acidic protein expression in response to 6-hydroxydopamine-induced denervation. Exp Brain Res 95:450–456.

Sherer TB, Betarbet R, Greenamyre JT (2002) Environment, mitochondria, and Parkinson's disease. Neuroscientist 8:192–197.

Sherer TB, Betarbet R, Kim JH, Greenamyre JT (2003) Selective microglial activation in the rat rotenone model of Parkinson's disease. Neurosci Lett 341:87–90.

Silverstein FE, Faich G, Goldstein JL, Simon LS, Pincus T, Whelton A, Makuch R, Eisen G, Agrawal NM, Stenson WF, Burr AM, Zhao WW, Kent JD, Lefkowith JB, Verburg KM, Geis GS (2000) Gastrointestinal toxicity with celecoxib vs nonsteroidal anti-inflammatory drugs for osteoarthritis and rheumatoid arthritis: the CLASS study: A randomized controlled trial. Celecoxib Long-term Arthritis Safety Study. JAMA 284:1247–1255.

Simard M, Nedergaard M (2004) The neurobiology of glia in the context of water and ion homeostasis. Neuroscience 129:877–896.

Singhrao SK, Neal JW, Rushmere NK, Morgan BP, Gasque P (2000) Spontaneous classical pathway activation and deficiency of membrane regulators render human neurons susceptible to complement lysis. Am J Pathol 157:905–918.

Smith WL, Garavito RM, DeWitt DL (1996) Prostaglandin endoperoxide H synthases (cyclooxygenases)-1 and -2. J Biol Chem 271:33157–33160.

Sofic E, Lange KW, Jellinger K, Riederer P (1992) Reduced and oxidized glutathione in the substantia nigra of patients with Parkinson's disease. Neurosci Lett 142:128–130.

Sofic E, Riederer P, Heinsen H, Beckmann H, Reynolds GP, Hebenstreit G, Youdim MB (1988) Increased iron (III) and total iron content in post mortem substantia nigra of parkinsonian brain. J Neural Transm 74:199–205.

Sofroniew MV (2005) Reactive astrocytes in neural repair and protection. Neuroscientist 11:400–407.

Spencer JP, Jenner P, Daniel SE, Lees AJ, Marsden DC, Halliwell B (1998) Conjugates of catecholamines with cysteine and GSH in Parkinson's disease: possible mechanisms of formation involving reactive oxygen species. J Neurochem 71:2112–2122.

Sriram K, Miller DB, O'Callaghan JP (2006) Minocycline attenuates microglial activation but fails to mitigate striatal dopaminergic neurotoxicity: role of tumor necrosis factor-alpha. J Neurochem 96:706–718.

Stokes AH, Hastings TG, Vrana KE (1999) Cytotoxic and genotoxic potential of dopamine. J Neurosci Res 55:659–665.

Stromberg I, Bjorklund H, Dahl D, Jonsson G, Sundstrom E, Olson L (1986) Astrocyte responses to dopaminergic denervations by 6-hydroxydopamine and 1-methyl-4-phenyl-1,2,3,6-tetrahydropyridine as evidenced by glial fibrillary acidic protein immunohistochemistry. Brain Res Bull 17:225–236.

Sudo S, Tanaka J, Toku K, Desaki J, Matsuda S, Arai T, Sakanaka M, Maeda N (1998) Neurons induce the activation of microglial cells in vitro. Exp Neurol 154:499–510.

Sulzer D, Zecca L (2000) Intraneuronal dopamine-quinone synthesis: a review. Neurotox Res 1:181–195.

Taylor DL, Diemel LT, Pocock JM (2003) Activation of microglial group III metabotropic glutamate receptors protects neurons against microglial neurotoxicity. J Neurosci 23:2150–2160.

Teismann P, Ferger B (2001) Inhibition of the cyclooxygenase isoenzymes COX-1 and COX-2 provide neuroprotection in the MPTP-mouse model of Parkinson's disease. Synapse 39:167–174.

Teismann P, Tieu K, Choi DK, Wu DC, Naini A, Hunot S, Vila M, Jackson-Lewis V, Przedborski S (2003) Cyclooxygenase-2 is instrumental in Parkinson's disease neurodegeneration. Proc Natl Acad Sci U S A 100:5473–5478.

Thomas M, Le WD (2004) Minocycline: neuroprotective mechanisms in Parkinson's disease. Curr Pharm Des 10:679–686.

Tse DC, McCreery RL, Adams RN (1976) Potential oxidative pathways of brain catecholamines. J Med Chem 19:37–40.

van Beek J, Elward K, Gasque P (2003) Activation of complement in the central nervous system: roles in neurodegeneration and neuroprotection. Ann N Y Acad Sci 992:56–71.

van Beek J, van MM, 't Hart BA, Brok HP, Neal JW, Chatagner A, Harris CL, Omidvar N, Morgan BP, Laman JD, Gasque P (2005) Decay-accelerating factor (CD55) is expressed by neurons in response to chronic but not acute autoimmune central nervous system inflammation associated with complement activation. J Immunol 174:2353–2365.

van der Goes A, Kortekaas M, Hoekstra K, Dijkstra CD, Amor S (1999) The role of anti-myelin (auto)-antibodies in the phagocytosis of myelin by macrophages. J Neuroimmunol 101:61–67.

Vane JR (1971) Inhibition of prostaglandin synthesis as a mechanism of action for aspirin-like drugs. Nat New Biol 231:232–235.

Volterra A, Meldolesi J (2005) Astrocytes, from brain glue to communication elements: the revolution continues. Nat Rev Neurosci 6:626–640.

Walker MC, Kurumbail RG, Kiefer JR, Moreland KT, Koboldt CM, Isakson PC, Seibert K, Gierse JK (2001) A three-step kinetic mechanism for selective inhibition of cyclo-oxygenase-2 by diarylhetero-cyclic inhibitors. Biochem J 357:709–718.

Wang MJ, Lin WW, Chen HL, Chang YH, Ou HC, Kuo JS, Hong JS, Jeng KC (2002) Silymarin protects dopaminergic neurons against lipopolysaccharide-induced neurotoxicity by inhibiting microglia activation. Eur J Neurosci 16:2103–2112.

Wang T, Pei Z, Zhang W, Liu B, Langenbach R, Lee C, Wilson B, Reece JM, Miller DS, Hong JS (2005) MPP+-induced COX-2 activation and subsequent dopaminergic neurodegeneration. FASEB J 19:1134–1136.

Warner TD, Mitchell JA (2004) Cyclooxygenases: new forms, new inhibitors, and lessons from the clinic. FASEB J 18:790–804.

Willard LB, Hauss-Wegrzyniak B, Danysz W, Wenk GL (2000) The cytotoxicity of chronic neuroin- flammation upon basal forebrain cholinergic neurons of rats can be attenuated by glutamatergic antagonism or cyclooxygenase-2 inhibition. Exp Brain Res 134:58–65.

Wilms H, Rosenstiel P, Sievers J, Deuschl G, Zecca L, Lucius R (2003) Activation of microglia by human neuromelanin is NF-kappaB dependent and involves p38 mitogen-activated protein kinase: implications for Parkinson's disease. FASEB J 17:500–502.

Xu J, Chalimoniuk M, Shu Y, Simonyi A, Sun AY, Gonzalez FA, Weisman GA, Wood WG, Sun GY (2003) Prostaglandin E2 production in astrocytes: regulation by cytokines, extracellular ATP, and oxidative agents. Prostaglandins Leukot Essent Fatty Acids 69:437–448.

Yamada T, McGeer PL, McGeer EG (1992) Lewy bodies in Parkinson's disease are recognized by antibodies to complement proteins. Acta Neuropathol (Berl) 84:100–104.

Yamamoto K, Arakawa T, Ueda N, Yamamoto S (1995) Transcriptional roles of nuclear factor kappa B and nuclear factor-interleukin-6 in the tumor necrosis factor alpha-dependent induction of cyclooxygenase-2 in MC3T3-E1 cells. J Biol Chem 270:31315–31320.

Yermakova AV, O'Banion MK (2001) Downregulation of neuronal cyclooxygenase-2 expression in end stage Alzheimer's disease. Neurobiol Aging 22:823–836.

Yoritaka A, Hattori N, Uchida K, Tanaka M, Stadtman ER, Mizuno Y (1996) Immunohistochemical detection of 4-hydroxynonenal protein adducts in Parkinson disease. Proc Natl Acad Sci U S A 93:2696–2701.

Zassler B, Weis C, Humpel C (2003) Tumor necrosis factor-alpha triggers cell death of sensitized potassium chloride-stimulated cholinergic neurons. Brain Res Mol Brain Res 113:78–85.

Zhang J, Perry G, Smith MA, Robertson D, Olson SJ, Graham DG, Montine TJ (1999) Parkinson's disease is associated with oxidative damage to cytoplasmic DNA and RNA in substantia nigra neurons. Am J Pathol 154:1423–1429.

Zimprich A, et al. (2004) Mutations in LRRK2 cause autosomal-dominant parkinsonism with pleomorphic pathology. Neuron 44:601–607.

SECTION VI

NUTRITION, INFLAMMATION AND CHRONIC DISEASE

CHAPTER 13

ESSENTIAL POLYUNSATURATED FATTY ACIDS, INFLAMMATION, ATHEROSCLEROSIS AND CARDIOVASCULAR DISEASES

MICHEL DE LORGERIL*

From the Laboratoire Nutrition, Vieillissement et Maladies Cardiovasculaires (NVMCV), Faculté de Médecine, Université Joseph Fourier, Grenoble, France

Abstract: Atherosclerosis is the primary cause of coronary and cardiovascular diseases (CVD). Epidemiological studies have revealed several important environmental (especially nutritional) factors associated with atherosclerosis. However, progress in defining the cellular and molecular interactions involved has been hindered by the etiological complexity of the disease. Nevertheless, our understanding of CVD has improved significantly over the past decade owing to the availability of new randomized trial data. In particular, the failure of antioxidant and anti-inflammatory treatments to consistently reduce the rate of CVD complications suggests that theories of atherosclerosis may have considerably exaggerated the importance of oxidized lipoprotein and vascular inflammation. In that context, one new and basic question is whether the biology of essential dietary lipids may help us understand the role of the inflammatory process in CVD. Essential dietary lipids of the omega-6 and omega-3 families are the precursors of major mediators of inflammation such as eicosanoids that regulate the production of inflammatory cytokines and the expression of some major inflammation genes. On the other hand, non-essential lipids

*NVMCV, UFR de Médecine et Pharmacie, Domaine de la Merci, 38706 La Tronche(Grenoble), France.
E-mail: michel.delorgeril@ujf-grenoble.fr

283

R. E. Harris (ed.), Inflammation in the Pathogenesis of Chronic Diseases, 283–297.
© 2007 *Springer.*

(omega-9 and saturated fatty acids) interfere with biological activities of essential lipids. Finally, essential omega-3 and omega-6 fatty acids have different, often antagonistic, effects on inflammation, and their effects can vary according to the type of cells and target organs involved, as well as their respective amounts in the diet. Because of the extreme complexity in the etiology of CVD, the best strategy may be to monitor the main features of dietary patterns, such as the Mediterranean diet, that are known to be associated with a low prevalence of both CVD and chronic inflammatory diseases

1.   INTRODUCTION

Coronary and cardiovascular diseases (CVD) remain the leading causes of morbidity and mortality in most developing and developed countries. Besides traditional risk factors such as hypercholesterolemia and hypertension, increased oxidant stress (or oxidized lipoproteins) and vascular inflammation have recently been considered as playing important roles in CVD [1–4]. However, in some studies, antioxidant and anti-inflammatory treatments had no protective effect against CVD [5–8]. Both nonsteroidal anti-inflammatory drugs (NSAIDs) and glucocorticoids were ineffective. Furthermore, arthritis patients on glucocorticoids had more CVD complications (after adjustment for disease severity and other confounders) than those not exposed to glucocorticoids [9]. This is not surprising, since glucocorticoids predispose to insulin resistance and metabolic syndromes, which are major risk factors for CVD [10]. In patients with established CVD, high-dose dexamethasone-eluting stents did not reduce neointimal proliferation instead causing restenosis within the stent and creating an experimental human model of accelerated coronary atherosclerosis [11]. Finally, NSAIDs have not only failed to prevent CVD complications in some controlled trials, but rather were associated with an increased risk [7, 8]. Thus, scientific and medical knowledge about the pathogenesis of atherosclerosis and CVD complications, with primary roles attributed to high cholesterol, oxidized lipoproteins and vascular inflammation, appears to be extremely confusing at present. Even the concept of inflammation in plaque instability (the triggering event of acute CVD complications) needs to be more clearly reformulated [12]. In this context, it is certainly important to examine the role of essential polyunsaturated fatty acids (PUFAs) as mediators of inflammation in the development of CVD.

2.   INFLAMMATION, ATHEROSCLEROSIS AND ESSENTIAL PUFAs

It is generally well accepted (although highly debatable) that inflammation plays a central role in atherosclerosis [1, 13]. All stages of the atherogenic process seem to be characterized by a dynamic interaction of inflammatory cells, cytokines and inflammatory eicosanoids in the arterial wall [1, 13, 14]. According to the most popular theory to date, the conventional risk factors for CVD, including oxidized low density lipoproteins (oxLDL), smoking, high blood glucose and high blood pressure, are harmful factors that initiate and promote the atherogenic process by triggering the inflammatory reaction within the arteries. The earliest detectable cellular event in atherosclerosis is assumed to be the attachment of monocytes to endothelial cells. This inflammatory response is facilitated by leukocyte adhesion molecules expressed on the surface of endothelial cells under the control of proinflammatory cytokines. OxLDLs are thought to promote the formation of chemoattractant cytokines by the endothelium which stimulates the migration of monocytes into the subendothelial space where they accumulate oxLDLs as macrophages and become foam cells [13]. Foam cells are a hallmark of fatty streaks, the first (but still reversible) stage of atherosclerosis. A later stage of inflammation is characterized by fibrosis, which is also a major feature of atherosclerosis [13]. Fibrosis results from the proliferation of smooth muscle cells after their migration from the muscular layer of the artery under the control of various mitogenic and growth factors, such as the platelet derived growth factor (PGDF) [13]. Fibrosis is a reparation process that contributes to irreversible sclerosis of the lesion and arterial stenosis; nevertheless, fibrosis *per se* is a stabilizing process and does not result in acute CVD complications. In fact, it is the disruption of the atherosclerotic plaque, with the subsequent potentially total obstruction of the lumen by thrombi that leads to acute CVD complications. According to current theory, macrophages are also the primary source of plaque vulnerability because they produce matrix metalloproteinases that break up collagen (the main component of fibrosis), weaken the fibrous cap of the plaque and favor contact between blood coagulation factors and the prothrombotic components of atherosclerotic plaque. Although it is generally well accepted, the inflammatory theory of atherosclerosis [1, 13, 14] appears to be quite speculative, as illustrated by the failure of most anti-inflammatory treatments to prevent CVD complications [7, 8]. Therefore, the theory needs additional supporting evidence to become more credible.

There is increasing interest in the effects of dietary fatty acids on immune parameters and on the inflammatory process. Initially, long chain omega-6 PUFAs, linoleic acid (LA) and particularly arachidonic acid (AA), were found to inhibit lymphocyte function [15, 16]. Later studies showed that omega-3 PUFAs also inhibited lymphocyte activity [17, 18]. Other non-essential dietary fatty acids (e.g., those in the omega-9 family) also influence inflammation. Recently, PUFAs of the omega-6 and omega-3 families have been found to have antagonistic effects on inflammation and CVD; omega-6 PUFAs are now seen as pro-inflammatory and omega-3 PUFAs as anti-inflammatory [19]. Arachidonic acid (AA), the major omega-6 PUFA in inflammatory cells, is the dominant substrate for eicosanoid synthesis giving rise to major pro-inflammatory mediators potentially involved in CVD complications [13, 14]. Blocking the first step of AA metabolism in platelets, at the level of the cyclo-oxygenase (COX) enzyme system (by aspirin for instance), results in inhibition of eicosanoid synthesis and platelet aggregation. However, only very low doses of aspirin (and not large anti-inflammatory doses) were shown to effectively reduce CVD complications [20]. In fact, there is ongoing controversy about the ability of low-dose aspirin to reduce CVD complications [21, 22]. What is the optimal dose? Which patients would maximally benefit from it? Is the effect seen in secondary prevention reproducible in primary prevention? In any case, since only very low doses were shown to be protective in certain (not all) studies [23], it is clear that the relative protection provided by low dose aspirin does not result from an anti-inflammatory effect but only from a specific anti-platelet effect. This raises some major questions about the inflammatory theory of atherosclerosis. First, as it has become clear that besides their role in hemostasis and thrombosis, platelets regulate a variety of inflammatory responses, especially through their interaction with the vascular endothelium [24], it is difficult to understand why large (anti-inflammatory) doses of aspirin were not effective in preventing CVD. Platelets represent an important link between inflammation, thrombosis and atherosclerosis, highlighting the concept of *atherothrombosis* in which thrombosis, in addition to being the consequence of plaque rupture, is also the starting point for stenosis progression through organization of residual thrombi [24]. However, apart from specific conditions such as accelerated coronary atherosclerosis after heart transplantation [25, 26], the availability of conclusive human data to support the "*atherothrombotic* theory" appears to be very limited. A second question relates to the role of inflammatory eicosanoids (from any source) in vascular inflammation and CVD. Why do substances blocking AA metabolism and the production of inflammatory eicosanoids and exhibiting potent anti-inflammatory effects (such as NSAIDs) have negative effects [7, 8] on CVD risk? A third crucial question relates to the significance of metabolic competition between the different families of PUFAs (omega-6, omega-9, and omega-3) and the vascular and anti-inflammatory effect of NSAIDs. Would COX inhibition have the same clinical effect in patients with different dietary intakes of omega-9, omega-6 and omega-3 fatty acids? In view of the complexity of these different questions, the present text aims at discussing certain aspects of the role of essential PUFAs in CVD through their pro- or anti-inflammatory properties.

3.   WHAT ARE ESSENTIAL PUFAs?

Essential PUFAs are fatty acids that contain two or more double bonds. They are named by identifying the number of double bonds and the position of the first double bond counted from the methyl terminus of the acyl chain. Thus, an 18-carbon fatty acid with two double bonds in the acyl chain and with the first double bond on carbon number 6 from the methyl terminus is termed 18:2 omega-6 (or 18:2n-6). The common name of this fatty acid is linoleic acid (LA) and it is the simplest member of the omega-6 family of PUFAs. LA can be further desaturated by insertion of a double bond between carbons 3 and 4 to yield alpha-linolenic acid (ALA or 18:3 omega-3 or 18:3n-3), the simplest member of the omega-3 family of fatty acids [27]. Plants, but not mammals, have the desaturase enzymes required to synthesize LA and ALA. For this reason, LA and ALA are termed "essential fatty acids", which means that they have to be supplied through our daily diet to cover our needs (Figure 1). Plant seed oils (and margarine) from corn, sunflower and soybean are rich in LA and are the main sources of LA in the Western diet. Nuts, canola oil and green leafy vegetables are the main sources of ALA in the

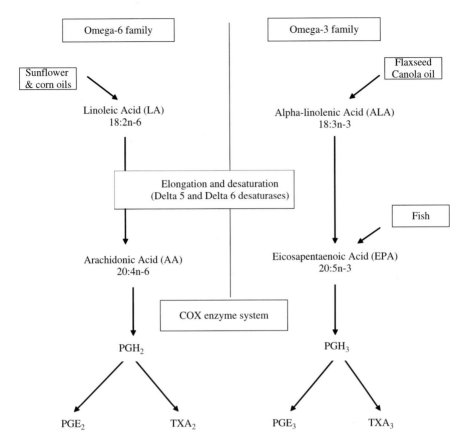

Figure 1. Schematic representation of the metabolization of 18-carbon fatty acids into longer chain fatty acids and subsequent eicosanoid metabolization under the effect of the COX system. Most AA in our body comes from LA (through endogenous biosynthesis), whereas most EPA comes from dietary intakes provided by fish. EPA can be further metabolized to produce DHA (see text). An alternative pathway for AA and EPA is the LOX system (see text). AA is arachidonic acid; EPA is eicosapentanoic acid; DHA is docosahexanoic acid; LA is linoleic acid; COX is cyclo-oxygenase and LOX is lipoxygenase

Western and Mediterranean diets [27]. LA is by far the main essential PUFA in the Western diet (average intake is between 12 and 20 grams per day), with an LA to ALA ratio of 20 or 25 according to recent studies. It has been clearly shown that the preferred LA to ALA ratio for the prevention of CVD should be 4 or lower, with a minimum ALA intake of about 2 grams per day [27]. In many countries, however, the ALA intake is lower than 1 gram per day. LA and ALA are the main PUFAs in the Western and Mediterranean diets and longer chain PUFAs (with 20 carbons or more) are consumed in small amounts: from 50 mg (often) to 500 mg (rarely) per day for AA (20:4n-6) and for the long chain omega-3 PUFAs mostly found in fish, eicosapentanoic acid (EPA, 20:5n-3) and docosahexanoic acid (DHA,

22:6n-3). Mammals are in theory able to synthesize EPA and DHA from ALA [19, 27]. In patients at high risk for CVD complications, high ALA intake resulted in a significant increase in blood and tissue EPA levels, whereas the increase in DHA was low and non-significant [27, 28]. Thus, DHA is often considered an "essential fatty acid" like LA and ALA, and it is prudent to provide for minimum amounts of it in our daily diet (at least 200 to 500 mg DHA per day depending on the associated amounts of ALA and EPA).

Unlike ALA (the precursor of EPA), oleic acid (18:1n-9) is consumed in substantial amounts in the typical Western diet and is not an essential fatty acid. Oleic acid is the precursor of eicosatreinoic acid (ETA, 20:3n-9), the main omega-9

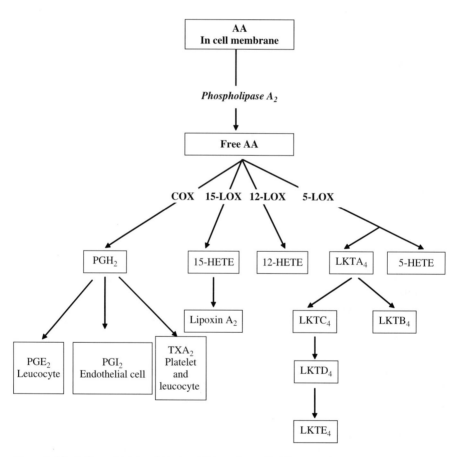

Figure 2. Metabolism of AA (arachidonic acid) in various cells. EPA can substitute for AA as a substrate for COX and LOX systems. This may result in the release of compounds that are generally less active (TXA$_3$ and LKTB$_5$ instead of TXA$_2$ and LKTB$_4$) than those produced from AA. There is one exception with PGI$_3$, which is as active as PGI$_2$ as an anti-platelet and vasodilating substance. TX is thromboxane, PGI$_2$ is prostacyclin and LKT is leukotriene

PUFA potentially involved in inflammation by competing with AA (and EPA) as substrates in the COX and LOX (lipoxygenase) enzyme systems. However, there is little ETA in cell membranes, probably because of the overwhelming competition from dietary LA and ALA for the relevant desaturase and elongase enzymes [29]. ETA is nevertheless assumed to decrease synthesis of leukotriene (LKT) B_4, a major inflammatory mediator, partly through a direct effect on $LKTA_4$ hydrolase (Figure 2). ETA is also a substrate for 5-LOX and may compete with AA for the formation of $LKTA_4$, especially in case of severe LA restriction leading to elevated ETA concentrations [29]. It is noteworthy that the Mediterranean diet is poor in LA and rich in oleic acid, which is another circumstance where ETA concentrations are relatively high compared with the LA-rich Western diet. Thus, whatever the nutritional context (severe LA restriction or Mediterranean diet), and in partial analogy to the situation with EPA, elevated ETA concentrations can alter the balance of eicosanoids produced by leukocytes toward a potentially less inflammatory mixture [29]. The effect of ETA on COX is less clear than on 5-LOX although inhibition of endothelial PGI_2 production has been ascribed to ETA [30]. This could, at least theoretically, increase the risk of thrombosis. Thus, a traditional Mediterranean diet with high intake of oleic acid and omega-3 PUFAs from both vegetable and marine sources and low intake of saturated fatty acids and LA may be the best compromise to reduce the risk of both inflammation and thrombosis. This has been confirmed in clinical trials [28, 31–33]. In any case, as emphasized by several major investigators in the field, the background omega-6 PUFA content of the diet is a key issue when fortifying diets with either omega-9 and/or omega-3 fatty acids for therapeutic or health-enhancing purpose [19, 27, 29].

4.   INFLAMMATORY EICOSANOID SYNTHESIS FROM ESSENTIAL PUFAs

A key link between PUFAs and inflammation is that the family of inflammatory mediators termed eicosanoids is generated from 20-carbon PUFAs released by cell-membrane phospholipids (Figure 2). Inflammatory cells typically contain a high proportion of omega-6 AA and low proportions of omega-3 EPA. In fact, the AA to EPA ratio is extremely dependent on the dietary habits of the populations examined [28, 29, 34]. In persons following a typical Western diet (with a high AA to EPA ratio), AA is the dominant substrate for eicosanoid synthesis. In contrast, in persons following a Mediterranean diet poor in omega-6 PUFAs (but rich in omega-9 oleic acid and omega-3 PUFAs), the relevance of AA and AA-derived eicosanoids is reduced. Eicosanoids include prostaglandins (PGs), thromboxanes (TXs), leukotrienes (LKTs), and many other less studied substances (Figure 2). AA is mobilized from cell membranes by phospholipases and subsequently acts as a substrate for the enzymes that synthesize eicosanoids. The metabolism of AA by COX gives rise to the 2-series PGs and TXs. However, when EPA is the substrate for COX instead of AA, the eicosanoids that are produced belong to 3-series PGs, the properties of which are very different (less inflammatory, less vasoconstrictive, less prothrombotic) from those of 2-series PGs [19]. Substances derived from ETA are less well-characterized and their physiological roles are not clearly determined.

There are two isoforms of COX: COX-1 is a constitutive enzyme and COX-2 is induced in inflammatory cells as a result of stimulation (for instance by cytokines produced by activated leukocytes) and accounts for the marked increase in eicosanoid production that occurs in activated cells. It is very important to understand that PGs are formed in a cell-specific manner (Figure 2). For instance, monocytes (and macrophages) produce large amounts of PGE_2 and PGF_2, neutrophils produce moderate amounts of PGE_2 and mast cells produce PGD_2. AA metabolism through the 5-lipoxygenase (5-LOX) pathway gives rise to hydroxyl and hydroperoxyl derivatives and to the 4-series LKTs. EPA metabolism by the 5-LOX pathway gives rise to 5-series LKTs, which have a considerably lower inflammatory effect than 4-series LKTs.

One of the major inflammatory AA-derived 2-series PGs is PGE_2. Its pro-inflammatory effects include fever, increased vascular permeability and vasodi-latation, as well as increased pain and edema. PGE_2 induces COX-2, up-regulates its own production by leukocytes, and induces the production of inflammatory cytokines (TNF, interleukins), which are other major mediators of inflammation that are able to recruit new leukocytes and again induce COX-2. However, PGE_2 also inhibits 5-LOX, decreasing the production of the 4-series LKTs, and induces 15-LOX, promoting the formation of lipoxins [35]. The latter mediators have potent anti-inflammatory effects [36, 37] indicating that the same compound, namely PGE_2, possesses both pro- and anti-inflammatory actions, whereas PGE_3 derived from EPA apparently is less active than PGE_2 [17–19]. This may explain some puzzling data showing benefits from PGE_2 in some inflammatory compartments, especially those where 4-series LKTs exert damaging effects [38]. In fact, $LKTB_4$, one of the major inflammatory AA-derived eicosanoids of the 4-series LKTs which increases vascular permeability is a potent chemotactic agent for leukocytes and increases the generation of reactive oxygen species and production of inflammatory cytokines. $LKTB_4$ was recently shown to play an important role in the atherosclerotic process (using the intima-media thickness as a surrogate marker of atherosclerosis) in certain patients with a specific polymorphism (variant 5-LOX genotypes) [39]. Interestingly, a protective effect of omega-3 PUFAs (and a deleterious effect of omega-6 PUFAs) was shown in that study, suggesting that long-chain omega-3 PUFAs may also be able to slow down the progression of the atherosclerotic process contrary to the results of large randomized trials where the protective effect of EPA+DHA appeared to be confined to myocardial anti-arrhythmic effects [40–42]. In addition, a recent study demonstrated that incorporation of EPA and DHA in the plaque might have a stabilizing (anti-inflammatory) effect thereby preventing acute ischemic events [43]. This suggests that EPA+DHA may inhibit the generation of metalloproteinases [44, 45], compounds that are potentially involved in plaque vulnerability and ulceration and subsequent thrombotic complications. Further studies are obviously needed to support this assertion.

The molecular biology of PGE_2 and 4-series LKTs illustrates the complexity of the health effects of eicosanoids and the necessity to be careful when using potent pharmacological agents to manage them. As shown with the anti-COX-2 (coxib) agents, the ultimate outcome may be less appealing than previously expected, e.g., an increased risk of CVD complications [7, 8].

The EPA-derived 3-series PGs and 5-series LKTs are considerably less inflammatory than those derived from AA [17–19]. Increased consumption of omega-3 PUFAs results in increased proportions of omega-3 PUFAs (especially EPA) in inflammatory cell phospholipids, at the expense of AA. This was shown to result in decreased production of PGE_2, TXB_2 and $LKTB_4$ by inflammatory cells and, at the same time, increased production of PGE_3, TXB_3 and $LKTB_5$. The functional significance is that the mediators derived from EPA are less potent than those derived from AA. It may be exaggerated, however, to say that EPA-derived eicosanoids are anti-inflammatory. Let it simply be said that they are less pro-inflammatory than the AA-derived eicosanoids.

Finally, recent studies have identified novel groups of mediators, termed E-series resolvins (for "*resolution phase interaction products*") when derived from EPA by COX-2, and D-series resolvins (or docosatrienes and neuroprotectins) when derived from DHA by COX-2, which appear to have anti-inflammatory properties, especially during the resolution phase of the inflammatory process [46]. The relevance of this specific anti-inflammatory activity for vascular inflammation associated with atherosclerosis remains to be elucidated.

Thus, the key "anti-inflammatory effect" of omega-3 PUFAs appears to be antagonism of AA, the major inflammatory PUFA (Table 1). But another major question is whether omega-3 PUFAs have anti-inflammatory effects that occur downstream of altered eicosanoid production.

5. OTHER ANTI-INFLAMMATORY EFFECTS OF OMEGA-3 PUFAs

Proposed mechanisms by which omega-3 PUFAs may have anti-inflammatory effects are shown in Table 1. In addition to competing with omega-6 PUFAs at various levels of PUFA metabolism, EPA and DHA have been shown to inhibit the production of cytokines by leukocytes and other inflammatory cells *in vitro* and *ex vivo* [47]. In clinical studies, EPA+DHA-rich fish oil supplementation resulted in decreased production of TNF and interleukins by leukocytes [48]. Also, diets enriched in ALA have been associated with reduced vascular inflammation and endothelial activation [49]. Which bioactive components (ALA itself or its metabolite, EPA, or both) inhibit endothelial activation is not clear. In fact, De Caterina et al. [50] showed that DHA and EPA significantly decrease cytokine-induced expression of adhesion molecules by endothelial cells. This has the functional effect of decreasing the binding of leukocytes, a crucial step of vascular inflammation and atherosclerosis [1, 13]. Interestingly, oleic acid (the precursor of the omega-9 PUFA ETA) was also shown to inhibit endothelial activation [51] and olive oil itself (the oil typically used around the Mediterranean Sea) had similar effects in middle-aged men [52].

Some of the anti-inflammatory effects of omega-3 PUFAs may also be exerted at the level of gene expression. Although the extent of these effects in humans *in vivo* is

Table 1. A summary of the main potential anti-inflammatory effects of omega-3 PUFAs

1.	The 18-carbon omega-3 ALA (18:3n-3) decreases the synthesis of pro-inflammatory AA from the omega-6 LA (18:2n-6) through competition at the level of their common elongation and desaturation pathways (Figure 1).
2.	The 20-carbon omega-3 PUFA EPA (20:5n-3) decreases the levels of AA in inflammatory cells. EPA replaces AA in membrane phospholipids (Figure 2).
3.	EPA decreases the production of AA-derived inflammatory eicosanoids by decreasing the release of AA from cell membranes and competing at the levels of the COX and LOX enzyme systems.
4.	EPA gives rise to a family of eicosanoid mediators that are analogs of those produced from AA (Figure 2) but are often less potent (less inflammatory).
5.	Omega-3 PUFAs reduce the production of inflammatory cytokines (including TNF and interleukins) by leukocytes and other cells involved in the inflammation process through decreased production of TXA_2 and $LKTB_4$ (see text).
6.	Omega-3 PUFAs induce production of the anti-inflammatory E-resolvins from EPA and D-resolvins from DHA (see text).
7.	The omega-3 PUFAs EPA and DHA alter the expression of inflammatory genes via inhibition of the non-specific transcription factor NF-?B (see text).

not yet clear, animal studies indicate potentially significant effects on the expression of a range of inflammatory genes. For instance, omega-3 PUFAs were shown to decrease the cytokine-mediated induction of expression of COX-2, TNFα and various interleukins in cultured chondrocytes and human cartilage explants [19]. Similar data were reported with DHA and vascular endothelial cells [50]. This effect on gene expression was independent of the effect on eicosanoid production; thus, omega-3 PUFAs may directly modulate the intracellular signaling pathway that leads to activation of one or more transcription factors such as nuclear factor κB (NF-κB) [19]. For instance, omega-3 PUFAs were shown to prevent NF-κB activation by TNFα and to decrease endotoxin-induced activation of NF-κB by leukocytes [51]. Thus, in addition to directly decreasing the production of inflammatory eicosanoids and leukocyte cytokines, omega-3 PUFAs act by altering the expression of inflammatory genes.

6.   ESSENTIAL PUFAs, COX, ASPIRIN AND COXIBS

Once mobilized from cell membrane phospholipids, 20-carbon PUFAs (either AA or EPA) are oxygenated into eicosanoids along various pathways including COX, LOX, P450 epoxygenase and (nonenzymatic) isoprostane synthesis. In addition, free PUFAs are available to exert direct effects on membrane receptors and ion channels, e.g. to deploy anti-arrhythmic effects in the ischemic myocardium [54].

As indicated above, the fate and distribution of AA or EPA metabolites depend on the cell type where they are formed. For example, leukocytes, endothelial cells, smooth muscle cells in the arterial wall, as well as platelets express PGE synthase and are thus all capable of producing proinflammatory PGE. Platelets also express TXA synthase and elaborate the prothrombotic and vasoconstrictive TXA_2. Endothelial cells express prostacyclin synthase and synthesize the antithrombotic and vasodilating PGI_2. In addition to cell-specific synthesis, the biological effects of eicosanoids are governed by cell-specific receptor-dependent signaling pathways that define biological responses. Pharmacological inhibition of eicosanoid synthesis has been the focus of intensive drug development, from aspirin to NSAIDs and specific coxibs. NSAIDs provide antipyretic, analgesic and anti-inflammatory properties but the relative degree of these effects varies markedly from one compound to another. NSAIDs also share the common side-effects of gastro-intestinal ulceration and renal function impairment.

With the recognition that aspirin inhibits platelet function via inhibition of thromboxane formation, the anti-thrombotic effects of NSAIDs gained unique therapeutic emphasis. Because endothelial PGI_2 also has an anti-platelet action, nonselective inhibition of COX attenuates the anti-platelet effect of aspirin. Thus, in view of the irreversible inhibition of thromboxane formation in platelets by aspirin and the differences in half-lives of platelet and endothelial COX, very low dose aspirin was found to provide optimal antithrombotic activity for prevention of thrombotic CVD complications [22, 23]. Finally, the recognition that there are two different COXs led to the straightforward view that COX-2 is specifically responsible for the adverse proinflammatory effects of eicosanoids and that selective COX-2 inhibitors (coxibs) would provide adequate analgesia and anti-inflammatory effects without the gastrointestinal side effects due to COX-1 inhibition and without platelet and endothelial cell effects [23]. Unfortunately, this clean mechanistic distinction between the COXs is an oversimplification [7]. In fact, inhibition of COX-2 appears to be associated with suppression of prostacyclin (PGI_3 from EPA and PGI_2 from AA) synthesis [55]. The complexity of the interactions between the different factors in arterial physiology is illustrated by the fact that suppression of COX-2 results in an increasing flux of AA towards the different LO pathways, with potential additional inflammatory effects. This may be especially important in the setting of inflammation in atherosclerotic plaque, as suggested by the study of Dwyer et al. [39] on the role of LKTs in plaque progression.

The consequences of COX-2 inhibition by coxibs recorded in some of the observational studies and randomized trials were therefore—perhaps not surprisingly—an increased risk of CVD complications [7, 8, 56, 57]. It is important to note that increased risks have been observed in populations at low risk for CVD complications [56, 57] and have also been found in some studies with nonselective NSAIDs [58]. This suggests that the increased risk of CVD complications associated with coxibs and other anti-inflammatory drugs may not be an effect of a specific class of drugs (such as the coxibs) but rather may be related to the indiscriminant inhibition of the inflammatory process itself.

Beyond the practical problems regarding the treatment of painful inflammatory chronic diseases such as arthritis, the controversy surrounding effects of coxibs on

CVD raises several major questions regarding the inflammatory theory of atherosclerosis. The main one is that it is difficult to accept that vascular inflammation is a prominent feature of CVD development if anti-inflammatory treatments (whatever the class of drugs) tested in randomized trials are not able to reduce the risk of CVD complications. In fact, a major question is whether we should not reconsider our conception of atherosclerosis and CVD complications. For instance, if arterial lesion fibrosis is a key factor in lesion stabilization, altering the process by any anti-inflammatory treatment may increase the risk of plaque ulceration and CVD complications.

The potential role of omega-3 PUFAs in vascular inflammation and CVD may help open new areas of investigation. From a biological point of view omega-3 PUFAs appear to have anti-inflammatory properties that make them good candidates to reduce vascular inflammation and prevent atherosclerosis (see Table 1). However, evidence from randomized trials supports the complex nature of PUFAs in modulating vascular inflammation and atherosclerosis. In clinical trials of CVD outcomes, omega-3-PUFAs administered at low dosages (less than 1 gram per day) reduced the risk of sudden cardiac death and ventricular arrhythmias [40, 41], and a combination of increased intake of omega-9 and omega-3 fatty acids and decreased intake of omega-6 PUFAs in a Mediterranean diet produced significant reductions in fatal and non-fatal CVD complications including ventricular arrhythmias [28, 31]. In mechanistic studies, the traditional Mediterranean diet produced significant anti-inflammatory effects associated with less endothelial dysfunction and lower vascular endothelial growth factor [32, 33]. The exact mechanisms of these effects remain to be elucidated, and the anti-inflammatory effects of low dosages of omega-3-PUFAs are not clear. Whether anti-inflammatory effects can be adequately balanced to prevent vascular inflammation without altering the reparation-fibrosis process that stabilizes atherosclerotic plaques is unknown, but these observed benefits should be used to establish a working hypothesis.

Taken together, the human data indicate that vascular inflammation is a complex multi-step process and atherosclerosis is a multifactorial disease. Considering only dietary lipids, it is clear that essential PUFAs of the omega-6 and omega-3 families, saturated fatty acids, as well as omega-9 fatty acids are collectively involved. Thus, to be effective and safe, any anti-inflammatory approach to prevent atherosclerosis and CVD should be prudent, preferably non-pharmacological, multifactorial, and primarily dietary. This is compatible with the well-accepted concept that CVD is a lifestyle disease that will require lifestyle (especially dietary) changes for prevention.

REFERENCES

1. Willerson JT, Ridker PM. Inflammation as a cardiovascular risk factor. Circulation 2004;109 (II): II-2-II-10.
2. Steinberg D, Parthasarathy S, Carew TE, et al. Beyond cholesterol: modification of low-density lipoprotein that increases its atherogenicity. N Engl J Med 1989;320:915–924
3. Palinski W, Rosenfeld ME, Ylä-Herttuala S, et al. Low density lipoprotein undergoes oxidative modification in vivo. Proc Natl Acad Sci U S A. 1989;86:1372–1376.
4. Ylä-Herttuala S, Palinski W, Rosenfeld ME, et al. Evidence for the presence of oxidatively modified low density lipoprotein in atherosclerotic lesions of rabbit and man. J Clin Invest. 1989;84:1086–1095.

5. Clarke R, Armitage J. Antioxidant vitamins and risk of cardiovascular disease. Review of large-scale randomised trials. Cardiovasc Drugs Ther 2002;16:411–5.
6. Asplund K. Antioxidant vitamins in the prevention of cardiovascular disease: a systematic review. J Intern Med 2002;251:372–92.
7. Antman EM, DeMets D, Loscalzo J. Cyclooxygenase inhibition and cardiovascular risk. Circulation 2005;112:759–70.
8. Hippisley-Cox J, Coupland C. Risk of myocardial infarction in patients taking cyclo-oxygenase-2 inhibitors or conventional non-steroidal anti-inflammatory drugs: population based nested case-control analysis. BMJ 2005;352:1366–72.
9. del Rincon I, O'Leary DH, Haas RW, Escalante A. Effect of glucocorticoids on the arteries in rheumatoid arthritis. Arthritis Rheum 2004;50:3813–22.
10. Brindley DN. Role of glucocorticoids and fatty acids in the impairment of lipid metabolism observed in the metabolic syndrome. Int J Obes Relat Metab Disord 1995;19 (1):S69–75.
11. Hoffmann R, Langenberg R, Radke P, et al. Evaluation of high-dose dexamethasone-eluting stent. Am J Cardiol 2004;15:193–5.
12. Cipollone F, Fazia M, Mezzetti A. Novel determinants of plaque instability. J Thromb Haemost 2005;3:1962–75.
13. Ross R. Atherosclerosis: an inflammatory disease. N Engl J Med 1999;340:115–126.
14. De Caterina R, Zampolli A. From Asthma to atherosclerosis: 5-lipoxygenase, leukotrienes, and inflammation. N Engl J Med 2004;350:4–7.
15. Offner H, Clausen J. Inhibition of lymphocyte response to stimulants induced by unsaturated fatty acids and prostaglandins in multiple sclerosis. Lancet 1974;2:1204–5.
16. Weyman S, Belin J, Smith AD, Thompson RHS. Linoleic acid as an immunosuppressive agent. Lancet 1975;2:33.
17. Santoli D, Phillips PD, Colt TL, et al. Suppression of interleukin-2-dependent human T lymphocyte growth in vitro by prostaglandin E and their precursor fatty acids. J Clin Invest 1990;85:424–32.
18. Purasiri P, McKechnie A, Heys SD, et al. Modulation in vitro of human natural cytotoxicity lymphocyte prolifderation response to mitogens and cytokine production by essential fatty acids. Immunology 1997;92:166–72.
19. Calder PC. Polyunsaturated fatty acids and inflammation. Biochem Soc Trans 2005;33:423–7.
20. Catella-Lawson F, Reilly MP, Kapoor SC, et al. Cyclo-oxygenase inhibitors and the anti-platelet effects of aspirin. N Engl J Med 2001;345:1809–17.
21. Cleland JFG. No reduction in cardiovascular risk with NSAIDs-including aspirin? Lancet 2002;359:92–3.
22. Bates ER, Lau WC. Controversies in antiplatelet therapy for patients with cardiovascular disease. Circulation 2005;111:267–71.
23. Patrono C, Garcia-Rodriguez LA, Landolfi R. Low dose aspirin for the prevention of atherothrombosis. N Engl J Med 2005;353:49–59.
24. Gawaz M, Langer H, May AE. Platelets in inflammation and atherogenesis. J Clin Invest 2005;115:3378–84.
25. de Lorgeril M, Loire R, Guidollet J, et al. Accelerated coronary artery disease after heart transplantation: the role of enhanced platelet aggregation and thrombosis. J Intern Med. 1993:233:343–50.
26. de Lorgeril M, Boissonnat P, Mamelle N, et al. Platelet aggregation and HDL cholesterol are predictive of acute coronary events in heart transplant recipients. Circulation 1994;89:2590–4.
27. de Lorgeril M, Salen P. Alpha-linolenic acid and coronary heart disease. Nutr Metab Cardiovasc Dis 2004;14:162–9.
28. de Lorgeril M, Renaud S, Mamelle N, et al. Mediterranean Alpha-linolenic rich-diet in secondary prevention of coronary heart disease. Lancet 1994;343:1454–9.
29. James MJ, Gibson RA, Cleland LG. Dietary polyunsaturated fatty acids and inflammation mediator production. Am J Clin Nutr 2000;71(suppl):343S-8S.
30. Lerner R, Lindstrom P, Berg A, et al. Development and characterisation of essential fatty acid deficiency in human endothelial cells. Proc Natl Acad Sci USA 1995;92:1147–51.

31. de Lorgeril M, Salen P, Martin JL, et al. Mediterranean diet, traditional risk factors, and the rate of cardiovascular complications after myocardial infarction: final report of the Lyon Diet Heart Study. Circulation 1999;99:779–85.

32. Esposito K, Marfella R, Ciotola M, et al. Effect of a Mediterranean-style diet on endothelial dysfunction and markers of vascular inflammation in the metabolic syndrome. A randomized trial. JAMA 2004;292:1440–6.

33. Ambring A, Johansson M, et al. Mediterranean-inspired diet lowers the ratio of serum phospholipids n-6 to n-3 fatty acids, the number of leukocytes and platelets, and vascular endothelial growth factor in healthy subjects. Am J Clin Nutr 2006;83:575–81.

34. Lands WEM. Impact of daily food choices on health promotion and disease prevention. World Rev Nutr Diet 2001;88:1–5.

35. Levy BD, Clish CB, Schmidt B, et al. Lipid mediator class switching during acute inflammation: signals in resolution. Nat Immunol. 2001;7:612–9.

36. Serhan CN, Jain A, Marleau S, et al. Reduced inflammation and tissue damage in transgenic rabbits overexpressing 15-lipoxygenase and endogenous anti-inflammatory lipid mediators. J Immunol. 2003;171:6856–65.

37. Bannenberg G, Moussignac RL, Gronert K, et al. Lipoxins and novel 15-epi-lipoxin analogs display potent anti-inflammatory actions after oral administration.Br J Pharmacol. 2004;143:43–52.

38. Vancheri C, Mastruzzo C, Sortino MA, Crimi N. The lung as a privileged site for the beneficial actions of PGE2. Trends Immunol. 2004;25:40–6.

39. Dwyer JH, Allayee H, Dwyer K, et al. Arachidonate 5-lipoxygenase promoter genotype, dietary arachidonic acid and atherosclerosis. N Engl J Med 2004;350:29–37.

40. Burr ML, Fehily AM, Gilbert JF, et al: Effects of changes in fat, fish, and fibre intakes on death and myocardial reinfarction: Diet and reinfarction trial (DART). Lancet 1989;334:757–761.

41. GISSI-Prevenzione Investigators: Dietary supplementation with n-3 polyunsaturated fatty acids and vitamin E after myocardial infarction: results of the GISSI-Prevenzione trial. Lancet. 1999;354:447–55.

42. Leaf A, Albert CM, Josephson M, et al. for the Fatty Acid Antiarrhythmia Trial Investigators: Prevention of fatal arrhythmias in high-risk subjects by fish oil n-3 fatty acid intake. Circulation 2005;112:2762–8.

43. Thies F, Garry JM, Yaqoob P, et al. Association of n-3 polyunsaturated fatty acids with stability of atherosclerotic plaques: a randomised controlled trial. Lancet. 2003;361:477–85.

44. Kim HH, Shin CM, Park CH, et al. Eicosapentanoic acid inhibits UV-induced MMP-1 expression in human dermal fibroblasts. J Lipid res 2005;46:1712–20.

45. Inhibitory effect of oleic acid and docosahexaenoic acids on lung metastasis by colon-carcinoma-26 cells are associated with reduced matrix metalloproteinases-2 and -9 activities. Int J Cancer 1997;73:607–12.

46. Serhan CN. Novel eicosanoid and docosanoid mediators: resolvins, docosatrienes, and neuroprotectins. Curr Opin Clin Nutr Metab Care 2005;8:115–21.

47. De Caterina R, Madonna R, Massaro M. Effects of omega-3 fatty acids on cytokines and adhesion molecules. Curr Atheroscler Rep 2004;6:485–91.

48. Ferrucci L, Cherubini A, Bandinelli S, et al. Relationship of plasma polyunsaturated fatty acids to circulating inflammatory markers. J Clin Endocrinol Metab 2006;2:439–446.

49. Zhao G, Etherton TD, Martin KR, et al. Dietary alpha-linolenic acid reduces inflammatory and lipid cardiovascular risk factors in hypercholesterolemic men and women. J Nutr 2004;134:2991–7.

50. De Caterina R, Liao JK, Libby P. Fatty acid modulation of endothelial activation. Am J Clin Nutr. 2000;71 (1):213S-23S.

51. Carluccio MA, Massaro M, Bonfrate C, et al. Oleic acid inhibits endothelial activation : a direct vascular antiatherogenic mechanism of a nutritional component in the Mediterranean diet. Arterioscl Thromb Vasc Biol 1999;19:220–8.

52. Yaqoob P, Knapper JA, Webb DH, et al. Effect of olive oil on immune function in middle-aged men. Am J Clin Nutr 1998;67:129–35.

53. Todd E, Novak, Tricia A, Babcock J, et al. NF-κB inhibition by ω-3 fatty acids modulates LPS-stimulated macrophage TNF-α transcription. Am J Physiol Lung Cell Mol Physiol 2003;284:L84-L89.

54. Leaf A, Kang JX, Xiao YF, et al. Clinical prevention of sudden cardiac death by n-3 polyunsaturated fatty acids and mechanism of prevention of arrhythmias by n-3 fish oils. Circulation 2003;107:2646–52.

55. McAdam BF, Catella-Lawson F, Mardini IA, et al. Systemic biosynthesis of prostacyclin by cyclooxygenase (COX)-2: the human pharmacology of selective inhibitors of COX-2. Proc Natl Acad Sci USA 1999;96:272–7.

56. Bresalier RS, Sandler RS, Quan H, et al. Cardiovascular events associated with rofecoxib in a colorectal adenoma chemopreventrion trial. N Engl J Med 2005;352:1092–102.

57. Solomon SD, McMurray JJ, Pfeffer MA, et al. Cardiovascular risk associated with celecoxib in a clinical trial for colorectal adenoma prevention. N Engl J Med 2005;352:1071–80.

58. Graham DJ, Campen D, Hui R, et al. Risk of acute myocardial infarction and sudden cardiac death in patients treated with cyclo-oxygenase 2 selective and non-selective non-steroidal anti-inflammatory drugs: nested case-control study. Lancet 2005;365:475–81.

CHAPTER 14

NUTRITIONAL INTERVENTION IN BRAIN AGING
Reducing the effects of inflammation and oxidative stress

FRANCIS C. LAU, BARBARA SHUKITT-HALE
AND JAMES A. JOSEPH
USDA-ARS, Human Nutrition Research Center on Aging at Tufts University, Boston, MA, USA

Abstract: It is estimated that by the year 2050 the elderly (aged 65 or older) population will double the population of children (aged 0–14) for the first time in history. The expansion of the elderly population has already taken a toll on health care systems. In order to alleviate the health care costs and increase the quality of living in the aging population, it is crucial to explore methods that may retard or reverse the deleterious effects of aging. Inflammation and oxidative stress play important roles in brain aging. Inflammatory markers, as well as cellular and molecular oxidative damage, increase during normal brain aging.

R. E. Harris (ed.), Inflammation in the Pathogenesis of Chronic Diseases, 299–318.
© 2007 *Springer.*

This increase is accompanied by the concomitant decline in cognitive and motor performance in the elderly population, even in the absence of neurodegenerative diseases.
Epidemiological studies have shown that consumption of diets rich in antioxidant and
anti-inflammatory agents, such as those found in fruits and vegetables, may lower the
risk of developing age-related neurodegenerative diseases such as Parkinson's disease and
Alzheimer's disease. Research from our laboratory suggests that dietary supplementation
with fruit or vegetable extracts can decrease the age-enhanced vulnerability to oxidative
stress and inflammation. Additional research suggests that the polyphenolic compounds
found in fruits such as blueberries may exert their beneficial effects through signal transduction and neuronal communication. Thus, nutritional intervention may exert therapeutic
protection against age-related deficits and neurodegenerative diseases

1.   INTRODUCTION

Aging is a slow process that is accompanied by the decline of motor and cognitive
performance [1]. The aging process also favors the occurrence of debilitating
neurodegenerative diseases. Alzheimer's disease (AD) and Parkinson's disease (PD)
are the most common neurodegenerative diseases found in the aged population [2].
Numerous studies have indicated that the incidence and prevalence of AD increase
after the age of 60 [3] and a 47% prevalence has been observed for patients over
the age of 85 [4]. As life expectancy increases so will the prevalence of these
neurodegenerative diseases. Although much research effort has been made, the
etiology of these diseases is not yet discovered, and treatments to retard or prevent
the progression of these diseases are years away.

In order to increase the quality of life among the aging population and decrease
the socioeconomic burden imposed by the aging population, it is necessary to
identify means to forestall or reverse age-related neuronal deficits. A large body of
evidence suggests that the aging brain may provide a fertile microenvironment for
the development of age-related neuronal deficits and neurodegenerative diseases [1].
Research from our laboratory has shown that diets supplemented with antioxidant-
rich fruits and vegetables are beneficial in forestalling and reversing the deleterious
effects of aging on neuronal functioning and behavior [5–12]. This protective effect
is postulated to be the result of the antioxidant and anti-inflammatory activities of
polyphenolic compounds found in these fruits and vegetables [13].

2.   INFLAMMATION

Inflammation in the central nervous system (CNS) plays an important role in
the observed behavioral and neuronal deficits in aging [14]. There is substantial
evidence indicating that neuroinflammation is elevated during normal brain
aging [15–18]. Glial cells mediate the endogenous immune system within the
microenvironment in the CNS [19]. Glial activation is the hallmark of inflammation in the brain [20]. Activated microglia produce inflammatory molecules such
as cytokines, growth factors, and complement proteins [21, 22, 23]. These proinflammatory mediators in turn activate other cells to produce additional signaling
molecules that further activate microglia in a positive feedback loop to perpetuate

and amplify the inflammatory signaling cascade [24]. It has been shown that activated glial cells increase in the normal aging brain which exhibits greater immunoreactivity in markers for both microglia and astrocytes [18, 25–27].

Although the events leading to the inflammatory response are not fully understood, microglia-mediated inflammation has been linked to the pathogenesis of several age-related neurodegenerative diseases such as AD and PD [28–31]. Activated microglia produce proinflammatory cytokines such as interleukin-1 (IL-1), interleukin-6 (IL-6) and tumor necrosis factor-α (TNF-α) [32, 33]. These cytokines have been found in the surrounding areas of amyloid plaques [34–37]. It has been suggested that these cytokines play important roles in the formation of senile plaques in AD brains because interleukins have been found to enhance the expression of amyloid precursor protein (APP) [38–40]. In a vicious cycle, β-amyloid peptides (Aβ) in turn stimulate the production of IL-1β, IL-6, and TNF-α [39,41–43]. An increase in reactive microglia has also been found in the striatum and substantia nigra of PD brains [44]. An increase in the production of proinflammatory cytokines interferon-γ (IFN-γ), IL-1α, and TNF-α in the substantia nigra of PD patients has been reported [45, 46]. Also, TNF-α immunoreactive glial cells have been detected in the substantia nigra of PD brains [47].

Activated microglia also produce high levels of free radicals such as superoxide and nitric oxide (through the activation of inducible nitric oxide synthase) [21, 29]. Therefore, inflammation in the CNS produces oxidative stress through the respiratory burst system of activated microglia [48–53].

3. OXIDATIVE STRESS

Oxidative stress results from the shift towards production of reactive oxygen species (ROS) in the equilibrium between ROS generation and the antioxidant defense system [54]. ROS are produced during normal aerobic metabolism [55, 56]. Approximately 2 to 5% of the oxygen consumed by a cell is subsequently reduced to free radicals [49, 57]. ROS production is normally kept in check by cellular defense systems [54, 58]. However, the antioxidant defenses are not entirely efficient. In fact, about 1% of the ROS escape elimination daily, leading to oxidative cellular damage [59]. The accumulation of oxidative damage results in an increase in oxidative stress in the aged population [55, 60].

The major source of ROS in mammalian cells comes from mitochondria [61–63]. An estimated 90% of the total O_2 consumed by the human body is used by mitochondria [57, 64]. Mounting evidence suggests that oxidants produced in the mitochondria cause oxidative damage in mitochondrial DNA, lipids, and proteins and that these damages accumulate with time and induce mitochondrial dysfunctions during the aging process [62, 65–69].

The degree of oxidative cellular damage can be experimentally determined by the quantification of end-products from nucleic acid damage, lipid peroxidation, and protein oxidation [69]. Oxidative damage to nuclear and mitochondrial DNA, protein, and lipids has been found to increase with normal aging in human brain tissues [49,70–72]. Animal studies have further shown that aging induces a significant increase in cellular hydrogen peroxide, the source of hydroxyl radicals [73]. Oxidative stress may also alter calcium homeostasis, cellular signaling cascades, and gene expression [74–79]. Therefore, the accumulation of oxidative damage throughout the life span contributes to the increased vulnerability to oxidative stress seen in the aging population [80, 81]. The observed oxidative damage during normal aging is elevated in neurodegenerative diseases such as AD [71,72,82] and PD [83, 84]. Oxidative stress may contribute to these age-related diseases by inducing the expression of proinflammatory cytokines through activation of the oxidative stress-sensitive nuclear factor kappa B (NF-κB) [48, 85]. NF-κB up-regulates the inflammatory response leading to a further increase in ROS [51], which results in a continuous increase in oxidative stress and inflammation, and thus, in the progression of these diseases.

4.   BRAIN AGING

The brain is especially vulnerable to oxidative damage because it consumes a large quantity of oxygen for its metabolism and consequently generates an elevated amount of ROS [49, 54]. The structural components of the brain, namely the polyunsaturated fatty acids, are readily peroxidizable by ROS. Furthermore, the presence of high levels of iron and ascorbate in the brain facilitates the catalysis of the lipid peroxidation reaction [49,86–88]. As mentioned above, the vulnerability of the brain to oxidative stress and inflammation is enhanced in aging [89, 90]. Oxidative stress and inflammation may interact in concert to induce the age-related neuronal and behavioral changes [1].

Normal brain aging produces behavioral deficits including both cognitive and motor behaviors [91–93]. Although the molecular basis for the observed decline in both cognitive and motor performance during aging remain to be determined, it is clear that both oxidative stress and inflammation are involved [94–96].

Cognitive deficits are measured by performance on tasks involving spatial learning and memory [91,97–100]. Brain regions responsible for the various types of memory functions are the hippocampus, prefrontal cortex, and the dorsomedial striatum [101–105]. Age-related deficits in motor performance, which include decreases in balance, muscle strength, and coordination [92], are thought to be the result of alterations in the striatal dopamine system [106], or in the cerebellum [107, 108].

Rodent studies have suggested that young animals exposed to oxidative stress show similar neuronal and behavioral changes to those seen in aged animals [105,109–111]. Similar changes in behavior have been elicited with exogenously introduced inflammatory mediators known to activate glial cells in the brain [95]. Intrahippocampal administration of lipopolysaccharide (LPS) has been shown to induce the up-regulation of inflammatory mediators resulting in the degeneration of hippocampal pyramidal neurons, accompanied by the impairments in working memory [112–114]. Chronic infusion of LPS into the ventricle of young rats has also replicated many of the behavioral, inflammatory, neurochemical, and neuropathological dysfunctions seen in the AD brains [95, 96, 112–114]. These studies indicate important roles for oxidative stress and inflammation in motor and cognitive deficits during normal and neurodegenerative aging.

Given these considerations, it is extremely important to increase endogenous antioxidant/anti-inflammatory protection to prevent the loss of neuronal and behavioral function in senescence. It appears that perhaps one way to accomplish this would be through nutrition. Substantial evidence suggests that nutritional antioxidants (nutraceuticals) may exert pharmacological benefits on certain neurodegenerative diseases by balancing the negative effects of ROS and inflammation [115–117]. There has been an increasing interest in the beneficial effects of nutritional antioxidants on combating the deleterious effects of oxidative stress and inflammation in aging and age-related neurodegenerative diseases [1, 9, 118–120]. Epidemiological studies have shown that nutritional antioxidants may forestall the onset of dementia [121–123]. The question arises, however, as to which of the nutritional antioxidants may be the most effective. It appears that some of the most beneficial can be derived from the large class of polyphenols known as flavonoids. These are particularly abundant in berryfruit.

5. BENEFICIAL EFFECTS OF FLAVONOIDS IN BERRYFRUITS

5.1. Flavonoids

Plants, including fruits and vegetables, synthesize polyphenolic compounds known as flavonoids. Flavonoids are chemically diverse. There have been more than 4000 derivatives of flavonoids identified in nature [124]. The term flavonoids, derived from the Latin word flavus which means yellow, was initially used to describe yellow-colored compounds with a flavone moiety and later used to designate plant polyphenols [125]. Flavonoids are comprised of a 15-carbon phenylpropanoid core that is highly modified by glycosylation, oxidation and alkylation [126]. Based on their structures, flavonoids are categorized into several subclasses [124]. Members of one of these classes, the anthocyanins, have received much attention recently due to their antioxidant, anti-inflammatory and anti-mutagenic benefits [127].

5.1.1. Anthocyanins

The term anthocyanin is derived from the Greek words anthos and kyaneos which translate to flower and blue respectively [128]. Anthocyanins are complex, glycosylated forms of their precursors, anthocyanidins. There are 17 known, naturally occurring anthocyanidins, but only six of them are commonly found in higher plants, and these are pelargonidin, peonidin, cyanidin, melvidin, petunidin, and delphinidin. There have been about 400 anthocyanins found in nature [128]. Blueberries (BBs) provide one of the highest sources of anthocyanins [129, 130]. In a study comparing 22 different fruits and vegetables, blueberries have been found to contain the highest antioxidant capacity as measured by the oxygen radical absorption capacity (ORAC) assay [131–133]. In fact, a comprehensive survey of common foods in the United States has found that wild blueberries rank second in total antioxidant capacity per serving among the 100 foods analyzed [134]. The positive correlation between anthocyanin content and ORAC antioxidant capacity which is found in blueberries makes them especially attractive for the study of their neutraceutical effects.

5.1.2. *Bioavailability of anthocyanins in rat brains*

Importantly, for this review it appears that the anthocyanins may have direct effects in the CNS. The beneficial effects afforded by anthocyanins depend largely on their permeability through the blood-brain barrier (BBB) [135]. Liquid chromatography-mass spectrometry studies of the distribution of anthocyanins in the brains of aged Fischer 344 (F344) rats showed that 10-week BB-supplementation resulted in the localization of glycosylated forms of cyanidin, malvidin and malvidin-3-O-α-arabinose in various brain regions, particularly in the hippocampus and cortex [136]. These findings suggest that the BBB may be permeable to anthocyanins which can localize in brain regions that are important in leaning and memory [136].

5.2. Blueberry Supplementation: Animal Studies

5.2.1. *Motor and cognitive behavioral improvements*

We have shown that short-term dietary supplementation (for 8 weeks) with spinach, strawberry or blueberry (BB) extracts in an AIN-93 diet was effective in reversing age-related deficits in neuronal and cognitive function in aged F344 rats, fed from 19 to 21 months of age [6]. However, only the BB-supplemented group demonstrated improved motor performance on tests such as rod walking and accelerating rotarod which measure balance and coordination. In contrast, none of the other supplemented groups showed improvement on these tasks as compared to the control group [6]. Short-term BB supplementation provided in a modified NIH-31 diet, which is more like a natural diet, has also been found to benefit age-related declines in behavioral parameters such as balance, coordination, and working and reference memory, as seen in F344 rats [137].

5.2.2. *Cell signaling*

The improvement by the BB supplementation observed in these rats may not have resulted directly from the antioxidant activity provided by BB. Assessment of the striatal level of the endogenous antioxidant enzyme glutathione (GSH) in BB-supplemented rats revealed no beneficial effect provided by the supplementation [6]. Also, the level of ROS in the striatal tissues from the BB-supplemented rats was only moderately reduced by the supplementation [6]. This small level of antioxidant activity provided by the supplemented diet may not be sufficient to account for the diet-induced significant improvement on motor and cognitive behaviors. Therefore, there may be other benefits, in addition to the antioxidant/anti-inflammatory effects, that contributed to the observed enhancement of motor and cognitive behaviors provided by BB supplementation. It is reasonable to postulate that the bioactive compounds in BB may act as signaling molecules [138].

5.2.2.1.   GTPase activity, calcium homeostasis, and dopamine release   Indeed, striatal slices from rats on a BB-supplemented diet showed increases in carbachol-stimulated GTPase activity and $^{45}Ca^{2+}$-recovery [6]. It has been shown that aging affects calcium homeostasis [139]. Thus, blueberry supplementation may mitigate the deleterious effect of aging on calcium homeostasis. Also, oxotremorine-induced dopamine (DA) release from striatal slices obtained from rats on a BB-supplemented diet was significantly increased [6, 137]. The loss in sensitivity of the DA neurotransmitter, as well as the adrenergic, the muscarinic, and the opioid system, has been linked to oxidative stress [140–143]. The oxidative stress-induced decline in neuronal functions has been demonstrated to cause deficits in motor functions [92, 93] and cognitive behaviors [97, 99]. The enhancement in DA release through BB supplementation may provide a direct link to the improved motor and cognitive behaviors seen in rats on the BB-supplemented diet [6, 137].

5.2.2.2.   MAPKs and PKC   A study using the APP/PS1 (amyloid precursor protein/presenilin-1) transgenic mice has revealed that BB may enhance neuronal signaling [144]. The APP/PS1 transgenic mouse was used as a murine model for AD because the mutations promote beta amyloid (Aβ) production and Alzheimer-like plaque deposit in several brain regions that are accompanied in middle age by cognitive deficits. In a long-term feeding experiment, four month-old transgenic and non-transgenic mice were given a BB-supplemented or control diet for eight months until they were 12 months old. After the eight-month feeding period, the mice were assessed for their memory performance in a Y-maze. The BB-supplemented trans-genic mice performed comparably to the non-transgenic mice but significantly better than the non-supplemented transgenic mice [144]. Although BB supplementation improved cognitive performance, it did not reduce the plaque burden in the BB-supplemented transgenic mice as there was no difference in the number of plaques between the BB-supplemented and non-supplemented transgenic mice [144]. This discrepancy may be due to enhanced neuronal signaling in BB-supplemented transgenic mice; the enhancement in neuronal communication may prevent or circumvent any putative deleterious effects of the amyloid plaques imposed upon behavior. Indeed, data from this study showed that the BB-supplemented transgenic mice exhibited higher levels of extracellular signal regulated kinases (ERK1/2) in the hippocampus than that of the non-supplemented transgenic mice. Also, a greater level of protein kinase C (PKC) was observed in the striatum and hippocampus of the BB-supplemented transgenic mice [144]. The ERK and PKC kinases have been shown to play an important role in mediating cognitive function, especially in conversion of short-term to long-term memory [145]. Therefore, the bioactive compounds in BB may serve as signaling mediators in addition to the antioxidant/anti-inflammatory effectors.

5.2.2.3. *NF-κB* The effects of BB supplementation on the level of oxidative stress-sensitive NF-κB expression have been examined [11]. In this study, young and aged male F344 rats were fed a BB-supplemented or a control diet for four months, after which time the rats were tested for their object recognition memory (ORM). After the behavioral tests, the rats were killed and the level of NF-κB protein expression was assayed in five different regions of the rat brains. An age-related decline in ORM was observed among the young and aged rats fed the control diet. Aged rats on the BB-supplemented diet showed an improvement in ORM as compared to that of the age-matched control rats. This enhancement in ORM seen in the BB-supplemented rats was accompanied by the reduction of age-induced increase in NF-κB expression to the young control level in the frontal cortex, hippocampus and the striatum. BB supplementation also reduced cerebellar NF-κB expression in BB-supplemented aged rats as compared to the age-matched control animals, but it did not restore the expression level to that of young controls. BB supplementation had no effect on the expression of NF-κB in the basal forebrain. The results indicated that BB supplementation attenuated the age-related elevation of NF-κB in a brain region-specific manner [11].

5.2.2.4. *Cerebellar noradrenergic function* Age-related changes in α-adrenergic function have been observed in the cerebellar noradrenergic system (NAS). These alterations may underlie certain deficits in motor learning observed in aged rats [108]. Investigation of α-adrenergic receptor function revealed that as high as 80% of the recorded cerebellar Purkinje cells from young rats responded to treatment with an α-adrenergic agonist producing enhancement of γ-amino butyric (GABA)-induced inhibition, in contrast to the 40% from old rats. However, this age-related decrease in α-adrenergic receptor function was restored by BB supplementation to the level seen in the young animals [146].

5.2.2.5. *Neurogenesis* The hippocampal neurons are capable of self renewal or neurogenesis. However, there is an age-related decline in neurogenesis which is accompanied by cognitive deficits [10, 147–149]. A short-term feeding experiment was conducted to determine whether BB supplementation could restore the age-related cognitive decline through enhanced neurogenesis [10]. In this study, 19-month-old male Fischer 344 rats were fed either a control or BB-supplemented diet for eight weeks. After being tested for their cognitive performance, the rats were injected with bromodeoxyuridine (BrdU), for 4 consecutive days, before they were processed for immunohistochemistry [10]. BrdU is a modified analog of thymidine that can be incorporated into nascent DNA during cell replication. Neurogenesis in the rat brains was quantified by counting the BrdU-positive cells obtained by immunostaining with anti-BrdU antibody [10]. BB supplementation significantly increased neurogenesis in the dentate gyrus of aged rat brains and improved cognitive performance of these animals by reducing reference and working memory errors [10]. There was negative correlation between the number of BrdU-positive neurons and the number of total memory errors [10]. Furthermore, BB supplementation enhanced the level of neurotrophic factor insulin-like growth factor 1 (IGF-1) and its receptor (IGF-1R). The level of mitogen-activated ERK was also increased by BB-supplementation. These increases in the signaling molecules were inversely correlated to the number of total memory errors. The results from this study clearly indicated that BB supplementation increased hippocampal plasticity and cognitive performance via concerted mechanisms involving neurogenesis, neurotrophic factor IGF-1 and its receptor, and MAP kinase signal transduction cascades [10].

5.2.3.   *Surgically-induced neurodegeneration*

5.2.3.1.   Kainic acid-induced neuroinflammation   Kainic acid (KA), an excito-toxin which produces neuronal lesions and induces an inflammatory response in the brain, was used to investigate the beneficial effects of BB supplementation on inflammation [150, 151]. This study used four-month old male F344 rats that were fed a control, 2% BB, or 0.015% piroxicam (PX, a non-steroidal anti-inflammatory drug, NSAID) diet for 8 weeks before they were subjected to intrahippocampal injection with Ringer's saline (R) or KA (300 ng in 0.5μ lR) via stereotaxic surgery. Ten days after the injection, rats were tested in the Morris water maze (MWM) for 4 days. After behavioral tests, rats were divided into two groups. One group was processed for immunohistochemical analysis of OX-6, a glial inflammatory marker. The other group was used to profile the expression of IL-1α, TNF-α, NF-κB and IGF-1 mRNA in the hippocampus.

Kainic acid produced an inflammatory response in the hippocampus as shown by increased hippocampal OX-6 activation. The BB supplementation reduced this inflammatory response; however it did not restore OX-6 activation to control levels [150].

The beneficial effects of the BB supplementation on behavioral performance were seen primarily on days 2 and 3, while the rats on the PX diet showed improved performance on day 4 which was the reversal day. The data indicated that BB and PX have differential effects on cognitive behavior. If both compounds had been fed to the rats in the same diet, they might have exerted a synergistic effect to improve memory better than either compound alone [150].

Also, BB- and PX-supplemented diets were found to improve performance in the rats injected with vehicle alone. These rats were not subjected to KA-induced oxidative stress and inflammation. This enhanced effect of the BB supplementation was consistent with previous studies. It is hypothesized that the bioactive compounds in blueberries may possess effects beyond antioxidant activity or anti-inflammation. They may serve as signaling molecules to facilitate neuronal communication and enhance neurogenesis.

Gene expression analysis showed that BB supplementation was able to restore the expression of NF-κB to the control level and reduce the expression of IL-1α and TNF-α (though not to the control level) in the hippocampus. On the other hand, BB supplementation elevated the expression of neuroprotective trophic factor

IGF-1 in KA-injected animals, suggesting that BB exerts its effect on inflammation and neurotrophic events through different cascades [151].

5.2.3.2.   Ischemia-induced stroke   The effect of BB supplementation on stroke by ischemia-induced brain damage was conducted in 45 day-old male Long-Evans rats [152]. Rats were fed a BB-supplemented or control AIN93G diet for six weeks prior to stroke-induction followed by hypoxia [152]. One week after the simulated stroke, the total neuronal damage in the ischemic hippocampus was assessed histologically. BB supplementation afforded a 57% neuroprotection as determined by the number of damaged neurons in the hippocampus [152]. However, the protection appeared to be selective for the C1 (66% neuroprotection) and C2 (68% neuroprotection) regions of the hippocampus. There was only a 9% neuroprotection in the C3 region of the hippocampus [152].

5.2.3.3.   6-OHDA-induced   nigrostriatal   dopaminergic   neuronal   damage Degeneration of dopaminergic neurons in the substantia nigra has been linked to age-related neurodegenerative Parkinson's disease [31]. A study was conducted to examine the beneficial effects of BB supplementation on the inflammatory response following striatal injection of 6-hydroxydopamine (6-OHDA) into rats fed a BB-supplemented or a control diet [153]. One week after striatal injection of 6-OHDA, a rapid but transient increase in OX-6 positive microglial cells from BB-supplemented rats was observed. However, one month post-injection, the number of OX-6 positive cells from the BB-supplemented rats was restored to the level of sham-injected rats while a significant increase in the number of OX-6 positive cells was observed in the control-fed 6-OHDA-injected rats [153]. An increase in the number of tyrosine hydroxylase (TH)-positive neurons was also found in BB-fed rats compared to control rats four weeks post-injection. These findings indicate that BB supplementation decreases neuroinflammation and facilitates the innervation of dopaminergic striatal neurons that have been surgically injured [153].

5.3.   Blueberry Treatment: Cell and Worm Studies

5.3.1.   *Muscarinic receptors in COS-7 cells*

Accumulating evidence suggests that there is age-related loss of sensitivity in muscarinic receptors of the brain (MAChRs). Loss of MAChRs has also been observed in neurodegenerative AD [154, 155] and we have shown that it is exacerbated by oxidative stress [156]. There is also strong evidence linking MAChRs to various aspects of amyloid precursor protein processing and vascular functioning [157, 158]. Moreover, the various MAChR subtypes may show differential susceptibility to oxidative stress. Indeed, we have shown that COS-7 cells transfected with MAChR subtypes M1, M2 or M4 showed greater oxidative stress susceptibility than those transfected with M3 or M5 when they were exposed to dopamine or Aβ [159]. However, chimeric M1 (M1M3i3) receptors, in which the variable i3 loop of the M3 receptor (M3i3) was replaced with the i3 loop of the M1 receptor, exhibited a reduction in dopamine sensitivity. This decrease in dopamine sensitivity was not seen in chimeric M3 (M3M1i3) receptors indicating that the variable i3 loop of the M3 receptor may be responsible for the observed decrease in oxidative stress sensitivity [159]. Results from BB-treated MAChR M1-transfected COS-7 cells revealed that BB-treatment protected these cells against dopamine- or Aβ-induced oxidative stress [12]. The findings indicate that BB may be used to mitigate the toxic effects of Aβ and dopamine seen in AD patients.

5.3.2. Anticancer activity in cancer cell lines

The beneficial effects of blueberries on antiproliferation and induction of apoptosis were examined with two human colon cancer cell lines [160]. The anticancer activities of phenolic compounds found in rabbiteye blueberries were systematically assessed. It was found that the phenolic acid fraction exhibited low levels of bioactivity while the anthocyanin fractions showed the highest antiproliferative effect [160]. The same fractions also demonstrated 3- to 7-fold increases in DNA fragmentation, suggesting that anthocyanins induced apoptosis in these cancer cells [160].

Extracellular matrix (ECM) proteolysis plays an important role in the process of cancer metastasis. Matrix metalloproteinases (MMPs) are the major mediators in the degradation of ECM. Therefore, regulation of MMP activity is crucial in the control of tumor metastasis [161]. The effects of three flavonoid-rich fractions (crude, anthocyanin, and proanthocyanin-enriched fraction) on MMP regulation in DU145 human prostate cancer cells were investigated [162]. Each fraction elicited a decrease in the activity of MMP-2 and MMP-9. However, cancer cells treated with the proanthocyanin-enriched fraction exhibited the greatest inhibition in MMP activity [162]. Therefore, blueberry flavonoids appear to inhibit cancer metastasis by blocking MMP activity.

5.3.3. Antioxidant/Anti-inflammatory effects on murine microglia

LPS-activated microglia provide an in vitro model for the study of mechanisms underlying inflammation-mediated neuronal damage. The antioxidant/anti-inflammatory effects of blueberry polyphenols were exemplified in mouse BV2 microglial cells. We found that incubation with BB significantly and dose-dependently inhibited the production of nitrite (a stable metabolite of nitric oxide) in LPS-conditioned media. This reduction was accompanied by a decline in the mRNA and protein expression of inducible nitric oxide synthase (iNOS) and cyclooxygenase-2 (COX-2) [163]. Furthermore, the proinflammatory cytokines IL-β and TNF-α from LPS-conditioned media were found to be reduced in a dose-responsive manner. Intracellular ROS levels were found to be attenuated by BB treatment [163]. These findings provided further evidence that the antioxidant and anti-inflammatory properties of blueberries may involve alterations in stress signaling.

5.3.4.   Longevity and thermotolerance in caenorhabditis elegans

It has been reported that a complex mixture of blueberry polyphenols was able to extend the lifespan and retard the age-related cellular damage in the nematode, C. elegans [164]. Results from this report indicated that the benefits of the blueberry polyphenols encompassed more than just antioxidant activity, since treatment with BB polyphenols also attenuated the deleterious effects of acute heat stress on the survival of nematodes. When BB polyphenols were separated into the three primary fractions (anthocyanin-, proanthocyanidin-, and hydroxycinnamic ester-enriched fraction), only the proanthocyanidin-enriched fraction produced significant increases in lifespan and thermotolerance similar to that of the starting BB polyphenol mixture [164]. The authors postulated that the beneficial effects of the blueberry polyphenols required activation of the calcium/calmodulin dependent protein kinase II (CaMKII) pathway that is important in osmotic stress resistance and independent of their antioxidant effects. Thus, in this particular model, the primary beneficial effect may be the regulation of osmotic stress resistance through activity of the osr-1 genetic pathway rather than oxidative stress per se. [164].

6.   CONCLUSIONS

Findings reviewed above suggest that oxidative stress and inflammation may be the major sources contributing to neuronal and behavioral deficits observed in the aging process and age-related neurodegenerative diseases [14,16, 68, 165–168]. A growing interest in dietary antioxidants has been heightened by the revelation that the plethora of natural antioxidants found in plant food matrices, such as fruits and vegetables, possess neuroprotective, cardioprotective, and chemoprotective properties [138,169–171].

In this regard, berryfruit may be especially potent in free radical quenching activity as assessed via the water-soluble ORAC index [132, 172, 173]. More importantly, it appears that berryfruit such as blueberries may also exert their antioxidant/anti-inflammatory effects by directly altering the oxidative and heat stress signaling pathways. Additionally, blueberries have been shown to increase the expression of MAP kinases [144], as well as neuronal signaling associated with learning and memory, that result in increases in neurogenesis, accompanied by increases in the levels of ERK and IGF-1 expression [10]. These alterations, coupled with increases in downstream mediators such as cAMP response element binding protein (CREB), might be mechanistically involved in the enhanced cognitive and motor behavioral performance in berryfruit-supplemented animals in senescence. Importantly, results from C. elegans indicate that [6], in addition to their antioxidant activities, blueberries may increase mean life span by increasing thermotolerance by regulation of osmotic stress. Thus, nutritional interventions with high antioxidant fruits such as berryfruits may prove to be a valuable asset in strengthening the brain against the ravages of time and retard or prevent the development of age-related neurodegenerative diseases.

REFERENCES

1. Joseph JA, Shukitt-Hale B, Casadesus G. Reversing the deleterious effects of aging on neuronal communication and behavior: beneficial properties of fruit polyphenolic compounds. Am J Clin Nutr 2005; 81:313S-316S.
2. Nicita-Mauro V. Parkinson's disease, Parkinsonism and aging. Arch Gerontol Geriatr Suppl 2002; 35 Suppl:225–38.
3. Di Matteo V, Esposito E. Biochemical and therapeutic effects of antioxidants in the treatment of Alzheimer's disease, Parkinson's disease, and amyotrophic lateral sclerosis. Curr Drug Targets CNS Neurol Disord 2003; 2:95–107.
4. Evans DA, Funkenstein HH, Albert MS, et al. Prevalence of Alzheimer's disease in a community population of older persons. Higher than previously reported. Jama 1989; 262:2551–6.
5. Bickford PC, Shukitt-Hale B, Joseph J. Effects of aging on cerebellar noradrenergic function and motor learning: nutritional interventions. Mech Ageing Dev 1999; 111:141–54.
6. Joseph JA, Shukitt-Hale B, Denisova NA, et al. Reversals of age-related declines in neuronal signal transduction, cognitive and motor behavioral deficits with blueberry, spinach or strawberry dietary supplementation. Journal of Neuroscience 1999; 19:8114–21.
7. Shukitt-Hale B, Smith DE, Meydani M, Joseph JA. The effects of dietary antioxidants on psychomotor performance in aged mice. Exp Gerontol 1999; 34:797–808.
8. Youdim KA, Shukitt-Hale B, MacKinnon S, Kalt W, Joseph JA. Polyphenolics enhance red blood cell resistance to oxidative stress: in vitro and in vivo. Biochim Biophys Acta 2000; 1523:117–22.
9. Galli RL, Shukitt-Hale B, Youdim KA, Joseph JA. Fruit polyphenolics and brain aging: nutritional interventions targeting age-related neuronal and behavioral deficits. Ann N Y Acad Sci 2002; 959:128–32.
10. Casadesus G, Shukitt-Hale B, Stellwagen HM, et al. Modulation of hippocampal plasticity and cognitive behavior by short-term blueberry supplementation in aged rats. Nutr Neurosci 2004; 7:309–16.
11. Goyarzu P, Malin DH, Lau FC, et al. Blueberry supplemented diet: effects on object recognition memory and nuclear factor-kappa B levels in aged rats. Nutr Neurosci 2004; 7:75–83.
12. Joseph JA, Fisher DR, Carey AN. Fruit extracts antagonize Abeta- or DA-induced deficits in Ca2+ flux in M1-transfected COS-7 cells. J Alzheimers Dis 2004; 6:403–11; discussion 443–9.
13. Rice-Evans CA, Miller NJ. Antioxidant activities of flavonoids as bioactive components of food. Biochemical Society Transactions 1996; 24:790–794.
14. Bodles AM, Barger SW. Cytokines and the aging brain – what we don't know might help us. Trends Neurosci 2004; 27:621–6.
15. Eikelenboom P, Veerhuis R. The role of complement and activated microglia in the pathogenesis of Alzheimer's disease. Neurobiol Aging 1996; 17:673–80.
16. O'Banion MK, Finch CE. Inflammatory mechanisms and anti-inflammatory therapy in Alzheimer's disease. Neurobiol Aging 1996; 17:669–71.
17. Gordon MN, Schreier WA, Ou X, Holcomb LA, Morgan DG. Exaggerated astrocyte reactivity after nigrostriatal deafferentation in the aged rat. J Comp Neurol 1997; 388:106–19.
18. Rozovsky I, Finch CE, Morgan TE. Age-related activation of microglia and astrocytes: in vitro studies show persistent phenotypes of aging, increased proliferation, and resistance to down-regulation. Neurobiol Aging 1998; 19:97–103.
19. Kreutzberg GW. Microglia: a sensor for pathological events in the CNS. Trends Neurosci 1996; 19:312–8.
20. Orr CF, Rowe DB, Halliday GM. An inflammatory review of Parkinson's disease. Prog Neurobiol 2002; 68:325–40.
21. Darley-Usmar V, Wiseman H, Halliwell B. Nitric oxide and oxygen radicals: a question of balance. FEBS Lett 1995; 369:131–5.
22. McGeer PL, McGeer EG. The inflammatory response system of brain: implications for therapy of Alzheimer and other neurodegenerative diseases. Brain Res Brain Res Rev 1995; 21:195–218.

23. Chen S, Frederickson RC, Brunden KR. Neuroglial-mediated immunoinflammatory responses in Alzheimer's disease: complement activation and therapeutic approaches. Neurobiol Aging 1996; 17:781–7.

24. Floyd RA. Neuroinflammatory processes are important in neurodegenerative diseases: an hypothesis to explain the increased formation of reactive oxygen and nitrogen species as major factors involved in neurodegenerative disease development. Free Radic Biol Med 1999; 26:1346–55.

25. Sheng JG, Mrak RE, Griffin WS. Enlarged and phagocytic, but not primed, interleukin-1 alpha-immunoreactive microglia increase with age in normal human brain. Acta Neuropathol (Berl) 1998; 95:229–34.

26. Sloane JA, Hollander W, Moss MB, Rosene DL, Abraham CR. Increased microglial activation and protein nitration in white matter of the aging monkey. Neurobiol Aging 1999; 20:395–405.

27. Conde JR, Streit WJ. Microglia in the aging brain. J Neuropathol Exp Neurol 2006; 65:199–203.

28. Akiyama H, Barger S, Barnum S, et al. Inflammation and Alzheimer's disease. Neurobiol Aging 2000; 21:383–421.

29. McGeer PL, McGeer EG. Inflammation and the degenerative diseases of aging. Ann N Y Acad Sci 2004; 1035:104–16.

30. Streit WJ. Microglia and Alzheimer's disease pathogenesis. J Neurosci Res 2004; 77:1–8.

31. Olanow CW, Tatton WG. Etiology and pathogenesis of Parkinson's disease. Annu Rev Neurosci 1999; 22:123–44.

32. Luterman JD, Haroutunian V, Yemul S, et al. Cytokine gene expression as a function of the clinical progression of Alzheimer disease dementia. Arch Neurol 2000; 57:1153–60.

33. Tarkowski E, Liljeroth AM, Minthon L, Tarkowski A, Wallin A, Blennow K. Cerebral pattern of pro- and anti-inflammatory cytokines in dementias. Brain Res Bull 2003; 61:255–60.

34. Bauer J, Ganter U, Strauss S, et al. The participation of interleukin-6 in the pathogenesis of Alzheimer's disease. Res Immunol 1992; 143:650–7.

35. Dickson DW, Lee SC, Mattiace LA, Yen SH, Brosnan C. Microglia and cytokines in neurological disease, with special reference to AIDS and Alzheimer's disease. Glia 1993; 7:75–83.

36. Rogers J, Webster S, Lue LF, et al. Inflammation and Alzheimer's disease pathogenesis. Neurobiol Aging 1996; 17:681–6.

37. Mrak RE, Griffin WS. Glia and their cytokines in progression of neurodegeneration. Neurobiol Aging 2005; 26:349–54.

38. Goldgaber D, Harris HW, Hla T, et al. Interleukin 1 regulates synthesis of amyloid beta-protein precursor mRNA in human endothelial cells. Proc Natl Acad Sci U S A 1989; 86:7606–10.

39. Del Bo R, Angeretti N, Lucca E, De Simoni MG, Forloni G. Reciprocal control of inflammatory cytokines, IL-1 and IL-6, and beta-amyloid production in cultures. Neurosci Lett 1995; 188:70–4.

40. Forloni G, Demicheli F, Giorgi S, Bendotti C, Angeretti N. Expression of amyloid precursor protein mRNAs in endothelial, neuronal and glial cells: modulation by interleukin-1. Brain Res Mol Brain Res 1992; 16:128–34.

41. Araujo DM, Cotman CW. Beta-amyloid stimulates glial cells in vitro to produce growth factors that accumulate in senile plaques in Alzheimer's disease. Brain Res 1992; 569:141–5.

42. Gitter BD, Cox LM, Rydel RE, May PC. Amyloid beta peptide potentiates cytokine secretion by interleukin-1 beta-activated human astrocytoma cells. Proc Natl Acad Sci U S A 1995; 92: 10738–41.

43. Tuppo EE, Arias HR. The role of inflammation in Alzheimer's disease. Int J Biochem Cell Biol 2005; 37:289–305.

44. McGeer PL, Itagaki S, Boyes BE, McGeer EG. Reactive microglia are positive for HLA-DR in the substantia nigra of Parkinson's and Alzheimer's disease brains. Neurology 1988; 38:1285–91.

45. Hirsch EC, Hunot S, Damier P, Faucheux B. Glial cells and inflammation in Parkinson's disease: a role in neurodegeneration? Ann Neurol 1998; 44:S115–20.

46. Hirsch EC, Hunot S, Hartmann A. Neuroinflammatory processes in Parkinson's disease. Parkinsonism Relat Disord 2005; 11 (1):S9-S15.

47. Boka G, Anglade P, Wallach D, Javoy-Agid F, Agid Y, Hirsch EC. Immunocytochemical analysis of tumor necrosis factor and its receptors in Parkinson's disease. Neurosci Lett 1994; 172:151–4.

48. Durany N, Munch G, Michel T, Riederer P. Investigations on oxidative stress and therapeutical implications in dementia. Eur Arch Psychiatry Clin Neurosci 1999; 249 (3):68–73.

49. Floyd RA, Hensley K. Oxidative stress in brain aging. Implications for therapeutics of neurodegenerative diseases. Neurobiol Aging 2002; 23:795–807.

50. Grimble RF. Inflammatory response in the elderly. Curr Opin Clin Nutr Metab Care 2003; 6:21–9.

51. Lane N. A unifying view of ageing and disease: the double-agent theory. J Theor Biol 2003; 225:531–40.

52. McGeer EG, McGeer PL. Inflammatory processes in Alzheimer's disease. Prog Neuropsychopharmacol Biol Psychiatry 2003; 27:741–9.

53. Emerit J, Edeas M, Bricaire F. Neurodegenerative diseases and oxidative stress. Biomed Pharmacother 2004; 58:39–46.

54. Halliwell B, Gutteridge JMC. Oxygen radicals and the nervous system. Trends in Neurosciences 1985; 8:22–26.

55. Beckman KB, Ames BN. The free radical theory of aging matures. Physiol Rev 1998; 78:547–81.

56. Droge W. Free radicals in the physiological control of cell function. Physiol Rev 2002; 82:47–95.

57. Wickens AP. Ageing and the free radical theory. Respir Physiol 2001; 128:379–91.

58. Freeman BA, Crapo JD. Biology of disease: free radicals and tissue injury. Lab Invest 1982; 47:412–26.

59. Berger MM. Can oxidative damage be treated nutritionally? Clin Nutr 2005; 24:172–83.

60. Sohal RS, Weindruch R. Oxidative stress, caloric restriction, and aging. Science 1996; 273:59–63.

61. Shigenaga MK, Hagen TM, Ames BN. Oxidative damage and mitochondrial decay in aging. Proc Natl Acad Sci U S A 1994; 91:10771–8.

62. Sastre J, Pallardo FV, Vina J. The role of mitochondrial oxidative stress in aging. Free Radic Biol Med 2003; 35:1–8.

63. Nohl H, Gille L, Staniek K. Intracellular generation of reactive oxygen species by mitochondria. Biochem Pharmacol 2005; 69:719–23.

64. Chance B, Sies H, Boveris A. Hydroperoxide metabolism in mammalian organs. Physiol Rev 1979; 59:527–605.

65. Brewer GJ. Neuronal plasticity and stressor toxicity during aging. Exp Gerontol 2000; 35:1165–83.

66. Linton S, Davies MJ, Dean RT. Protein oxidation and ageing. Exp Gerontol 2001; 36:1503–18.

67. Balazy M, Nigam S. Aging, lipid modifications and phospholipases–new concepts. Ageing Res Rev 2003; 2:191–209.

68. Bokov A, Chaudhuri A, Richardson A. The role of oxidative damage and stress in aging. Mech Ageing Dev 2004; 125:811–26.

69. Junqueira VB, Barros SB, Chan SS, et al. Aging and oxidative stress. Mol Aspects Med 2004; 25:5–16.

70. Mecocci P, MacGarvey U, Kaufman AE, et al. Oxidative damage to mitochondrial DNA shows marked age-dependent increases in human brain. Ann Neurol 1993; 34:609–16.

71. Smith CD, Carney JM, Starke-Reed PE, Oliver CN, Stadtman ER, Floyd RA, Markesbery WR. Excess brain protein oxidation and enzyme dysfunction in normal aging and in Alzheimer disease. Proc. Natl. Acad. Sci. 1991; 88:10540–10543.

72. Marcus DL, Thomas C, Rodriguez C, et al. Increased peroxidation and reduced antioxidant enzyme activity in Alzheimer's disease. Exp Neurol 1998; 150:40–4.

73. Cavazzoni M, Barogi S, Baracca A, Parenti Castelli G, Lenaz G. The effect of aging and an oxidative stress on peroxide levels and the mitochondrial membrane potential in isolated rat hepatocytes. FEBS Lett 1999; 449:53–6.

74. Perez-Campo R, Lopez-Torres M, Cadenas S, Rojas C, Barja G. The rate of free radical production as a determinant of the rate of aging: evidence from the comparative approach. J Comp Physiol [B] 1998; 168:149–58.

75. Dalton TP, Shertzer HG, Puga A. Regulation of gene expression by reactive oxygen. Annu Rev Pharmacol Toxicol 1999; 39:67–101.

76. Davies KJ. Oxidative stress, antioxidant defenses, and damage removal, repair, and replacement systems. IUBMB Life 2000; 50:279–89.

77. Annunziato L, Pannaccione A, Cataldi M, et al. Modulation of ion channels by reactive oxygen and nitrogen species: a pathophysiological role in brain aging? Neurobiol Aging 2002; 23:819–34.
78. Hughes KA, Reynolds RM. Evolutionary and Mechanistic Theories of Aging. Annu Rev Enzymol 2005; 50:421–425.
79. Waring P. Redox active calcium ion channels and cell death. Arch Biochem Biophys 2005; 434:33–42.
80. Halliwell B. Role of free radicals in the neurodegenerative diseases: therapeutic implications for antioxidant treatment. Drugs Aging 2001; 18:685–716.
81. Rego AC, Oliveira CR. Mitochondrial dysfunction and reactive oxygen species in excitotoxicity and apoptosis: implications for the pathogenesis of neurodegenerative diseases. Neurochem Res 2003; 28:1563–74.
82. Lovell MA, Ehmann WD, Butler SM, Markesbery WR. Elevated thiobarbituric acid-reactive substances and antioxidant enzyme activity in the brain in Alzheimer's disease. Neurology 1995; 45:1594–601.
83. Dexter DT, Holley AE, Flitter WD, et al. Increased levels of lipid hydroperoxides in the parkinsonian substantia nigra: an HPLC and ESR study. Mov Disord 1994; 9:92–7.
84. Spencer JP, Jenner P, Daniel SE, Lees AJ, Marsden DC, Halliwell B. Conjugates of catecholamines with cysteine and GSH in Parkinson's disease: possible mechanisms of formation involving reactive oxygen species. J Neurochem 1998; 71:2112–22.
85. Munch G, Schinzel R, Loske C, et al. Alzheimer's disease–synergistic effects of glucose deficit, oxidative stress and advanced glycation endproducts. J Neural Transm 1998; 105:439–61.
86. Marklund SL, Westman NG, Lundgren E, Roos G. Copper- and zinc-containing superoxide dismutase, manganese-containing superoxide dismutase, catalase, and glutathione peroxidase in normal and neoplastic human cell lines and normal human tissues. Cancer Res 1982; 42:1955–61.
87. Halliwell B. Reactive oxygen species and the central nervous system. J Neurochem 1992; 59:1609–23.
88. Floyd RA. Antioxidants, oxidative stress, and degenerative neurological disorders. Proc Soc Exp Biol Med 1999; 222:236–45.
89. Joseph JA, Denisova N, Fisher D, Bickford P, Prior R, Cao G. Age-related neurodegeneration and oxidative stress: putative nutritional intervention. Neurol Clin 1998; 16:747–55.
90. Joseph JA, Denisova N, Fisher D, et al. Membrane and receptor modifications of oxidative stress vulnerability in aging. Nutritional considerations. Ann N Y Acad Sci 1998; 854:268–76.
91. Bartus RT. Drugs to treat age-related neurodegenerative problems. The final frontier of medical science? J. Am. Geriat. Soc. 1990; 38:680–695.
92. Joseph JA, Bartus RT, Clody D, et al. Psychomotor performance in the senescent rodent: reduction of deficits via striatal dopamine receptor up-regulation. Neurobiol Aging 1983; 4:313–9.
93. Kluger A, Gianutsos JG, Golomb J, et al. Patterns of motor impairment in normal aging, mild cognitive decline, and early Alzheimer's disease. J. Gerontol. 1997; 52:28–39.
94. Shukitt-Hale B. The effects of aging and oxidative stress on psychomotor and cognitive behavior. Age 1999; 22:9–17.
95. Hauss-Wegrzyniak B, Vannucchi MG, Wenk GL. Behavioral and ultrastructural changes induced by chronic neuroinflammation in young rats. Brain Res 2000; 859:157–66.
96. Hauss-Wegrzyniak B, Vraniak P, Wenk GL. The effects of a novel NSAID on chronic neuroinflammation are age dependent. Neurobiol Aging 1999; 20:305–13.
97. Ingram DK, Jucker M, Spangler EL. Behavioral manifestations of aging. 1994; 2:149–170.
98. Muir JL. Acetylcholine, aging, and Alzheimer's disease. Pharmacol. Biochem. Behav. 1997; 56:687–696.
99. Shukitt-Hale B, Mouzakis G, Joseph JA. Psychomotor and spatial memory performance in aging male Fischer 344 rats. Exp. Gerontol. 1998; 33:615–624.
100. West RL. An application of pre-frontal cortex function theory to cognitive aging. Psych. Bull. 1996; 120:272–292.
101. Devan BD, Goad EH, Petri HL. Dissociation of hippocampal and striatal contributions to spatial navigation in the water maze. Neurobiol. Learn. Mem. 1996; 66:305–323.

102. McDonald RJ, White NM. Parallel information processing in the water maze: Evidence for independent memory systems involving dorsal striatum and hippocampus. Behav. Neural Biol. 1994; 61:260–270.

103. Oliveira MGM, Bueno OFA, Pomarico AC, Gugliano EB. Strategies used by hippocampal- and caudate-putamen-lesioned rats in a learning task. Neurobiol. Learn. Mem. 1997; 68:32–41.

104. Zyzak DR, Otto T, Eichenbaum H MG. Cognitive Decline Associated with Normal Aging in Rats: A Neuropsychological Approach. Learning and Memory 1995; 2:1–16.

105. Forster MJ, Dubey A, Dawson KM, Stutts WA, Lal H, Sohal RS. Age-related losses of cognitive function and motor skills in mice are associated with oxidative protein damage in the brain. Proc Natl Acad Sci U S A 1996; 93:4765–9.

106. Joseph JA. The putative role of free radicals in the loss of neuronal functioning in senescence. Integ. Physiol. Behav. Sci. 1992; 27:216–227.

107. Bickford P, Heron C, Young DA, Gerhardt GA, De La Garza R. Impaired acquisition of novel locomotor tasks in aged and norepinephrine-depleted F344 rats. Neurobiol Aging 1992; 13:475–81.

108. Bickford P. Motor learning deficits in aged rats are correlated with loss of cerebellar noradrenergic function. Brain Res 1993; 620:133–8.

109. Joseph JA, Erat S, Rabin BM. CNS effects of heavy particle irradiation in space: behavioral implications. Adv. Space Res. 1998; 22:209–216.

110. Joseph JA, Shukitt-Hale B, McEwen J, Rabin BM. CNS-induced deficits of heavy particle irradiation in space: the aging connection. Adv Space Res 2000; 25:2057–64.

111. Shukitt-Hale B, Casadesus G, McEwen JJ, Rabin BM, Joseph JA. Spatial learning and memory deficits induced by exposure to iron-56-particle radiation. Radiat Res 2000; 154:28–33.

112. Hauss-Wegrzyniak B, Dobrzanski P, Stoehr JD, Wenk GL. Chronic neuroinflammation in rats reproduces components of the neurobiology of Alzheimer's disease. Brain Res 1998; 780:294–303.

113. Hauss-Wegrzyniak B, Willard LB, Del Soldato P, Pepeu G, Wenk GL. Peripheral administration of novel anti-inflammatories can attenuate the effects of chronic inflammation within the CNS. Brain Res 1999; 815:36–43.

114. Yamada K, Komori Y, Tanaka T, et al. Brain dysfunction associated with an induction of nitric oxide synthase following an intracerebral injection of lipopolysaccharide in rats. Neuroscience 1999; 88:281–94.

115. Cui K, Luo X, Xu K, Ven Murthy MR. Role of oxidative stress in neurodegeneration: recent developments in assay methods for oxidative stress and nutraceutical antioxidants. Prog Neuropsychopharmacol Biol Psychiatry 2004; 28:771–99.

116. Kim HP, Son KH, Chang HW, Kang SS. Anti-inflammatory plant flavonoids and cellular action mechanisms. J Pharmacol Sci 2004; 96:229–45.

117. Joseph JA, Fisher DR, Bielinski D. Blueberry extract alters oxidative stress-mediated signaling in COS-7 cells transfected with selectively vulnerable muscarinic receptor subtypes. J Alzheimer's Dis 2005; 9.

118. Vaya J, Aviram M. Nutritional Antioxidants: Mechanisms of Action, Analyses of Activities and Medical Applications. Curr Med Chem – Imm, Endoc & Metab Agents 2001; 1:99–117.

119. Youdim KA, Spencer JP, Schroeter H, Rice-Evans C. Dietary flavonoids as potential neuroprotectants. Biol Chem 2002; 383:503–19.

120. Youdim KA, Joseph JA. Phytochemicals and brain aging: a mutiplicity of effects. In: Rice-Evans C, Packer L, eds. Flavonoids in health and disease. New York: Marcel Dekker, Inc., 2003;205–231.

121. Deschamps V, Barberger-Gateau P, Peuchant E, Orgogozo JM. Nutritional factors in cerebral aging and dementia: epidemiological arguments for a role of oxidative stress. Neuroepidemiology 2001; 20:7–15.

122. Engelhart MJ, Geerlings MI, Ruitenberg A, et al. Dietary intake of antioxidants and risk of Alzheimer disease. Jama 2002; 287:3223–9.

123. Solfrizzi V, Panza F, Capurso A. The role of diet in cognitive decline. J Neural Transm 2003; 110:95–110.

124. Hu HL, Forsey RJ, Blades TJ, Barratt ME, Parmar P, Powell JR. Antioxidants may contribute in the fight against ageing: an in vitro model. Mech Ageing Dev 2000; 121:217–30.

125. Cotelle N. Role of flavonoids in oxidative stress. Curr Top Med Chem 2001; 1:569–90.

126. Turnbull JJ, Nakajima J, Welford RW, Yamazaki M, Saito K, Schofield CJ. Mechanistic studies on three 2-oxoglutarate-dependent oxygenases of flavonoid biosynthesis: anthocyanidin synthase, flavonol synthase, and flavanone 3beta-hydroxylase. J Biol Chem 2004; 279:1206–16.

127. Bagchi D, Sen CK, Bagchi M, Atalay M. Anti-angiogenic, antioxidant, and anti-carcinogenic properties of a novel anthocyanin-rich berry extract formula. Biochemistry (Mosc) 2004; 69:75–80, 1 p preceding 75.

128. Kong JM, Chia LS, Goh NK, Chia TF, Brouillard R. Analysis and biological activities of anthocyanins. Phytochemistry 2003; 64:923–33.

129. Francis FJ. Food colorants: Anthocyanins. Crit. Rev. Food Sci. Nutr. 1989; 28:273–314.

130. Mazza G, Kay CD, Cottrell T, Holub BJ. Absorption of anthocyanins from blueberries and serum antioxidant status in human subjects. J Agric Food Chem 2002; 50:7731–7.

131. Wang H, Cao G, Prior RL. Total antioxidant capacity of fruits. J Agric Food Chem 1996; 44:701–705.

132. Prior RL, Cao G, Martin A, et al. Antioxidant capacity as influenced by total phenolic and anthocyanin content, maturity and variety of Vaccinium species. J Agric Food Chem 1998; 46:2586–2593.

133. Kalt W, Ryan DA, Duy JC, Prior RL, Ehlenfeldt MK, Vander Kloet SP. Interspecific variation in anthocyanins, phenolics, and antioxidant capacity among genotypes of highbush and lowbush blueberries (Vaccinium section cyanococcus spp.). J Agric Food Chem 2001; 49:4761–7.

134. Wu X, Beecher GR, Holden JM, Haytowitz DB, Gebhardt SE, Prior RL. Lipophilic and hydrophilic antioxidant capacities of common foods in the United States. J Agric Food Chem 2004; 52:4026–37.

135. Youdim KA, Shukitt-Hale B, Joseph JA. Flavonoids and the brain: interactions at the blood-brain barrier and their physiological effects on the central nervous system. Free Radic Biol Med 2004; 37:1683–93.

136. Andres-Lacueva C, Shukitt-Hale B, Galli RL, Jauregui O, Lamuela-Raventos RM, Joseph JA. Anthocyanins in aged blueberry-fed rats are found centrally and may enhance memory. Nutr Neurosci 2005; 8:111–20.

137. Youdim KA, Shukitt-Hale B, Martin A, Wang H, Denisova N, Joseph JA. Short-term dietary supplementation of blueberry polyphenolics: beneficial effects on aging brain performance and peripheral tissue function. Nutritional Neuroscience 2000; 3:383–97.

138. Williams RJ, Spencer JP, Rice-Evans C. Flavonoids: antioxidants or signalling molecules? Free Radic Biol Med 2004; 36:838–49.

139. Landfield PW, Eldridge JC. The glucocorticoid hypothesis of age-related hippocampal neurodegeneration: role of dysregulated intraneuronal calcium. Ann N Y Acad Sci 1994; 746:308–21; discussion 321–6.

140. Jaffee E, Hoyer L, Nachman R. Synthesis of von Willebrand factor by cultured human endothelial cells. Proc. Natl. Acad. Sci. USA 1974; 71:1906–1913.

141. Egashira T, Takayama F, Yamanaka Y. Effects of bifemelane on muscarinic receptors and choline acetyltransferase in the brains of aged rats following chronic cerebral hypoperfusion induced by permanent occlusion of bilateral carotid arteries. Jap. J. Pharmacol. 1996; 72:57–65.

142. Joseph JA, Roth GS, Strong R. The striatum, A microcosm for the examination of age-related alterations in the CNS: A selected review. Rev. Biologic. Res. 1990; 4:181–199.

143. Kornhuber J, Schoppmeyer K, Bendig C, Riederer P. Characterization of [3H] pentazocine binding sites in post-mortem human frontal cortex. J. Neural. Trans. 1996; 103:45–53.

144. Joseph JA, Arendash G, Gordon M, Diamond D, Shukitt-Hale B, Morgan D. Blueberry supplementation enhances signaling and prevents behavioral deficits in an Alzheimer disease model. Nutr Neurosci 2003; 6:153–62.

145. Micheau J, Riedel G. Protein kinases: which one is the memory molecule? Cell Mol Life Sci 1999; 55:534–48.

146. Bickford PC, Gould T, Briederick L, et al. Antioxidant-rich diets improve cerebellar physiology and motor learning in aged rats. Brain Res. 2000; 866:211–217.

147. Kuhn HG, Dickinson-Anson H, Gage FH. Neurogenesis in the dentate gyrus of the adult rat: age-related decrease of neuronal progenitor proliferation. J Neurosci 1996; 16:2027–33.

148. Gage FH, Kempermann G, Palmer TD, Peterson DA, Ray J. Multipotent progenitor cells in the adult dentate gyrus. J Neurobiol 1998; 36:249–66.

149. Drapeau E, Mayo W, Aurousseau C, Le Moal M, Piazza PV, Abrous DN. Spatial memory performances of aged rats in the water maze predict levels of hippocampal neurogenesis. Proc Natl Acad Sci U S A 2003; 100:14385–90.

150. Shukitt-Hale B, Carey A, Simon LE, et al. Fruit polyphenols prevent inflammatory mediated decrements in cognition. Soc. Neurosci. Abs. 2004; 30:565.5.

151. Lau FC, Shukitt-Hale B, Joseph JA. Effect of blueberry supplementation on gene expression in the hippocampus of kainic acid-treated and control rats. Soc. Neurosci. Abs. 2004; 30:565.6.

152. Sweeney MI, Kalt W, MacKinnon SL, Ashby J, Gottschall-Pass KT. Feeding rats diets enriched in lowbush blueberries for six weeks decreases ischemia-induced brain damage. Nutr Neurosci 2002; 5:427–31.

153. Stromberg I, Gemma C, Vila J, Bickford PC. Blueberry- and spirulina-enriched diets enhance striatal dopamine recovery and induce a rapid, transient microglia activation after injury of the rat nigrostriatal dopamine system. Exp Neurol 2005; 196:298–307.

154. Roth GS, Joseph JA, Mason RP. Membrane alterations as causes of impaired signal transduction in Alzheimer's disease and aging. Trends Neurosci 1995; 18:203–6.

155. Fowler CJ, Cowburn RF, Joseph JA. Alzheimer's, ageing and amyloid: an absurd allegory? Gerontology 1997; 43:132–42.

156. Joseph JA, Villalobos-Molina R, Yamagami K, Roth GS, Kelly J. Age-specific alterations in muscarinic stimulation of K(+)-evoked dopamine release from striatal slices by cholesterol and S-adenosyl-L-methionine. Brain Res 1995; 673:185–93.

157. Rossner S, Ueberham U, Schliebs R, Perez-Polo JR, Bigl V. The regulation of amyloid precursor protein metabolism by cholinergic mechanisms and neurotrophin receptor signaling. Prog Neurobiol 1998; 56:541–69.

158. Elhusseiny A, Cohen Z, Olivier A, Stanimirovic DB, Hamel E. Functional acetylcholine muscarinic receptor subtypes in human brain microcirculation: identification and cellular localization. J Cereb Blood Flow Metab 1999; 19:794–802.

159. Joseph JA, Fisher DR, Carey A, Szprengiel A. The M3 muscarinic receptor i3 domain confers oxidative stress protection on calcium regulation in transfected COS-7 cells. Aging Cell 2004; 3:263–71.

160. Yi W, Fischer J, Krewer G, Akoh CC. Phenolic compounds from blueberries can inhibit colon cancer cell proliferation and induce apoptosis. J Agric Food Chem 2005; 53:7320–9.

161. Stetler-Stevenson WG. The role of matrix metalloproteinases in tumor invasion, metastasis, and angiogenesis. Surg Oncol Clin N Am 2001; 10:383–92, x.

162. Matchett MD, MacKinnon SL, Sweeney MI, Gottschall-Pass KT, Hurta RA. Blueberry flavonoids inhibit matrix metalloproteinase activity in DU145 human prostate cancer cells. Biochem Cell Biol 2005; 83:637–43.

163. Lau FC, Bielinski DF, Joseph JA. Inhibitory effect of blueberry extract on the production of inflammatory mediators in LPS-activated BV2 microglia. Age 2006; 28:46.

164. Wilson MA, Shukitt-Hale B, Kalt W, Ingram DK, Joseph JA, Wolkow CA. Blueberry polyphenols increase lifespan and thermotolerance in Caenorhabditis elegans. Aging Cell 2006; 5:59–68.

165. Simonian NA, Coyle JT. Oxidative stress in neurodegenerative diseases. Ann. Rev. Pharmacol. Toxicol 1996; 36:83–106.

166. Hughes DA. Dietary antioxidants and human immune function. Nutrition Bulletin 2000; 25:35–41.

167. Ischiropoulos H, Beckman JS. Oxidative stress and nitration in neurodegeneration: cause, effect, or association? J Clin Invest 2003; 111:163–9.

168. McGeer PL, McGeer EG. Inflammation and neurodegeneration in Parkinson's disease. Parkinsonism Relat Disord 2004; 10 (1):S3–7.

169. Esposito E, Rotilio D, Di Matteo V, Di Giulio C, Cacchio M, Algeri S. A review of specific dietary antioxidants and the effects on biochemical mechanisms related to neurodegenerative processes. Neurobiol Aging 2002; 23:719–35.

170. Cornwell T, Cohick W, Raskin I. Dietary phytoestrogens and health. Phytochemistry 2004; 65:995–1016.
171. Willcox JK, Ash SL, Catignani GL. Antioxidants and prevention of chronic disease. Crit Rev Food Sci Nutr 2004; 44:275–95.
172. Cao G, Sofic E, Prior RL. Antioxidant capacity of tea and common vegetables. J. Agric. Food Chem. 1996; 44:3426–3431.
173. Prior RL, Cao G. Analysis of botanicals and dietary supplements for antioxidant capacity: a review. J AOAC Int 2000; 83:950–6.

INDEX